Believe It or Not

Michael S. Kramer

Believe It or Not

The History, Culture, and Science
Behind Health Beliefs and Practices

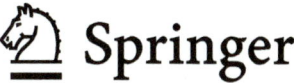 Springer

Michael S. Kramer
Faculty of Medicine and Health Sciences
McGill University
Montreal, QC, Canada

ISBN 978-3-031-46021-0   ISBN 978-3-031-46022-7   (eBook)
https://doi.org/10.1007/978-3-031-46022-7

This Springer imprint is published by the registered company Springer Nature Switzerland AG
The registered company address is: Gewerbestrasse 11, 6330 Cham, Switzerland

Paper in this product is recyclable.

Preface

As a physician, epidemiologist, and devout skeptic, I have been an avid collector of "medical myths" during a professional career spanning more than four decades. I always wanted to research these myths but did not have the time to do them justice while carrying out the tasks for which I earned my salary: research, teaching, clinical work, and administrative responsibilities. The COVID epidemic and my recent retirement from McGill University gave me the opportunity to pursue the project.

Before starting, of course, I needed to find out what others had already written. Every new research project should start with a review of the published literature, and the same is true for a new non-fiction book. I read a dozen or so books on medical myths; most of the books and authors were unknown to me.

What I found convinced me that I was on the right track. For example, several existing books argue that common colds couldn't possibly be caused by exposure to cold air, because colds are caused by respiratory viruses. None considered the possibility of **joint causation**, that is, that colds might be caused by combined exposure to the cold virus **and** cold air. In fact, very few diseases or other health outcomes have a single cause: a factor that is both necessary and sufficient to induce the outcome. Single necessary and sufficient causes exist for a few genetic diseases (like Huntington disease, a rare form of brain degeneration that affects young and middle-aged adults) and for rare infectious agents like Ebola virus. But most genetic and infectious diseases involve an interplay between the genetic defect or infectious agent and other factors involving both the host (the person affected) and the environment. This is even more obviously true for cancer, heart disease, diabetes, and other chronic diseases. It is no longer possible to doubt that cigarette smoking is a cause of lung cancer, while recognizing that most smokers, even heavy smokers, do *not* develop lung cancer, and that occasional cases of lung cancer occur among non-smokers.

The word *myth* can have two quite different meanings: (1) a shared tradition or story, like the Oedipus myth in Greek mythology; and (2) a belief that can be falsified, such as the earth is flat. Most previous books have focused on "busting" the second type of myth: explaining why the myths are untrue, often in a clear and accessible style. I wanted to write something different by exploring the possibility that some longstanding health beliefs might actually be true.

But I am also interested in the first meaning of myth, especially the history and culture surrounding it. When and where did the health belief or practice originate?

What cultural or religious factors led to its origin, its spread to other geographical areas, and its persistence over time? How does the belief or practice vary among countries, and within countries according to age, education, ethnicity, and urban vs rural location? As I discovered in researching the health beliefs and practices I review in this book, some have been around for thousands of years, others only a few decades. For many of them, the historical and cultural influences are as fascinating as the scientific evidence favoring or undermining them.

Finally, previous "myth-busting" books have not attempted rigorous and systematic evaluations of the scientific evidence for and against each of the beliefs and practices they discuss. Some cite published studies, but it is unclear whether the authors came to their conclusions as a *result* of the published evidence, or if they selectively sought and cited studies that supported a position to which they had already arrived!

What is required for a scientifically rigorous assessment of any health belief or practice is a *systematic review*, which I define and explain in Chap. 2. To my knowledge, this book is the first to attempt such an assessment. When systematically reviewing the published evidence, it is important to consider the methodological strengths and weaknesses of the studies reviewed. These strengths and weaknesses often have little to do with how recently the study was published, the journal in which it appeared, or the university at which the principal author works.

Carrying out an original systematic review on any one of the health beliefs and practices I discuss would require many months, or even years, of my time and effort. Not only would such an undertaking ignore the excellent work of others who have carried out systematic reviews of the topics I include in the book, but the time required to do that for all the topics would exceed my remaining life expectancy! I will therefore rely heavily on recently published systematic reviews whenever possible. When I am unable to find any, I will acknowledge that fact and cite and assess the best individual studies I can find on the topic, say why I selected them, and explain how they justify the inferences I make.

I can assure you that by the time you read this book, some of its content will be out of date. In the year and a half between the time I began (April 2021) and completed (August 2023) the book, I felt obliged to update my literature search. Although the changes were not earth-shattering, some of the text was substantially revised in the light of new references.

The transience of knowledge should not discourage you, however; it lies at the very heart of science.

How to Read the Book

The first chapter of this book reviews the principles of scientific inference of cause and effect and provides the conceptual basis for evaluating individual research studies. The second chapter moves beyond individual studies to consider the entire body of published research on the topics reviewed: how to sum up the combined evidence based on systematic reviews, where available, of the best research. These first two chapters are dense and should not be quickly skimmed, except by readers with formal training in epidemiologic and clinical research methods. I have done my best to minimize the technical jargon and to "translate" complicated epidemiologic and statistical concepts in an understandable way for a well-educated general audience.

The subsequent chapters of the book deal with specific health beliefs and practices and can be read in any order, much like an encyclopedia. The topic chapters are divided into sections related to infection, skin and eye conditions, foods and beverages, and pregnancy and childhood. You should feel free to skip around within and between sections, however, to focus on those health beliefs and practices in which you are most interested. Each topic chapter begins with an Introduction that traces the historical and geographical origins of the belief or practice, including the cultural and religious factors that have favored its adoption and persistence. The second section of each topic chapter summarizes the information available on the current prevalence of the beliefs and practices that are the focus of the chapter, that is, *who believes*. In this section, I prioritize systematic reviews or individual studies of variations in the prevalence of the belief or practice across and within countries and according to age, education, ethnicity, and other factors. In the third section of each topic chapter, I provide a detailed evidence review of the published studies supporting or undermining the belief or practice: in other words, *why* you should believe it or not. Readers who read this section may find it helpful to refer back to Chaps. 1 and 2. For those who do not want or need in-depth information on the published studies, I summarize the key evidence points in a textbox placed just before the detailed review. I conclude each topic chapter with a brief summary.

Montreal, QC, Canada   Michael S. Kramer

Acknowledgments

I received encouragement and valuable advice from many persons in planning, organizing, writing, and editing this book. These persons include colleagues at McGill University, as well as family and friends. I would particularly like to cite a few of them:

My wife Claire not only supported the need for the book, but also read every word. Although untrained in science, she is an unabashed but constructive critic. She made many insightful suggestions about how to "translate" difficult scientific concepts into language that is accessible to educated lay readers.

My daughter Elise is a practicing optometrist who excels at expressing complex medical concepts and terms that her patients and the general public can understand. She too read every word of the book and suggested major improvements in content and style. She also contributed to the content and interpretation of the chapters on myopia and eye strain.

Contents

Part I   How to Evaluate Scientific Evidence

1   How Science Helps Decide What to Believe   3
   What Is Science?.   3
   Scientific Inference   5
      Experiments Versus Observational Studies.   6
      Bias and Precision.   8
   How Should Science Influence Health Beliefs?   10

2   Summing Up: Synthesizing the Scientific Evidence.   11
   Why Synthesize the Evidence?.   11
   Systematic Review   12
   Reviewing the Evidence on Health Beliefs and Practices   14
   How to Read the Rest of This Book   15

Part II   Infection

**3   Dodging the Draft: Does Avoiding the Cold Reduce the
Risk of Catching a Cold?**   19
   Introduction.   19
      What Is a Cold?.   19
      Historical Origins   20
   Current Beliefs About the Cause of the Common Cold   21
   Detailed Review of the Scientific Evidence   23
      Seasonality   23
      Effects of Exposure to Cold Temperature.   23
      Effects of Cold Weather on Virus Infectivity and the
      Immune Response.   25
      Effects of Indoor Crowding and Ventilation   26
   Summary.   27
   References.   27

4   Dietary Supplements and Common Viral Infections:
     "Boosting" the Immune System or the Manufacturers' Profits?   29
     Introduction   29
        Nutrition and Health   30
        Nutrition and Infection   30
     Dietary Supplements: How Commonly Are They Used?
     Who Uses Them?   33
     Detailed Review of the Scientific Evidence   35
        Vitamin A   36
        Vitamin D   36
        Vitamin C   37
        Vitamin E   38
        Omega-3 Fatty Acids   38
        Flavonoids   38
        Zinc   39
        Probiotics   39
     Summary   40
     References   41

5   Common Sense or Nonsense? Non-Drug Treatments for
     the Common Cold   45
     Introduction   45
        Historical Origins   46
     Who Uses These Cold Remedies?   48
     Detailed Review of the Scientific Evidence   49
        Bedrest and Exercise   49
        Supplemental Fluids   50
        Humidifiers and Vaporizers   51
        Nasal Irrigation   51
     Summary   51
     References   52

Part III   Skin and Eye Conditions

6   Duct (or Duck) Tape for Treating Warts: A Quack Remedy?   55
     Introduction   55
        A Brief History of Duct (or Duck) Tape   55
     Who Uses or Recommends Duct Tape to Remove Warts?   56
     Detailed Review of the Evidence   57
     Summary   59
     References   60

7   *Aloe Vera*: Does It Work? A Burning Question   61
     Introduction   61
        History   61
     How Are Burns Currently Treated?   62
     Detailed Review of Scientific Evidence   63

Summary.. 64
References.. 65

8   Diet and Acne: Should Teenagers Avoid Pizza and Chocolate? 67
Introduction.. 67
Current Beliefs About Diet and Acne 69
Detailed Review of Scientific Evidence 70
   Glycemic Index.. 70
   Chocolate 70
   Vitamin D 72
   Long-Chain Polyunsaturated Fatty Acids (LCPUFAs)........... 72
   Other Nutrients 73
   Zinc... 74
   Fatty or Oily Foods.................................... 75
Summary.. 75
References.. 76

**9   I Can See Clearly Now: Do Glasses Make You More
Nearsighted?** 79
Introduction.. 79
   Ethnic and Geographic Differences and Temporal Trends.......... 80
Current Beliefs About Wearing Glasses 82
Detailed Review of Scientific Evidence: What Slows Progression of
Myopia? 83
Summary.. 86
References.. 86

10 Eye Strain and Headache: A Change in Viewpoint 89
Introduction.. 89
   A Brief History 90
   Why Should Refractive Errors Cause Headache?................ 91
Current Beliefs About and Prevalence of Eye Strain Headaches 91
Detailed Review of Scientific Evidence 93
   Do Refractive Errors Cause Eye Strain and Headache?........... 93
   Does Correction of Refractive Errors Reduce Eye Strain and
Headache?.. 96
Summary.. 96
References.. 97

Part IV   Foods and Beverages

11 The Benefits of Intermittent Fasting: Detox or Redux? 101
Introduction.. 101
   Voluntary Fasting: A Brief History........................ 102
Current Beliefs and Practices About Intermittent Fasting 103
Detailed Review of Scientific Evidence 105
Summary.. 107
References.. 107

12 Preventing or Treating a Hangover: Dilution or Delusion? 109
    Introduction... 109
        Historical and Cultural Overview 110
    Current Beliefs and Practices 111
    What Works? Detailed Review of Scientific Evidence................ 113
    Summary... 115
    References... 116

13 "Natural" Remedies to Improve Sleep: Perchance a Dream? 119
    Introduction... 119
    Current Beliefs and Practices 120
    Detailed Review of Scientific Evidence: Do "Natural"
    Remedies Work?.. 121
        Herbal Teas and Extracts...................................... 122
        Milk... 125
        Dietary Supplements.. 126
        Aroma Therapy... 126
    Summary... 127
    References... 127

14 The Bitter Truth About Artificial Sweeteners 131
    Introduction... 131
        History of Artificial Sweeteners 131
    Current Practices and Beliefs 133
    Detailed Review of Scientific Evidence 136
        General Principles... 136
        Changes in Body Weight, Fat, and Other Cardio-Metabolic
        Risk Factors... 137
        Dental Health 138
        Cancer... 139
        Adverse Effects on Offspring Due to Exposure During Pregnancy..... 140
        Other Adverse Health Outcomes................................. 140
    Summary... 140
    References... 141

15 The "Hype" About Sugar and Children's Behavior 143
    Introduction... 143
        How Common Is "Hyper" Behavior?............................... 144
    Sugar Intake and Behavior: Knowledge and Beliefs 145
    Detailed Review of the Scientific Evidence 146
    Summary... 148
    References... 148

16 Organic Foods: A Healthier Alternative? 151
    Introduction... 151
        The History of Organic Farming............................... 152
    Current Beliefs and Practices Concerning Organic Food
    Consumption... 153

Detailed Review of the Evidence on Health Benefits of
Organic Foods.   155
   Do Organic Foods Taste Better?.   156
   Do Organic Foods Provide Lower Exposure to Chemical
   Contaminants?.   157
   Do Organic and Conventional Foods Differ in Bacterial
   Contamination?.   158
   Do Organic Foods Have a Better Nutrient Content?.   158
   Does Organic Food Consumption Improve Health?.   159
   Summary.   160
   References.   160

17   Protein Supplements: Bulk or Bilk?   163
   Introduction.   163
     Protein Supplements to Increase Muscle Mass and Strength:
     A Brief History   165
   Current Beliefs and Practices Concerning Protein Supplements   165
   Detailed Review of Scientific Evidence   167
     Protein Supplements in Healthy Adults   168
     Protein Supplements in the Elderly.   170
   Summary.   172
   References.   172

18   Prevention and Treatment of Jet Lag: What Works?   175
   Introduction.   175
   Current Beliefs and Practices: Who Gets Jet Lag and What Do
   They Do About It?   177
   Detailed Review of Scientific Evidence on Prevention or Treatment of
   Jet Lag.   178
   Summary.   180
   References.   180

19   High Sugar Consumption and Diabetes Risk: A Sweet Lie   183
   Introduction.   183
     Historical Background   184
   Current Beliefs and Behaviors Concerning Sugar Consumption and
   Diabetes.   185
   Detailed Review of Evidence on Sugar Consumption and Risk of
   Diabetes.   186
   Summary.   188
   References.   189

Part V   Pregnancy and Childhood

20   Born Too Soon: What's in a Number?   193
   Introduction.   193
     When Does Pregnancy Begin?   193
     How Long Does Pregnancy Last?.   194

Review of Scientific Evidence 195
History and Cultural Origins. 197
References. 198

21 Take Your Shots? Parents' Fear of Adverse Effects of Vaccines 199
Introduction. 199
    Historical Context 199
Parents' Beliefs About the Risks and Benefits of Vaccination 201
    Qualitative Studies 201
    Quantitative Studies 202
Detailed Review of Scientific Evidence Behind Parents' Beliefs. 205
    Autism. 205
    Adverse Effects on the Immune System 207
Summary. 209
References. 209

22 Does Teething Cause Fever, Rash, and Other Signs of Illness? 213
Introduction. 213
    Historical Perspective 213
What Do Parents and Health Providers Believe About Teething? 215
    Parents. 215
    Health Care Professionals. 215
Systemic Consequences of Teething: Detailed Review of the
Evidence 217
Summary. 219
References. 219

**23 No Tylenol? No Problem! Beliefs About Fever and Its
Treatment in Children** 221
Introduction. 221
    Historical Perspective 222
Beliefs About Fever and Its Treatment in Children 223
    Parents. 223
    Health Care Professionals. 224
    Do Educational Interventions Reduce Fever Phobia?. 225
Detailed Review of Evidence on Treating Fever in Children 226
    The Biology of Fever 226
    Review of Published Evidence 228
Summary. 229
References. 230

Index. 233

About the Author

Michael S. Kramer completed most of his early schooling in Miami, Florida. He left Miami to pursue his undergraduate studies at the University of Chicago, then moved to Yale, where he completed medical school, a residency in pediatrics, and a research fellowship in clinical epidemiology. Following his education and professional training, he moved north to accept a faculty position at the McGill University Faculty of Medicine in Montreal, Canada, where he spent his entire academic career of 42 years and is now Professor Emeritus. He practiced clinical pediatrics for nearly 25 years, but most of his time has been devoted to research and teaching.

Dr Kramer has published over 500 scientific articles and has won numerous national and international awards for his research. He served as a member of expert committees of the World Health Organization (WHO), the U.S. Institute of Medicine, and the Council of Canadian Academies. He helped establish the Canadian Perinatal Surveillance System in 1995 and from 2003 to 2011 was Scientific Director of the Institute of Human Development, Child and Youth Health at the Canadian Institutes of Health Research, Canada's national health research funding agency. In 2011, he was elected to Fellowship in the Royal Society of Canada. Dr Kramer's systematic review of the scientific evidence on the optimal duration of exclusive breastfeeding led directly to new infant feeding recommendations by WHO in 2001. His research on preterm birth helped draw attention to labor induction and elective cesarean delivery as drivers of the rise in preterm birth from the 1980s to the early 2000s. That research contributed to obstetric guidelines to restrict provider-initiated early delivery, which helped reverse the trend. Dr Kramer was recently cited as among the most impactful 0.01% of the world's researchers across all scientific fields. His book written for the general public, entitled *Beyond Parenting Advice: How Science Should Guide Your Decisions on Pregnancy and Child-Rearing*, was published by Springer Nature in late 2021.

Dr Kramer is married and has three children and six grandchildren. He plays violin and is an avid chamber musician. He also enjoys a variety of outdoor activities, including cycling, hiking, tennis, and skiing.

How Science Helps Decide What to Believe

> *"The most costly of all follies is to believe passionately in the palpably not true. It is the chief occupation of mankind."*
>
> H. L. Mencken

What Is Science?

Before explaining what science is, I will start by discussing what it is not. Science is not technology. Yes, developing new technologies requires scientific training and knowledge. Conversely, many scientific advances benefit from, and may even require, technologic innovation. Technology is a tool that enables good science—not an end in itself, but a means to an end. The Large Hadron Collider (the giant nuclear accelerator located near Geneva, Switzerland) creates high-speed collisions of subatomic particles. But it is scientific hypotheses that lead to the design of specific experiments using the collider, and analysis of the data from those experiments, that lead to new knowledge about the fundamentals of matter.

If you ask school-age children or most adults without formal scientific education to define science, they are likely to mention white coats, laboratory glassware, or high-tech machines. They rarely invoke the testing of hypotheses through carefully designed and conducted experiments or other studies.

If science is not technology, neither is it unquestioned and untested belief in the truth of a proposition. The so-called natural remedies are derived from natural sources and are therefore *believed* to be safe. Because of their long history, popularity, and apparent safety, natural remedies can be sold in pharmacies and grocery stores at any price the market will bear. But you are probably unaware that the companies manufacturing natural remedies are not required to demonstrate that they are

M. S. Kramer, *Believe It or Not*, https://doi.org/10.1007/978-3-031-46022-7_1

effective, that is, that they actually work. People who buy these products do so out of faith: the ***belief*** that the products are effective. Because the manufacturers are not legally required to demonstrate efficacy, they don't even try. They have nothing to gain from science and everything to lose.

In contrast, drugs and vaccines cannot be legally marketed in most countries unless they have been approved by national health agencies on the basis of rigorous scientific studies that demonstrate both safety and effectiveness. These rigorous studies are called randomized controlled trials, or RCTs, and I will have much more to say about them later in this chapter. National health agencies do allow the sale of some drugs without evidence of efficacy from RCTs. Such drugs can be purchased "over the counter" without a prescription and were "grandfathered" in after long periods of prior use without major safety concerns. Medicines for the common cold are examples of such drugs.

Beliefs are often based on anecdote. For example, some people are unshakably convinced that their colds are *always* caused by exposure to cold air. Every time they come down with a sneeze and cough, they reflect back on the previous few days (or hours) and recall, "Oh, yeah, I went out on Monday when my hair was still wet" or "My office was freezing cold yesterday." The same reasoning is applied to prevention ("I haven't had a single cold since I started taking vitamin C tablets") and successful recovery ("Every time I have a bad cold, my doctor prescribes antibiotics, and my cold gets better within a few days"). I have devoted chapters to these beliefs about colds in the next section of the book.

These examples demonstrate a very strong cognitive bias: *"post hoc ergo propter hoc"* (after this, therefore because of this), which also known as the post hoc fallacy. But just as the rooster's morning crow doesn't cause the sun to rise, a correct temporal sequence (or, more likely, biased recollection) of events is weak evidence of causality. For example, *any* treatment taken for a cold will appear to be beneficial when it is taken at the peak of symptoms, since down is the only direction possible after a peak! Anecdotes tend to become reinforced by similar episodes that recur, or are selectively recalled, another type of cognitive bias called *confirmation bias*. Eventually, these reinforced beliefs become established in society at large as "folk wisdom."

What about the role of serendipity, a beneficial chance occurrence? Serendipity has enjoyed a rich history in science. But as Louis Pasteur famously said, chance favors the prepared mind. One often-cited medical example of serendipity is Alexander Fleming's discovery of the antibacterial properties of *Penicillium*, a common bread mold that had contaminated one of Fleming's bacteria-containing culture dishes that he had mistakenly left open. Fleming noticed a clear halo (where bacterial growth had been inhibited) surrounding the mold. The serendipitous discovery of penicillin, which is produced by the mold, ushered in the modern era of antibiotic treatment of infections. But observations like Fleming's are not in themselves scientific. They generate hypotheses when, in Pasteur's words, the mind is suitably prepared. Those hypotheses then lead to experiments and other studies to test the hypotheses—that is, science. When scientific tests convincingly support a hypothesis, it is said to be confirmed ("proven").

Scientific Inference

Not all scientific inferences are cause-and-effect. Some studies have a predictive purpose, such as quantifying the probability of having a fetus affected by Down's syndrome (a birth defect also called trisomy 21, a third copy of the 21st chromosome), based on measurements of various hormones and proteins in the blood during the second trimester of pregnancy. The number of study women, the methods used to recruit them, and their age and other factors will affect the accuracy of the prediction. But no cause-and-effect relationship is inferred. The hormones and proteins measured are not causes of Down's syndrome, but rather, biological markers that help predict its occurrence and thereby help the clinician decide whether or not to recommend a more expensive test based on fetal DNA in the mother's blood or a riskier test like amniocentesis (obtaining and analyzing a sample of amniotic fluid to examine the fetus's chromosomes).

Other scientific inquiries have a descriptive goal. Some population health studies, for example, describe geographic differences or temporal trends in occurrence of health events. Are certain types of cancer more common in some states or provinces than in others? Have a country's hysterectomy rates risen or fallen over time? As mentioned in the Preface to this book, a major section of each of the book's topic chapters is devoted to the current and past prevalence of the beliefs and practices that are the focus of the chapter. That section is primarily based on descriptive studies. No cause-and-effect relationships are inferred from descriptive studies, but they may lead to new causal hypotheses about *why* the observed geographic or temporal differences have occurred. Those hypotheses can then be tested in subsequent studies.

It may surprise you to learn that most scientific questions bearing on health beliefs involve causes and consequences. Does eating oily food and chocolate cause acne? Will vaccination increase the risk of infections caused by bacteria or viruses not related to those vaccinated against? Will going outdoors in the winter with wet hair increase your risk of catching a cold?

As shown in Fig. 1.1, such questions have two essential ingredients: a hypothesized cause and a hypothesized effect. In health research, we call these the *exposure* and *outcome*, respectively. The hypothesis is that the exposure causes a change in the outcome. The process of causal inference is thus: formulate a hypothesis about an exposure and its effect on outcome, design a study to test that hypothesis, analyze and interpret the data that result from the study, and infer the validity of—that is, confirm or refute—the hypothesis.

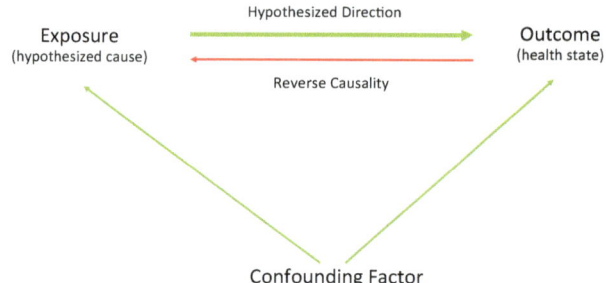

Fig. 1.1 The essentials of causal inference. The study exposure is the hypothesized cause of the outcome, and the outcome is the health state on which an effect of exposure is hypothesized. Arrows point from causes to effects. The direction of an arrow also denotes temporal sequence; the tail occurs earlier in time than the head. Green arrows denote known or hypothesized causal directions, while the red arrow from outcome to exposure denotes reverse causality: the study outcome precedes and causes the exposure. A confounding factor is an underlying (antecedent) cause of both the exposure and outcome and biases the apparent effect of exposure on outcome. It needs to be adjusted ("controlled") for to remove the bias

Experiments Versus Observational Studies

It is important to distinguish two broad types of studies bearing on human health. The first type is called an *experiment*. An experiment means that the researcher actively intervenes to change the exposure and then observes the outcome in the study participants. In health research, the intervention is often a treatment intended to improve the study participant's health, either by preventing an illness or lessening its impact—sometimes even curing it. The outcome is the health state: an illness or some measure of discomfort or disability due to the illness. A *controlled experiment* is a study in which two treatments are compared, or an active treatment is compared to an inactive placebo. The *"control"* part is key to the comparison. It provides another group of participants in whom the outcome (disease or no disease, average blood pressure, cure or no cure) can be compared to the outcome observed in the active treatment group.

The controlled experiment is analogous to a laboratory study in experimental animals. One group of animals receives the active treatment, the other group receives an inactive placebo or another active treatment. Two main differences distinguish animal and human experiments: a scientific one and an ethical one.

The scientific difference is that the animals who receive both treatments are usually genetically identical mice, rats, fruit flies, etc. Humans, thankfully, are not genetically identical, unless they are monozygotic (from a single fertilized egg) twins, triplets, etc. The question then becomes: How can a researcher ensure that the two groups of human participants receiving the two different treatments are identical in all respects *other than* receipt of the active versus the control treatment?

The answer is randomization. Letting the flip of a coin or a computer-generated random sequence of numbers determine which participants receive which treatment does not guarantee that each participant is equivalent to every other participant in the two study groups. Instead, it guarantees *exchangeability*. Exchangeability means that the two groups are virtually identical *on average* and would have been equally similar had those receiving the active and control treatments been switched—in other words, had they received the opposite treatment. This type of human experiment is called a *randomized controlled trial*, or RCT. As mentioned earlier in this chapter, the RCT design is required for licensing new drugs. The RCT is the "gold standard" for making causal scientific inferences, not only in drug studies but in all human health research.

The ethical difference between human experiments (RCTs) and animal experiments goes beyond the legal and moral necessity to obtain human participants' informed consent. That necessity applies to all human studies, not just RCTs. But it is unethical to administer interventions that are known or suspected to be harmful to human beings, even if they consent to those interventions. We cannot randomize children to be exposed to lead versus a placebo or to physical punishment versus "time out" approaches to discipline.

Instead, studies of the effects of hypothesized harmful exposures must be non-experimental by design. We call these *observational studies*. Of course, RCTs also require observations; all participants must be observed to see if and when then they develop the outcome hypothesized to be caused or prevented by the active intervention. But in observational studies, the researcher does not intervene. He or she merely observes both the exposure (treatment) and the outcome and then compares the outcomes in groups of exposed and unexposed participants. Observational studies are also used to investigate exposures that are not known to be harmful, including common health behaviors and treatments chosen by the participants or their care givers. The key feature of observational studies that distinguishes them from RCTs is the lack of exchangeability of exposed and unexposed participants that randomized treatment allocation provides. Table 1.1 compares and contrasts the main features of experimental and observational studies.

Table 1.1 Comparison of experimental and observational human health studies

Experimental studies	Observational studies
Researcher intervenes to change exposure	No intervention by researcher
Interventions often referred to as treatments	Exposure is observed, not assigned, by researcher
Treatment is hypothesized to prevent or ameliorate an illness	Exposure may be hypothesized as harmful or beneficial, may be a treatment
Two or more treatments usually compared:	Two or more exposures usually compared:
• Experimental (new) treatment • One or more control treatments • Most rigorous design randomly allocates treatment to participants (randomized controlled trial, RCT)	• Main exposure of interest • Non-exposure or control exposure
Health outcome is observed	Health outcome is observed

As shown in Fig. 1.1, the inference that exposure causes a change in outcome critically depends on knowing the temporal sequence of exposure and outcome. Whether a study is experimental or observational, it is essential that participants have not yet developed the outcome at the time they are exposed. An outcome that precedes the exposure cannot have been caused by that exposure.

Bias and Precision

In the context of causal inference in human health studies, bias refers to an observed association between exposure and outcome that differs *systematically* (that is, not merely by chance) from the true causal effect of exposure on outcome. In other words, the researcher is likely to observe an association in the absence of a true effect, fail to observe an association in spite of a true effect, or observe an association that is stronger or weaker than the true effect. I will focus on the two most important sources bias: confounding and reverse causality. Both are illustrated in Fig. 1.1.

Confounding occurs when a third factor (neither the exposure nor the outcome) biases the association between the study exposure and outcome. The bias occurs because, as shown by the arrows in Fig. 1.1, the confounding third factor is an underlying (antecedent) cause of both the exposure and the outcome. For example, let's say we knew nothing about the fact that cigarette smoking causes lung cancer. A clever researcher carries out an observational study of 100 cases of lung cancer and 100 controls without lung cancer; this is called a case-control study. The researcher carefully interviews and examines the 100 cases and 100 controls. Of the 100 cases, 30 are found to have yellow fingers on their dominant hand, whereas only 3 of the 100 controls have this finding. It would be incorrect to infer that yellow fingers cause lung cancer, because (as we now know) both the yellow fingers and the lung cancer are caused by smoking cigarettes. This bias can be reduced or eliminated by measuring and adjusting for the confounding factor through one of several statistical techniques. For example, if we analyze smokers and non-smokers separately, we will find none of the non-smoking cases or controls to have yellow fingers but a similarly high proportion of smokers with yellow fingers both among cases and controls.

The second important source of bias is *reverse causality*. It is illustrated by the red arrow in Fig. 1.1. This bias occurs when the outcome actually precedes and causes the exposure, rather than the reverse. It is particularly likely to occur in what are called cross-sectional studies, because exposure and outcome are ascertained at the same moment (cross-section) of time. For example, many of the studies investigating whether a large number of hours per day spent in front of a television or computer screen causes obesity are based on a cross-sectional design in which particpants are weighed and measured and are interviewed about how many hours per day they spend watching television or using a computer. If those measurements and interviews occur around the same time, we have no way of knowing if a positive association reflects the causal effect of screen time on causing obesity or the causal effect of obesity on screen time. Either direction is biologically plausible. The only way to be sure of inferring the correct direction is to design a *longitudinal (prospective)* study in which eligible participants have a normal body weight at baseline when the hypothesized cause, prolonged screen time, is also measured. The participants are then followed up over time, and the proportion of *new* cases of obesity is compared in those with and without prolonged screen time at baseline.

Confounding and reverse causality biases are much more likely in observational studies than in randomized trials (RCTs). Because "association does not prove causation," it is sometimes claimed that causal inference *requires* a randomized trial. But bias can occur even in randomized trials. For example, confounding can occur if the treatment received is not well concealed from participants or care givers (we say they are not "blinded") and leads to other co-interventions that affect the trial outcome.

Conversely, well-designed observational studies that consistently show strong associations with a dose–response relation (for example, higher risks of the outcome in participants with higher levels of exposure), as well as confirmation in repeated studies in different settings, often provide sufficient evidence of causation to take action. That cigarette smoking causes lung cancer can no longer be debated, despite the efforts of tobacco companies to undermine the "merely observational" evidence base. The reduced lung cancer risk in ex-smokers, the fall in lung cancer incidence in countries that have succeeded in reducing their smoking rates, and the rise in incidence in other countries with increased smoking provide strong evidence of causality despite the "observational" design of the studies demonstrating the association. Similar arguments can be made for prone sleeping position as a cause for the sudden infant death syndrome, or SIDS.

Precision is different from bias. Like bias, insufficient precision can lead to an error in the estimate of an exposure-outcome association, whether that estimate comes from an observational study or an RCT. Unlike bias, however, precision is the degree of uncertainty about the magnitude of association due to chance variation. Imprecision, or low precision, leads to an estimate that is not systematically too high or too low, but one that shows a wide range of statistical uncertainty around the observed estimate. It is usually due to a small sample size and often prevents detection of a true association or effect. The observed association or effect is called *statistically non-significant*. In other words, it may be entirely attributable to chance. For example, if our above-mentioned study of lung cancer and yellow fingers had included only ten cases and ten controls, we might have observed three cases and no controls with yellow fingers. That would be a statistically non-significant result, because the sample size of only 20 total participants might well yield a difference of this magnitude (three out of ten vs. zero out of ten) solely by chance even if yellow fingers had no true association with lung cancer. This "false-negative" finding has nothing to do with confounding by cigarette smoking. It is merely a consequence of an insufficient sample size, that is, imprecision.

How Should Science Influence Health Beliefs?

What you believe is your decision. Your belief may be based on folk wisdom, cultural or religious influences, or your own personal experience. Deciding what you believe requires a choice among alternatives. First, you should list the realistic alternatives. You may well want to weigh the evidence among those alternatives, which can require quantifying (or at least ranking) their respective benefits, risks, efforts, and costs. You then must attach your own values to those benefits, risks, and costs. Finally, you should choose the alternative that maximizes the overall value of your choice for you, for your child, for your family, and for society. Different people may well arrive at different decisions. Although the true health benefits and risks of a given decision are often the same for most people, some people tend to be more risk-averse than others. And you may not be willing to spend the effort or money required by some of the alternatives.

How should you assess the risks and benefits of alternative decision choices? Unfortunately, conformity with "expert" recommendations is not an ideal recipe for deciding what to believe and act on. Different experts (or expert groups) may well disagree. Many expert recommendations are based on minimizing risks for everyone, even when the risks are already extremely low and even when considerable effort is required to reduce them further. What about conformity with your family, neighborhood, or church? Social interactions can lead to a "herd effect" by which communities defined by geographic, cultural, religious, or socioeconomic backgrounds encourage similar or even identical decisions by members of the community. Instead of following expert advice or your group's norm, however, you may want to know more about the scientific basis underlying that advice and those norms. If you seek the evidence (or lack thereof) for risk and harm of your health beliefs, this book is for you.

Key Evidence Points
- A key aspect of science is the rigorous testing of cause-and-effect hypotheses about the relation of an exposure (postulated cause) and outcome (postulated effect).
- The randomized controlled trial (RCT) is the human analog of an animal experiment and is the scientific "gold standard" for testing causal hypotheses in human health.
- Biases are systematic errors that can lead to erroneous causal inferences, especially in observational (non-experimental) studies.
- The major sources of bias are confounding by underlying causes of both the exposure and outcome, and reverse causality, whereby the outcome precedes and causes the exposure, rather than the reverse.

Summing Up: Synthesizing the Scientific Evidence

2

Why Synthesize the Evidence?

If you are reading this book, you want access to the best scientific evidence before deciding which commonly held health beliefs to adhere to and which to ignore. In today's world, access usually means online access. Most people start with an Internet search, selecting one or a few summaries from sources they believe to be reliable and unbiased or that seem useful. But a simple Google search won't cut it, because you and other people without epidemiologic or other training in research methodology are not usually able to sift through the mountain of "hits" and separate the grain from the chaff. The most recent study also does not suffice—it almost never replaces all those that precede it. It is true that knowledge increases over time, but the process is not linear. Sometimes it is two steps forward, one step backward.

Even for doctors and other health providers, keeping up with the best evidence is tough. Clinicians often rely on reviews published in their specialty's journals; some even subscribe to a regular (monthly, for example) review service that summarizes topics in the diagnosis and treatment of conditions relevant to their practice. Similarly, governments, insurance companies, and other organizations responsible for health systems or policy also depend on up-to-date scientific evidence. They often seek reviews in scientific journals and publications by professional societies and government agencies.

Unfortunately, most conventional reviews are narrative descriptions. That is, they tell a story in a way that is digestible for the intended audience. Their readability is a strong point, but they are seriously flawed in one important respect: they are shaped by the reviewer's choices. They are therefore almost always selective, incomplete, and unverifiable. In other words, they tend to be biased. The reviewer may be biased by her prior opinion, or she may make an honest appraisal rooted in her past experience, augmented by a recent literature search. But the reader has no way of knowing how she selected the studies cited in her review. Selective citation of published studies can lead to serious bias in reviewing scientific evidence. This is

© The Author(s), under exclusive license to Springer Nature Switzerland AG 2023
M. S. Kramer, *Believe It or Not*, https://doi.org/10.1007/978-3-031-46022-7_2

often referred to as "cherry picking," a colloquial expression for bias due to selective citation of studies when reviewing the evidence.

You may well ask, "But isn't the reviewer an expert in the field? If so, why shouldn't I trust her?" The answer is simple. Two expert reviewers can and often do disagree with each other. Both of their reviews are readily available, either from Professor Google or via a library search. What are you, as an intelligent and thoughtful member of the general public seeking a review of the published evidence, supposed to do when faced with two (or five!) conflicting expert reviews? That is the problem.

A personal anecdote will illustrate the problem. In 1995, I was meeting with potential Belarusian obstetrician and pediatrician collaborators to discuss a large randomized controlled trial (RCT) we were planning to conduct in their country, Belarus. The RCT's goal was to assess the impact of a breastfeeding promotion intervention on infant feeding practices and the health of the offspring. At that 1995 meeting, I was discussing the strengths of the RCT design with my collaborators, reviewing many of the arguments I made in Chap. 1 of this book. I asked them how they decide between two different treatment options for their patients. "We ask an expert," they replied. "But," I countered, "what if you ask two different experts, and the two give opposite advice?" "Then we'd ask a third expert," they responded, "a bigger expert." That response got a few assenting nods, but also a good laugh from the attendees. The episode underlines the problem of reliance on expert opinion.

The truth is conflicting views or interpretations of the evidence are the rule, not the exception. Expert judgments are not mere mechanical, arithmetical manipulations. Rather, they must consider the quality of the studies: their potential for bias, their size, and their representativeness. Quality assessments are both time-consuming and subjective.

What is the alternative? What should *you* do when faced with conflicting expert opinion? Or even in the absence of conflict, should you follow the crowd, that is, the shared opinion of your friends, family, church, or yoga class (what I referred to as the herd effect in Chap. 1)? My suggestion is to distrust expert opinion, no matter how "big" the expert, and also to distrust your "herd." The preferred alternative is called a *systematic review*, which I describe in the following section.

Systematic Review

Unlike a conventional review, a systematic review is a research study in its own right. In fact, it can require greater effort and time than a new, independent study. Like an individual research study, it should attempt to test a specific scientific hypothesis: often, a causal hypothesis that a specific treatment or other exposure affects one or more subsequent health outcomes. For example, we might want to review the published evidence comparing the effects on subsequent aggressive child behavior of physical punishment, "time out" in the bedroom, or removal of privileges in school-age children who exhibit some undesirable behavior. Systematic reviews are also useful for descriptive and predictive studies.

Like an individual research study, a systematic review benefits from a formal *protocol* written beforehand. The protocol states the objective(s) of the review: usually, the causal question to be addressed. The protocol also details the bibliometric methods (which electronic databases, keywords, and logic) to be used in searching the literature for published studies and the criteria by which studies will be included in or excluded from the review. It should also indicate how the reviewer(s) will assess the quality and validity of each study meeting the inclusion criteria. Finally, the protocol should describe the methods to be used to synthesize the evidence from the collected studies. These include both qualitative synthesis (a descriptive summary of the characteristics, strengths, and weaknesses of the assembled studies) and, if justified, a quantitative pooling of data and statistical analysis across studies (called a *meta-analysis*).

Many of the published systematic reviews I cite in this book are limited to a narrative description of the studies reviewed, summarizing their designs, geographic settings, and main results in text and tables, perhaps also commenting on their individual strengths and weaknesses. Others provide that information but also include a meta-analysis. Some narrative systematic reviews omit meta-analysis because they judge the characteristics or results of the studies to be too heterogeneous to pool, but most do not state the reasons for the omission.

A systematic review takes far more time to complete than a conventional review and may require research funding (a grant). It also requires expertise in research methods, statistical analysis, and the substantive area under review. Although a single author may have expertise in all of these areas, a collaborative team is often necessary. Moreover, collaboration is helpful to enhance the validity of the many judgments needed on study eligibility and quality, and of the data extracted for meta-analysis. Table 2.1 compares and contrasts systematic and conventional reviews.

Table 2.1 Systematic vs. conventional review of published scientific evidence

Systematic review	Conventional review
Addresses a specific scientific hypothesis	Often topic-driven, not hypothesis-driven
Benefits from a formal protocol that specifies objectives and methods: • Inclusion/exclusion criteria • Bibliometric methods • Assessment of study quality • Data extraction from included studies • Meta-analysis, if justified	Narrative description, no prior protocol, no formal methods, no meta-analysis
Very time-consuming, may require funding	Requires skill and time, usually unfunded
Requires expertise in research methods, statistics, and substantive area (collaboration)	Requires expertise in substantive area
Less susceptible to reviewer bias	Often biased by selective citation ("cherry picking")

Reviewing the Evidence on Health Beliefs and Practices

In the remainder of this book, I will apply the principles laid out in the first two chapters. The areas covered will be divided into four main sections: health beliefs and practices regarding infections, skin and eye conditions, foods and beverages, and pregnancy and childhood. The four sections contain several chapters, each covering a single topic related to health beliefs and practices.

I do not review every health belief and practice. Many have been thoroughly debunked by existing books and online resources. Instead, I focus on those I have encountered during my 45-year career as a physician and medical researcher, and that I found intriguing. I wanted to understand their historical and cultural origins; to discover who currently subscribes to them; and to undertake a rigorous and systematic review of the scientific *evidence for and against* them. My intent is to provide you with a complete and unbiased source of the science underlying the beliefs. After reading my analysis of each belief or practice, you may or may not agree with my inferences, but I can promise that you will learn about its history and societal influences, as well as the scientific evidence bearing on its validity. As mentioned in the Preface to this book, your doctor or other health provider is *unlikely* to be familiar with this evidence and may be surprised to learn from you about your inferences!

In line with the arguments made in this chapter, I will heavily rely on systematic reviews. These will not be *my* systematic reviews. Since you have made it this far, you will appreciate that even a single original systematic review relevant to any of the 21 topic chapters that comprise the remainder of this book is a major undertaking that could require as much of my time and effort as this entire book. The time required to carry out an original systematic review of all topics in this book would far exceed my remaining life expectancy. Moreover, such an undertaking would ignore the thought and work that other researchers have put into publishing their systematic reviews.

You may now believe that the conclusions of a systematic review are an objective, almost arithmetic, summary of the evidence. That would be nice, but systematic reviews unfortunately cannot avoid subjectivity. Subjective choices are made in searching the published literature, deciding the eligibility criteria for studies to be included, which studies meet those criteria, the quality of the included studies, and whether or not to pool (meta-analyze) the results across studies. It is not rare for two systematic reviews on the same topic to reach different conclusions. But systematic reviews have a major strength: it is usually far easier to understand *why* they disagree than it is with conventional reviews.

I will therefore base my assessment of the evidence on systematic reviews whenever possible. For health beliefs on which I am unable to find systematic reviews, I will not conduct my own. Instead, I will mention their absence and summarize the results of what I believe to be the best individual studies on the topic, as well as the major outstanding issues requiring resolution. I will also comment on the overall strengths and weaknesses of published studies in the topic area and on how to fill the major evidence gaps.

Most published health research studies are conducted by researchers living and working in high-income, Western settings, although some have examined within-country ethnic or socioeconomic differences in associations between exposures/treatments and outcomes. High-quality research from some Asian and Latin American countries has also become increasingly common in recent years. But the evidence base remains weak for many areas of the world, especially the Middle East and sub-Saharan Africa. I will try to identify ethnocultural gaps in the evidence base and speculate about why the published literature might, or might not, apply to people in different geographic areas or ethnocultural groups.

Finally, the evidence I review should influence, and in many cases already has influenced, recommendations for clinical practice, health policy, and education. But you are probably more interested in health beliefs and practices that affect you and your family. You should therefore consider how you and your family value the benefits, risks, effort, and costs associated with following each belief and practice. In this book, I attempt to quantify the estimated benefits and risks. Those estimates are statistical *probabilities* of good and bad outcomes, respectively. But weighing the estimates and deciding whether the effort and cost of maximizing the benefits and minimizing the risks are worth expending, depend on *your values*—not mine and not even society's.

Key Evidence Points
- Conventional reviews of published evidence are highly susceptible to bias due to selective citation ("cherry picking").
- In contrast, *systematic reviews* use rigorous methods to find all relevant studies, evaluate their strengths and weaknesses, and (if justified) pool their results.
- Ideally, systematic reviews of the scientific evidence should inform your health beliefs and practices, especially where that evidence is complex and conflicting.
- The benefits and risks associated with alternative choices based on specific beliefs and practices can often be estimated from systematic reviews, but *your* values of those benefits and risks, as well as the effort and costs required to achieve them, are likely to vary from those of others.

How to Read the Rest of This Book

As mentioned in the Preface, you can read this book by selecting chapters of particular interest to you. Now that you've read the first two chapters and understand the basic scientific and epidemiologic concepts discussed therein, you can skip around and limit your reading to those topics that are important to you.

Each of the remaining chapters is organized in a similar fashion. It begins with an Introduction that provides a background and context for the topic, including the historical, cultural, and religious origins of the health belief or practice under discussion. The second section of each topic chapter summarizes the information available on the prevalence of the beliefs and practices comprising the chapter, that is, *who believes*. In this section, I prioritize systematic reviews or individual studies of variations in the prevalence of the belief or practice across and within countries, over time, and according to age, education, ethnicity, and other factors. In the third section of each topic chapter, I provide a detailed review of the scientific evidence supporting or undermining the belief or practice, including the quality of published studies: in other words, why you should believe it or not. You may find it useful to refer back to Chaps. 1 and 2 when reading this section. For those of you who do not want or need the detailed review, I provide a bulleted summary of the evidence just before it. I conclude each topic chapter with a brief summary text.

Part II

Infection

Dodging the Draft: Does Avoiding the Cold Reduce the Risk of Catching a Cold?

3

Introduction

What Is a Cold?

The "common cold" is indeed common; it is the most frequent human infectious disease. Adults often average 2–5 colds per year, children average 6–10, and infants and toddlers in day care, even more. In clinical terms, a cold is limited to the upper respiratory tract: the nose, eyes, and throat, although it can also mildly affect the larynx (voice box) and trachea (windpipe). The symptoms of a cold are runny or stuffy nose, sneezing, tearing, sore throat, and cough. Mild fever, reduced appetite, headache, muscle soreness, and weakness are more general (systemic) symptoms, but they are generally far less severe and of shorter duration than with influenza ("the flu").

Colds are viral infections, and several distinct families of viruses have been identified as the causative infectious agents [1]. The most common are rhinoviruses in older children and adults and, in young children, the respiratory syncytial virus. Although coronaviruses are now widely known as the causative agents of COVID-19 and SARS, they are also the causes of milder colds limited to the upper respiratory tract. Influenza virus can also cause mild cold symptoms, rather than the more severe illness typically associated with the flu. Adenoviruses are another family of viruses causing the common cold.

None of these viruses has specific features that allow clinicians to identify which virus is responsible for the cold. A viral culture or other laboratory test is required for such identification, although identifying the infectious agent is not necessary or helpful for managing the infections. No treatment has been clearly established to lessen the severity or shorten the duration of cold symptoms, including antiviral medications that can be helpful in influenza or COVID-19. Pain relievers like acetaminophen (Tylenol) and non-steroidal anti-inflammatory drugs like ibuprofen (Advil, Motrin) and naproxen (Naprosyn, Aleve) can help reduce headache, sore throat, muscle soreness, and fever.

Historical Origins

Colds have probably contributed to human suffering throughout the history of our species. They are described in the Egyptian Ebers papyrus, the oldest known medical text, written over 35 centuries ago and named after the nineteenth-century German Egyptologist Georg Ebers. In the English language, the linking of the illness (*a* cold) with environmental temperature (***the*** cold) dates back at least to the sixteenth century [2]. This link thus arose well before germs (bacteria, viruses, fungi) became established as the causative agents of infectious diseases. The rationale for the link is likely the similarity between symptoms of exposure to cold air (runny nose and eyes, shivering) to those of upper respiratory tract infections, as well as the higher incidence during winter (cold) months in temperate regions.

It is remarkable, to me at least, that the semantic link between a cold and the cold is not limited to the English language. In Spanish, the word for a cold is *resfriado* (or, less commonly, *resfrio*); *tener un resfriado* (to have a cold) clearly contains the adjective root (*frio*) denoting a cold temperature. In Italian, to have a cold is *essere raffreddato*, clearly linked to the adjective *freddo* denoting cold temperature. In German also, the word for a cold (*Erkältung*) contains the adjective *kalt*, meaning cold temperature. At first glance, French might seem to be an exception (*Vive la différence!*): the word for cold (*rhume*) contains no elements of the adjective (*froid*) used to describe cold weather. But a deeper dive shows that French has not escaped the general trend. *Attraper froid* (catch a cold) is a more common expression among francophones around the globe than *attraper un rhume*!

Given its long history and widespread geographic distribution, the link between cold weather and the common cold is ensconced in folk wisdom and is a generally held health belief. This belief takes several forms. The obvious one is related to cold environmental temperature. But other forms include the perceived need to dress warmly to avoid "catching cold" (note here the absence of the indefinite article, *a*); avoiding drafts of cool air from an open window or door (see Fig. 3.1), or from an air conditioner or fan; moving from a hot environment to a cooler one "too rapidly," i.e., without gradual adaptation; wearing wet clothes for a prolonged time; and my personal favorite, venturing outdoors with wet hair.

The reasons for the persistence of these beliefs and the firmly held conviction with which they are defended across the world are incompletely understood. You might think that the general public would have abandoned them when the germ theory of infectious diseases was established by Pasteur, Koch, and others in the late nineteenth century. Viruses were discovered at that time as infectious agents that, unlike bacteria, passed through filter paper and required dividing cells to grow. It was not until the electron microscope was invented in the 1930s that viruses could be visualized, however, and not until the 1950s that cold viruses were identified.

Fig. 3.1 Defying the risks of a cold

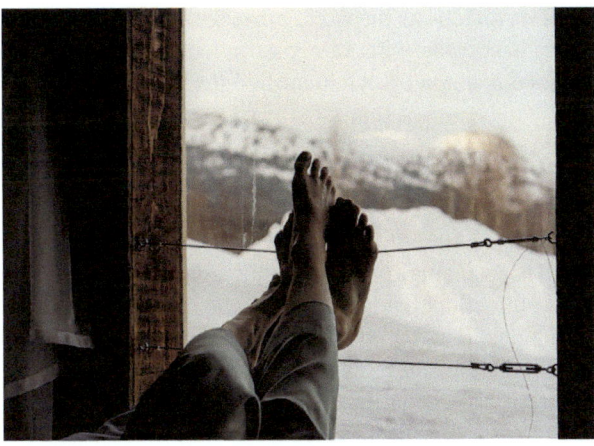

Current Beliefs About the Cause of the Common Cold

I was unable to find any systematic reviews or high-quality individual studies documenting current beliefs about cold exposure as a cause of the common cold. In the absence of such studies, I will fall back on my own clinical experience—flawed though it may be. In the course of working in a children's hospital emergency department, I saw hundreds of children with colds. Most of their parents were aware that viruses can cause the common cold. But some of them minimized the role of contagion, that is, "catching" a cold from another infected child or family member, firmly maintaining their belief in the causal role of cold air, insufficient clothing, sudden drop in environmental temperature, or wet clothes or hair.

Part of the problem here is what is understood as a "cause" by the general public. Many mistakenly believe that causation requires that all persons exposed to a causal agent will experience the outcome that is hypothesized to be the effect of that exposure; in other words, the exposure is *sufficient* to cause the effect. They also believe that exposure to the hypothesized cause is *necessary* to cause that outcome. In fact, it is rarely true that causes are both necessary and sufficient to achieve an outcome.

Some rare genetic diseases do fulfill both criteria. For example, Huntington's disease is inherited from a parent and *always* leads to brain degeneration and the consequent movement, mood, and cognitive decline that characterize the disease. Conversely, one *cannot* develop Huntington's disease without genetic mutation. In other words, the mutation is both necessary and sufficient to cause the disease.

For infectious diseases, however, the microbial agent (bacterium, virus, or fungus) is necessary but rarely sufficient to cause the infection. Tuberculosis provides a good example. Koch identified the responsible bacterium in 1882, but it was well known even then that most persons exposed to the bacterium did *not* get infected. Moreover, many of those who are infected are able to limit their infection without becoming ill (the so-called latent infection). A good recent example is COVID-19. Many persons exposed to infected family members, friends, or coworkers remain uninfected, and those who are infected may not have any symptoms of the disease.

These examples do not argue against causality. Other factors besides the causative infectious agent influence who contracts the disease and, among those infected, who gets ill and who dies from the infection. These other factors are also *causes* of the infection; they may include older age (well-known with COVID-19), genetic susceptibility, poor nutrition, and impaired immune function. None of these factors is necessary or sufficient on its own to cause infection, but one or more of them may be required, *along with* the necessary infectious agent, to lead to infection and illness.

The same argument for multiple causes holds for the common cold. In other words, belief in the dangers of "the cold" does not exclude respiratory viruses as the infectious agents of the common cold. A virus is necessary to cause a cold, but it may not be sufficient. The relevant scientific question here is whether exposure to cold temperatures *increases* a person's risk of contracting a cold when exposed to the causative virus. Answering that scientific question requires a careful review of the scientific evidence.

Key Evidence Points
- The common cold shows a very consistent pattern of increased frequency during the winter at temperate latitudes in the Northern and Southern Hemispheres.
- The seasonal pattern is less consistent at tropical latitudes.
- Studies in human participants do *not* indicate increased risks of colds due to chills brought on by cold air or water immersion.
- No studies were found bearing on brief drafts or venturing outside while perspiring or with wet hair.
- The low humidity that characterizes heated indoor environments in winter has been shown to increase replication and transmission of cold and influenza viruses.
- Some laboratory studies suggest impaired immune responses to cold and influenza viruses at low temperatures, but studies in human participants are unconvincing.
- Indoor crowding and poor ventilation are associated with an increased risk of colds in winter.

Detailed Review of the Scientific Evidence[1]

Seasonality

One of the most important pieces of evidence supporting a causal effect of exposure to cold air or cold weather on the risk of colds is seasonality. Are colds more frequent in the winter than in the summer? If so, does the seasonality effect vary by latitude? In other words, is the seasonal effect stronger in temperate locations far from the equator than the effect in more tropical locations? As we shall see shortly, the answer to all of these questions is "yes."

In temperate latitudes in both the Northern and Southern Hemispheres, the common cold and other respiratory infections are far more frequent in winter than in summer. This effect has been documented in separate studies of hospitalized children in Germany [3] and in Argentina [4] that included identification of individual respiratory virus species, as well as in a systematic review limited to respiratory syncytial virus [5]. Similar findings (but without virus identification) were reported in a study of general practitioner consultations for upper and lower respiratory infections over a 10-year period among the elderly in the UK [6].

A more recent global systematic review that included viral identification focused on lower respiratory tract infections (pneumonia, bronchiolitis, tracheobronchitis, and croup) [7]. The authors observed a similar pronounced seasonal pattern (increase in frequency of infection during colder months) in temperate regions but a far weaker pattern in the tropics. A separate recent systematic review limited to influenza virus observed very similar patterns in temperate versus tropical locations [8].

Effects of Exposure to Cold Temperature

Many people are already convinced about the causal effect of exposure to cold temperature. A major source of bias in causal inference is the logical fallacy known as post hoc, *ergo propter hoc* (Latin for "after this, therefore because of this"), also referred to as the post hoc fallacy. As discussed in Chap. 1, inferring that an exposure that precedes an outcome caused that outcome merely because of its temporal precedence is like inferring that the rooster's pre-dawn crowing causes the sun to rise. For the common cold, this logical fallacy is very common. During the winter, anyone who comes down with a cold can think back to a recent draft or chill, insufficient dress, or leaving the house with wet hair or while perspiring.

For those who fervently believe that chills are responsible for colds, or at least *their* colds, such exposures are far more likely to be recalled and blamed than they are among skeptics or agnostics about the role of chills. This phenomenon has been well documented by cognitive psychologists; it is called *confirmation bias*. Confirmation bias is the tendency to interpret information in a way that is consistent

---

[1] Readers who prefer to skip the Detailed Review should proceed to the Summary at the end of the chapter.

with one's existing beliefs. If you believe in the chill theory, that theory is confirmed by recollection of a recent chill. If you do not believe in the theory, you are not only less likely to recall a recent chill but also more likely to reject its etiologic importance even if you recall it. When combined with the post hoc fallacy, confirmation bias is a potent source of erroneous causal inference.

In seeking rigorous scientific studies that answer the key questions, I found few systematic reviews, but some of the individual basic science and human participant studies are of high scientific quality. None of the studies bear on exposure to cold drafts, sudden changes in temperature, wearing thin versus heavy clothing, or venturing out into the cold while sweating or with wet hair.

I did succeed, however, in finding three controlled human experimental studies that attempted to test the "chill theory." The first was a 1958 study comparing three different treatment conditions among 428 young healthy adult volunteers [9]. Control participants were placed in a room kept at 80 °F (27 °C) and 30% relative humidity for 4 h, dressed in shorts and socks (plus brassieres or halters in the women). One chilled group was similarly dressed but kept in a room at 60 °F (15.5 °C) and 80% relative humidity. The third group spent 2 h in a room maintained at 10 °F (−12 °C) and 80% relative humidity, dressed in street clothes, overcoat, hat, and gloves. Participants in all three groups received an instillation in each nostril of 0.2 mL of filtered nasal secretions from patients suffering from colds, either just before going into their assigned room or immediately after leaving. (Research ethics were a lot looser in 1958!) The method of allocating the 428 participants is not mentioned but was unlikely to have been randomized, especially since the third group was half the size of the other two—probably because it was difficult to recruit volunteers for that one! Outcomes were based on symptoms reported to research staff who were unaware of ("blinded" to) group assignment when the participants returned to the research laboratory 1, 2, 3, and 5 days after their treatment. The participants themselves could not, of course, be blinded. About one-third of the participants in all three groups developed symptoms that met preestablished criteria for a cold. In other words, neither of the chilling conditions increased the risk of a cold.

The second experimental human study recruited 49 male prisoner volunteers deliberately infected (via nasal instillation or small-particle aerosol) with a single strain of rhinovirus [10]. The participants were each exposed to a control or chill treatment. The chill treatments varied in type. In one type, the room was maintained at 4–10 °C and 50% relative humidity for 1–2 h, and participants were dressed in shorts and undershirts. In the second type of chilling, participants were immersed in a bath maintained at 32 °C for 4–6 h. The timing of the chill treatment was also varied: at the time of inoculation with the virus, during the incubation period (the day after inoculation, before becoming ill), and during the illness. The control group was kept in a room maintained at 23 °C. The method of treatment allocation is not mentioned but was clearly not randomized. Given the small and variable number of participants receiving each treatment, it is hardly surprising that no differences were observed among the treatment groups in the proportion who developed illness, the proportion in whom rhinovirus was detected, or the participants' antibody response.

The third human experimental study was a bona fide randomized trial of sudden foot cooling [11]. Johnson and Eccles randomized 90 of 180 healthy young adults to a single immersion of both of their feet in a bowl of water maintained (with ice, if necessary) at 10 °C for 20 min. The 90 randomized to the control intervention kept on their shoes and socks and placed their feet in an empty bowl for 20 min. No live viruses were administered, and no viral identification tests were performed. The primary outcome was the sum of cold symptom scores recorded in a diary over 4–5 days of follow-up after the experimental or control intervention. The total symptom score was significantly higher in the experimental group, but the control intervention was far from being a true placebo, and participants were obviously not blinded to the intervention they received. Given the subjective nature of the outcome and the non-blinding of participants, this trial provides no useful evidence on the effect of chilling on risk of catching a cold.

Effects of Cold Weather on Virus Infectivity and the Immune Response

If chills are not responsible for the higher risk of colds in the winter, what other factors might play a role? Might a lower temperature, either outdoors or indoors, enhance the virus's ability to replicate (multiply)? Or even if it has no effect on the virus, might it depress the host's immune response to the virus and thereby increase the risk of infection?

Foxman and colleagues reported enhanced replication of rhinovirus in cultured airway cells from mice at 33 °C than at normal body temperature (37 °C) [12]. The 33° temperature is the same as that measured in the human nose, where rhinoviruses are known to adhere and initiate infection. This enhanced viral replication appeared to be mediated by the cells' impaired synthesis of interferon, an important antiviral protein. Similar findings were reported by Boonarkart and coworkers in human kidney cells infected with influenza virus. Both enhanced viral replication and reduced interferon synthesis were observed at 25 °C (vs. 37°), but at 33°, only viral replication was affected [13].

Do these effects in cells raised in laboratory conditions translate into increased infection risk or severity in intact humans exposed to cold temperatures? Based on the narrative review by Castellani and colleagues, studies of immune responses in cold-exposed human participants have yielded equivocal results [14].

Cold outdoor temperatures in winter do not adequately reflect conditions indoors. Homes, offices, and other buildings are likely to be heated to (or near to) outdoor summer temperatures, but humidity is far lower in winter. Outdoor air in winter may be quite humid, especially in places like Northern Europe with high rainfall in winter. But the humidity drops markedly indoors, because warm air can hold far more water vapor than cold air. The heated air has the same water *content* as the outdoor air but a much lower *relative humidity* (that is, relative to completely saturated warm air). Shaman and Kohn observed that influenza virus in aerosol droplets was far less likely to survive, and less likely to infect susceptible guinea pigs, in humid air than in dry air [15]. Similarly, Noti and colleagues studied simulated coughs (from a nebulizer of aerosols containing influenza virus) and their ability to infect susceptible dog kidney cells grown in laboratory culture [16]. Infectivity of the virus dropped off considerably over a 5-h period in a room maintained at 20% relative humidity versus that observed in a room at 45% relative humidity.

Effects of Indoor Crowding and Ventilation

In temperate climates, people spend less time outdoors during the cold winter months than they do in summer. As has been confirmed in the COVID-19 pandemic, respiratory viruses are far more transmissible indoors than outdoors. Colds and other respiratory virus infections are primarily transmitted by droplets and aerosols, in which coughing, sneezing, singing, or even speaking leads to droplets or mists that contain live virus. These droplets and aerosols are capable of traveling at least a meter or two from the person who projects them. Transmission by touch (hands, hugs, kisses) can also occur, as can touching objects or surfaces contaminated by infected persons.

Jaakkola and Heinonen studied nearly 900 office workers in a single building in Helsinki, Finland [17]. Workers who shared their office with one or more coworkers had a 35% increased risk of two or more self-reported colds in the previous year than those with an office to themselves, after statistically adjusting (controlling) for age, sex, young children at home, and cigarette smoking.

Al-Khatib and Tabakhna surveyed 200 randomly selected households living in homes contained in a Palestinian refugee camp [18]. Prevalent (at the time of the survey) self-reported cold symptoms were significantly more frequent among households with a higher number of occupants and with more occupants per bedroom, but these associations were not adjusted for smoking or ventilation.

Sun and colleagues carried out two similar studies 10 years apart in about 3000 students living in a dozen college dormitories in Tianjin, China, a large coastal city near Beijing [19, 20]. Both studies comprised two phases: (1) a questionnaire-based survey of colds experienced in the previous 12 months and (2) ventilation rates measured in the dormitory rooms. Students living in six-person dorm rooms were twice as likely to report frequent (six or more episodes) colds in the previous year as those living in three-person rooms, even after statistically adjusting for age, sex, time spent in the room, and exposure to tobacco smoke. An inverse dose–response association was observed between the room ventilation rate per person in winter and the proportion of students with six or more reported colds: the higher the ventilation rate, the lower the risk of frequent colds.

Summary

The common cold has been recognized throughout human history. The semantic link between exposure to *the* cold and an increased risk of catching *a* cold is found not only in the English language, but also in Spanish, Italian, German, and French. And although I was not able to identify reliable epidemiologic studies that quantitate specific beliefs, many people believe that their colds occur when they are exposed to cold temperatures, sudden drops in temperature, cold drafts, wearing thin clothing in winter, or going outside in winter while perspiring or with wet hair. These beliefs are prevalent even among persons who know that viruses can cause the common cold. Yet, many physicians have mistakenly "debunked" such beliefs merely by citing evidence that viruses are the infectious agents.

The marked increase in occurrence of the common cold in temperate regions and the less consistent seasonal variation in tropical regions indicate that *something* about cold weather does indeed increase the risk of catching a cold. Studies in human participants do not demonstrate an increased risk of colds due to chills brought on by exposure to cold air or water immersion, although no studies were found bearing on exposure to brief drafts or venturing outside while perspiring or with wet hair. The low humidity that characterizes heated indoor environments in winter has been shown to increase replication and transmission of cold and influenza viruses. Some laboratory studies suggest impaired immune responses to cold and influenza viruses at low temperatures, but studies in human participants have reported equivocal results. Indoor crowding and poor ventilation are significantly associated with an increased frequency of colds in winter. Although more evidence is needed, cold weather is clearly associated with an increased risk of catching a cold, but that increased risk is probably a consequence of the drier indoor air, indoor crowding, and reduced ventilation characteristic of indoor life in colder climates.

References

1. Eccles R. Understanding the symptoms of the common cold and influenza. Lancet Infect Dis. 2005;5(11):718–25.
2. Online Etymology Dictionary. etymonline.com.
3. du Prel JB, Puppe W, Gröndahl B, Knuf M, Weigl JA, Schaaff F, Schmitt HJ. Are meteorological parameters associated with acute respiratory tract infections? Clin Infect Dis. 2009;49(6):861–8.
4. Viegas M, Barrero PR, Maffey AF, Mistchenko AS. Respiratory viruses seasonality in children under five years of age in Buenos Aires, Argentina: a five-year analysis. J Infect. 2004;49(3):222–8.
5. Tang JW, Loh TP. Correlations between climate factors and incidence—a contributor to RSV seasonality. Rev Med Virol. 2014;24(1):15–34.
6. Hajat S, Bird W, Haines A. Cold weather and GP consultations for respiratory conditions by elderly people in 16 locations in the UK. Eur J Epidemiol. 2004;19(10):959–68.

7. Li Y, Reeves RM, Wang X, Bassat Q, Brooks WA, Cohen C, Moore DP, Nunes M, Rath B, Campbell H, Nair H, RSV Global Epidemiology Network; RESCEU Investigators. Global patterns in monthly activity of influenza virus, respiratory syncytial virus, parainfluenza virus, and metapneumovirus: a systematic analysis. Lancet Glob Health. 2019;7(8):e1031–45.
8. Dave K, Lee PC. Global geographical and temporal patterns of seasonal influenza and associated climatic factors. Epidemiol Rev. 2019;41(1):51–68.
9. Dowling HF, Jackson GG, Spiesman IG, Inouye T. Transmission of the common cold to volunteers under controlled conditions. III. The effect of chilling of the subjects upon susceptibility. Am J Hyg. 1958;68(1):59–65.
10. Douglas RG, Lindgren KM, Couch RB. Exposure to cold environment and rhinovirus common cold: failure to demonstrate effect. N Engl J Med. 1968;279:742–7.
11. Johnson C, Eccles R. Acute cooling of the feet and the onset of common cold symptoms. Fam Pract. 2005;22(6):608–13.
12. Foxman EF, Storer JA, Fitzgerald ME, Wasik BR, Hou L, Zhao H, Turner PE, Pyle AM, Iwasaki A. Temperature-dependent innate defense against the common cold virus limits viral replication at warm temperature in mouse airway cells. Proc Natl Acad Sci U S A. 2015;112(3):827–32.
13. Boonarkart C, Suptawiwat O, Sakorn K, Puthavathana P, Auewarakul P. Exposure to cold impairs interferon-induced antiviral defense. Arch Virol. 2017;162(8):2231–7.
14. Castellani JW, M Brenner IK, Rhind SG. Cold exposure: human immune responses and intracellular cytokine expression. Med Sci Sports Exerc. 2002;34(12):2013–20.
15. Shaman J, Kohn M. Absolute humidity modulates influenza survival, transmission, and seasonality. Proc Natl Acad Sci U S A. 2009;106(9):3243–8.
16. Noti JD, Blachere FM, McMillen CM, Lindsley WG, Kashon ML, Slaughter DR, Beezhold DH. High humidity leads to loss of infectious influenza virus from simulated coughs. PLoS One. 2013;8(2):e57485.
17. Jaakkola JJ, Heinonen OP. Shared office space and the risk of the common cold. Eur J Epidemiol. 1995;11(2):213–6.
18. Al-Khatib IA, Tabakhna H. Housing conditions and health in Jalazone Refugee Camp in Palestine. East Mediterr Health J. 2006;12(1–2):144–52.
19. Sun Y, Wang Z, Zhang Y, Sundell J. In China, students in crowded dormitories with a low ventilation rate have more common colds: evidence for airborne transmission. PLoS One. 2011;6(11):e27140.
20. Yang F, Sun Y, Wang P, Weschler LB, Sundell J. Spread of respiratory infections in student dormitories in China. Sci Total Environ. 2021;777:145983.

Dietary Supplements and Common Viral Infections: "Boosting" the Immune System or the Manufacturers' Profits?

4

Introduction

It will not surprise you to learn that the presumed link between nutrition and health can be traced back to Hippocrates, the fifth-century BC ancient Greek physician often referred to as the father of medicine. The link is summarized by a quote that is often attributed to Hippocrates: "Let food be thy medicine and medicine be thy food." Like many such quotes, its source can be questioned.

Beyond the assumption that anything said 2500 years ago must be true (especially if it was said by Hippocrates!), precious little was known about medicine, and even about nutrition, until the Enlightenment during the seventeenth and eighteenth centuries. In 1747, James Lind, a Scottish physician working on a British naval ship, carried out what may have been the first controlled (albeit not randomized) trial of a medical treatment when he divided 12 sailors who had developed scurvy during their voyage into six groups of two sailors each. Scurvy is a disease characterized by swollen, bleeding gums, and poor wound healing. It had a high fatality rate, killing more British sailors than did sea battles with the French and Spanish navies. Despite the tiny sample size of Lind's trial (the concept of "statistical significance" was unknown at the time), the only two sailors whose condition improved were those given oranges and lemons. Scurvy is now known to be caused by a deficiency of vitamin C, but it and other vitamins were not identified until the twentieth century. Other vitamin deficiency diseases like rickets (insufficient vitamin D), beriberi (thiamine, vitamin B_1), pellagra (niacin, vitamin B_3), and night blindness (vitamin A) were also identified around the same time.

Vitamins are essential micronutrients, meaning that they are required for survival and health, cannot be synthesized by the human organism, and must therefore be consumed in food or dietary supplements in "micro" quantities, that is, measured in milligrams or micrograms. They are organic compounds containing carbon linked to hydrogen, oxygen, and nitrogen. Inorganic essential micronutrients, usually referred to as minerals, include iron, zinc, copper, and magnesium. Vitamins and minerals began to be produced and sold as supplements in the 1930s and 1940s and are often combined as "multivitamins."

Nutrition and Health

Nowadays, we hear a lot about the importance of good nutrition, with frequent pleas for healthy eating from physicians, nutritionists, other health care practitioners, and public health authorities. So-called healthy diets can refer to the overall quantity of food, to dietary macronutrients (energy, fat, carbohydrates, and protein measured in calories, grams, and ounces), micronutrients (vitamins and minerals), dietary fiber, or the variety and balance among the nutrients consumed.

It is also often unclear what aspect of health is believed to be impacted by these aspects of the diet. Is it prevention of heart disease, high blood pressure, and stroke? Is it cancer? Is it obesity and diabetes? Is it mental illness, cognitive function, or mood? Does it imply an increase in life expectancy? Fewer hospitalizations? Fewer days lost from work, school, or leisure activities? Fewer infections or other episodic illnesses? Without improved specificity about both the exposure (which aspect of the diet) and the outcome (which aspect of health), any inferences about the effect of diet on health are too broad to be useful.

The adverse effects of obesity on the heart, circulatory system, metabolism (diabetes), and longevity are well documented and non-controversial. So too are the effects of obesity and high fat intake on certain cancers, such as breast and colorectal cancer. The benefits of a high-fiber diet in reducing the risks of colorectal cancer and diverticulitis are also well established. Micronutrient deficiencies, such as rickets with insufficient vitamin D intake and impaired vision due to inadequate intake of vitamin A, are seen much less frequently today than in the past but are still endemic in certain regions of the world. The same can be said for iron and vitamin B_{12} deficiencies, especially in strict vegetarian populations.

But in the absence of true micronutrient deficiencies, other beneficial effects of dietary supplements, which are highly touted by the multibillion-dollar supplement industry, are not necessarily supported by rigorous scientific studies such as placebo-controlled randomized trials. Vitamin and mineral supplements in doses below those known to be toxic can be sold legally without evidence of any health benefit. Their manufacturers therefore have no incentive to fund studies testing their beneficial effects (Fig. 4.1).

Nutrition and Infection

This chapter will focus on one category of potential benefits of dietary supplements: reducing the risk of infectious diseases like the common cold, influenza, and other viral respiratory infections. Infectious diseases also include viral gastroenteritis,

Fig. 4.1 Do these dietary supplements help prevent common viral infections?

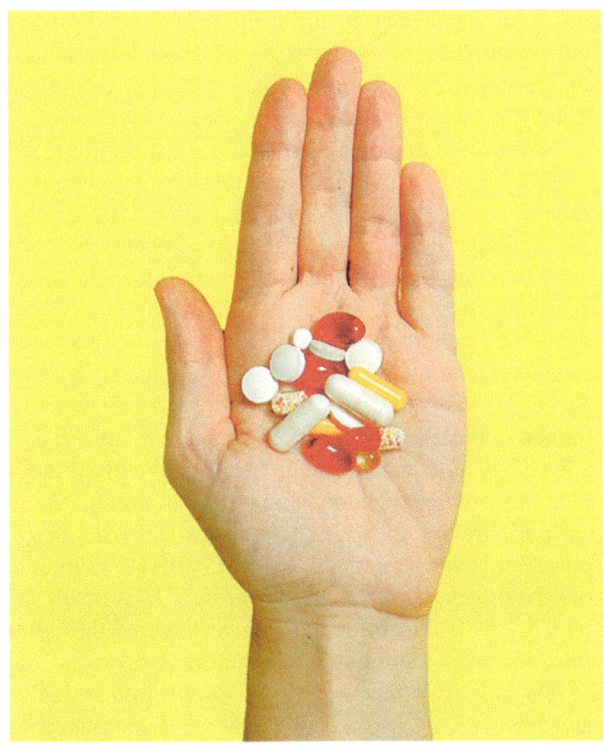

which is characterized by diarrhea, sometimes preceded by nausea and vomiting, and is often (but erroneously) referred to as "stomach flu." The supplements that I will review in relation to common viral infections include vitamins, minerals, other micronutrients, herbal supplements, and probiotics.

The relationship between nutrition and infection has been amply demonstrated in famine settings. As early as 1810, JF Menkel described the atrophy (wasting and disappearance) of the thymus (a lymphatic organ in the chest) in malnourished patients [1]. Jewish physicians working in the Warsaw ghetto during World War II also observed atrophy of lymphoid tissues, along with loss of positivity to tuberculosis skin tests and low white blood cell counts, in residents suffering from starvation during the siege imposed by the Nazi army [2].

In a series of epidemiologic and clinical studies in Guatemalan children in the 1950s, Scrimshaw and colleagues demonstrated that the causal links between nutrition and infection were reciprocal [3]. The Guatemalan studies showed that frequent infection in infants and young children, and especially gastroenteric infection (diarrhea), had adverse effects on nutritional status, as reflected in reduced growth. The adverse effects on growth were manifested first by reduced weight gain, which could be reversed over time if the children consumed a normal diet. But reductions in length gain were only partially reversible, leading to permanent stunting (short stature). Severe malnutrition led to increases in both the incidence and severity of infection, including death from infection. Feeding supplementation studies in undernourished Guatemalan and Mexican preschool children observed reduced incidence and percentage of days ill from respiratory and gastrointestinal infection [3].

At the other end of the nutrition spectrum, Wood and colleagues' recent umbrella review examined associations of obesity with common infections [4]. An umbrella review is a review of systematic reviews, rather than of individual studies. The authors separated studies of incidence (occurrence of new infections) from those of complications *among* persons already infected. The studied complications include hospitalization, mechanical ventilation, intensive care unit (ICU) admission, and death. For infection incidence, the authors observed a 30% increased risk of pneumonia in general and of influenza-associated pneumonia in particular among obese participants. In studies of overall influenza infection (not limited to influenza pneumonia), obesity was observed to increase the risks of hospital admission, ICU admission, and death between two- and threefold in three of the systematic reviews. In another review included under the "umbrella," the risk increases were more modest and limited to adults. Complication risk increases of 20–100% were also observed in obese patients with COVID-19, although one of the included reviews observed a paradoxical *reduction* in risk of death in obese versus normal-weight patients with that infection. No reviews of the common cold or gastrointestinal infection were identified by the umbrella review.

The adverse effects of severe malnutrition and of obesity on the immune system are thus well established. But how do these effects relate to dietary supplements? Do supplements reduce the risk of common infections like colds, influenza, and gastroenteritis? In the absence of vitamin, mineral, or other micronutrient deficiencies, do supplements further reduce the risks? In other words, if "enough" is necessary, is more even better?

I am not sure why, but in the latter part of the twentieth century, the adverse effects of dietary deficiencies resulted in the following notion: If deficiency is harmful to health, then consumption of additional (supplemental) nutrients, especially micronutrients, must be beneficial. This "more is better" philosophy resulted in an explosion of the dietary supplement industry, including macronutrients and especially protein supplements, micronutrients (vitamins, minerals, and omega-3 and other essential long-chain polyunsaturated fatty acids, or LCPUFAs), and herbal products. In 1994, the U.S. Congress passed a new law, the Dietary Supplement Health and Education Act, designed to ensure that these supplements were safe, that is, did not contain harmful "mega-doses" of micronutrients and were not adulterated with harmful contaminants. The law did not require scientific evidence that the supplements were beneficial for health—only that they were not harmful. Moreover, the law did not forbid or discourage manufacturers from making claims of benefit. Vague claims by manufacturers and lay "nutritionists" that such supplements "boost the immune system" (whatever that means) preceded the 1994 law, but the fact that such a boost does not require scientific evidence to back up the claims has at least boosted the dietary supplement industry!

Dietary Supplements: How Commonly Are They Used? Who Uses Them?

I was not able to locate a systematic review of studies comparing differences in prevalence of use of vitamins, minerals, and other supplements across different countries or temporal trends in use over time. In the absence of such a review, I sought out rigorous epidemiologic studies from individual countries and regions.

Data on the use of nutritional supplements are available from two main sources: supplement manufacturers and government agencies. The manufacturers hire experienced survey companies to carry out market surveys to find out how many people are using the supplements; the main reasons why they are used; which ones are used the most; differences by age, sex, and country of use; and trends in these data over time. Their purpose is to gauge the past business success and future potential (that is, financial profits) of these products. Government agencies are interested in these same data, but for the purpose of assessing health behaviors in the populations for which they are responsible. The data might not be comparable from the two sources, however, since people are more likely to volunteer to participate in a government health survey in which their weight, nutritional status, blood pressure, and other health measures are assessed than to help rich companies get richer. Moreover, people who volunteer for supplement manufacturers' market surveys are almost certainly more likely to use supplements and to believe in their health benefits. In other words, they are likely to be a biased sample of the general population.

The U.S. Centers for Disease Control and Prevention's (CDC's) National Health and Nutrition Examination Survey (NHANES) began in the 1960s: on a periodic basis (every few years) at first and annually since 1999. NHANES is currently based on approximately 5000 participants per year, who are nationally representative of the U.S. population. The survey includes both questionnaire-based, self-reported histories and behaviors, as well as direct measures obtained by trained and standardized examiners. Although the general focus has remained health and nutrition, the specific content has evolved over time to include new topics.

The most recent report of dietary supplement use was based on the NHANES surveys of 2017–2018 [5]. More than half of the adult participants 20 years or older reported consumption of supplements within the month prior to their interview, and the rate was higher in women (64%) than in men (51%). Reported use increased with age in both sexes and was highest in women 60 years or older. The main types of supplements used were multivitamins-minerals, followed by vitamin D and omega-3 fatty acids. Other common types of supplements consumed included vitamin C, botanical (herbal) products, calcium, and vitamin B_{12}. The authors also compared the 2017–2018 survey data to those collected in 2007–2008, that is, a decade earlier. The consumption increased in all age groups over this period, continuing a trend previously reported from NHANES since the late 1980s [6].

Consumer marketing survey data are also available from the supplement manufacturer members of the Council for Responsible Nutrition (CRN), which has carried out online dietary supplement surveys in adults over the last 20 years. Their 2017 survey data show similar trends over time and similar differences by sex and age as those reported by the CDC [7]. The absolute percentages are considerably higher than those reported by the CDC, probably reflecting the online methodology and selective participation by supplement users. CRN data also show higher rates of supplement use by health-conscious participants: higher in those who try to eat a balanced diet, maintain a healthy weight, visit a doctor regularly, exercise regularly, and don't smoke. In other words, supplements were more likely to be consumed by those least likely to benefit from them!

Data from the 2004 Canadian Community Health Survey were based on nearly 35,000 respondents and also included children [8]. For the children, 30–40% used vitamin and mineral supplements on a regular basis, falling to about 25% during adolescence, and then rising steadily among adults with increasing age. As in the U.S. surveys, supplement use was higher among women than among men at all ages, with 60% of women over 70 years taking regular supplements versus 45% of men in that age group. Supplement use also increased with higher income and more advanced education and was higher in those who were food secure (could afford the food they needed) than in those who were food insecure. These Canadian data again suggest that those taking regular supplements were less likely to benefit from them than those who were not.

Two Finnish surveys were based on random samples of elderly adults 75, 80, 85, 90, and 95 years of age in 1999 (2500 participants) and 2009 (1600 participants) living in Helsinki [9]. Participants reported on consumption of vitamins, minerals, and fish oil or other omega-3 fatty acid products in the 2 weeks prior to interview. Half of the respondents reported recent supplement use in the 1999 survey; that fraction had risen to two-thirds in the 2009 survey. Most of the increase over the 10-year interval between surveys was due to increases in use of vitamin D and calcium supplements. In both surveys, supplement use was higher in women than men, and higher supplement use was associated with more advanced education.

An Asian survey was based on nearly 1000 younger adults, 19–44 years of age, who participated in the Taiwan Nutrition and Health Survey carried out in 2005–2008 [10]. As in the Western countries mentioned above, Taiwanese women were more likely to use vitamin or mineral supplements than men: 40% versus 27%. Also as seen in the West, supplement use was higher among respondents with higher income and more advanced education. The only major differences in types of supplements taken versus those reported from Western settings were the inclusion of traditional Chinese medicines and herbs, which were nonetheless used by fewer respondents than standard multivitamins, minerals, and fish oil products.

Finally, the European Prospective Investigation into Cancer and Nutrition (EPIC) is a longitudinal (follow-up) study of nutrition and cancer in ten European countries that enrolled over half a million middle-aged and elderly adults who were not necessarily nationally representative [11]. A subsample of 36,000 participants were selected for a 24-h dietary recall at baseline that included questions about their use of nutritional supplements. As in the representative surveys reviewed above, prevalence of use was higher in women than men and increased with age in all ten countries. But use varied widely from one country to another, with a marked north-south gradient. Prevalence of use was tenfold higher in Denmark (66%) than in Greece

(6.7%). Scandinavian countries had the highest rates of use, southern Mediterranean countries the lowest use, while rates were intermediate in the Netherlands, Germany, and France.

In summary, micronutrient supplement use is common across much of the world, is higher in adult women than men, increases with age, and is associated with high income, advanced education, and behaviors such as healthy weight, regular exercise, and non-smoking. Persons who are most likely to use these supplements appear least likely to need them. In the next section of this chapter, I will review the evidence concerning the effect of nutrition in general, and of dietary supplement use in particular, on the incidence, duration, and severity of common viral infections.

Key Evidence Points
- Vitamin A supplements reduce the risks of measles and gastrointestinal infection in preschool children living in countries with a high prevalence of vitamin A deficiency.
- Vitamin C and D supplements have very small effects in preventing respiratory infections, but vitamin D treatment of adults with COVID-19 can help prevent severe outcomes.
- Insufficient evidence is available for vitamin E and omega-3 fatty acids.
- Zinc supplementation reduces the risk of both diarrhea and pneumonia in young children living in low- and middle-income countries. In adults living in high-income settings, zinc supplements do not prevent respiratory infections but can reduce their duration.
- Flavonoids appear to lower the risk of contracting respiratory infections by about one-third but not the number of sick days due to such infections. Curcumin may help prevent death in adults infected with COVID-19, but larger trials are needed.
- Probiotics do not significantly reduce the duration of diarrhea in children with gastroenteritis but are modestly effective in preventing gastroenteritis and colds. This benefit may not be worth the expense and effort of daily probiotic supplements.

Detailed Review of the Scientific Evidence[1]

Before reviewing the published evidence on dietary supplements and common viral infections, I will begin by discussing several important issues bearing on research design. As reviewed above, dietary supplement use is highly associated with high income, advanced education, and healthy lifestyle habits involving weight, physical activity, and smoking. These associations make it difficult, if not impossible, to infer a causal effect of diet and nutrition on infection risk using observational

---

[1] Readers who prefer to skip the Detailed Review should proceed to the Summary at the end of the chapter.

studies. For example, one recent large observational study in the U.S. and U.K. examined the association of diet quality, as reflected by fruit and vegetable intake, with risk of COVID-19 infection [12]. Participants were recruited through the general and social media and self-reported their pre-pandemic dietary information and follow-up COVID-19 symptoms via smartphones; they were therefore unblinded. It seems highly likely that participants with "healthy diets" would under-report their illness symptoms.

In other words, randomized, placebo-controlled trials are essential to avoid confounding by these known, as well as unknown, factors that are underlying causes of both supplement use and infection. Fortunately, such trials have been numerous for vitamins, minerals, and other supplements and provide a solid basis for recommendations regarding their use.

Vitamin A

Imdad and colleagues' recent Cochrane review analyzed randomized trials of vitamin A supplementation in children between 6 months and 5 years of age living in low- and middle-income countries [13]. That review analyzed 47 trials in over 1.2 million children and observed a 50% reduction in risk of measles infection, a 15% reduction in risk of diarrheal disease, and a 12% reduction in death from diarrheal disease, but no reduction in risk of non-measles respiratory infection. Two systematic reviews have examined vitamin A supplementation for treatment of children with pneumonia, rather than its prevention. Neither Wu and colleagues' 2005 Cochrane review of six RCTs [14] nor Mathew's more recent (2010) non-Cochrane review of nine RCTs [15] observed a reduction in mortality, illness duration, or risks of hospitalization or other complications.

Because of the findings of the Cochrane review of prevention trials, vitamin A supplementation is recommended for infants and preschool children living in low- and middle-income countries with a high prevalence of vitamin A deficiency. Vitamin A deficiency is rare in high-income countries, however, and I am unaware of any evidence suggesting a need for vitamin A supplements in those settings.

Vitamin D

Vitamin D is important for bone health, since it enhances calcium absorption, but also plays a role in immune function. Ultraviolet (UV) light absorbed by the skin is necessary for converting cholesterol to vitamin D, which is why vitamin D is sometimes called the "sunshine vitamin." Vitamin D deficiency is of particular concern in dark-skinned individuals, because the melanin pigment in skin absorbs much of the UV light. In many high-income countries, commercially sold milk is now fortified with vitamin D, but milk and other dietary sources of vitamin D may not provide sufficient dietary intake to ensure adequate vitamin D status when sunlight exposure is low.

Jolliffe and colleagues carried out a recent systematic review and meta-analysis of vitamin D supplementation in relation to acute respiratory tract infection [16]. The review included 45 randomized trials in over 70,000 participants ranging in age from infants to elderly adults. Most of the trials were placebo-controlled and double-blind. The supplemented group had a slight (9%) but statistically significant reduction in risk of one or more episodes of infection but no reduction in more serious outcomes like hospitalizations, emergency department visits, or work or school absences. A recent systematic review by Hosseini and coworkers focused on COVID-19 in adults and included 9 randomized trials and 14 observational studies [17]. Vitamin D supplements given as prevention did not reduce the risk of developing COVID-19, but supplements given to treat persons already infected with the virus resulted in a reduced risk of death and intensive care unit (ICU) admission, even among the randomized trials.

Vitamin C

As reviewed in the Introduction section of this chapter, vitamin C is the vitamin responsible for the dramatic effect of lemons and oranges in the first known controlled clinical trial: James Lind's landmark eighteenth-century experiment to cure scurvy in British navy sailors on a long-term sea voyage. Even if vitamins (including vitamin C) weren't discovered until the early twentieth century, we now know that vitamin C is essential for making collagen, a structural protein required for maintaining the skin, gums, and blood vessels and for wound healing. It is also an anti-oxidant that supports the immune system, and especially the migration and function of white blood cells, by combatting the oxidant stress associated with infection.

Linus Pauling was a brilliant Nobel double laureate (Chemistry in 1954 and Peace in 1962) without any particular training in biology or medicine. Nonetheless, his 1970 book, *Vitamin C and the Common Cold*, led to a controversy about the possible benefits of mega-doses of the vitamin that Pauling claimed both helped prevent and treat the common cold [18]. The normally recommended daily allowance (RDA) for vitamin C is about 75 mg per day in adults and correspondingly lower doses in children. The mega-doses advocated by Pauling and his followers were of the order of 1 g (1000 mg) per day, or even several grams per day. These doses are 10–100 times the RDA for vitamin C. These high doses are probably not dangerous, however; excess vitamin C is not stored in the body but is rapidly excreted in the urine.

Hemilä and Chalker's 2013 Cochrane review of 29 randomized trials in over 11,000 participants observed a very modest 5% reduction in risk of catching a cold in the vitamin C group versus the placebo group [19]. That 5% reduction was further lowered to 3% in the 24 trials of participants in the general community but increased to a 52% reduction in five trials among 600 marathon runners, skiers, or soldiers engaging in subarctic exercises. In seven treatment (rather than prevention) trials with over 3000 participants, vitamin C supplementation begun after onset of cold symptoms did not significantly reduce the duration or severity of the cold symptoms.

Vitamin E

Vitamin E has both anti-oxidant and anti-inflammatory activity. Shokri-Mashhadi and colleagues' recent narrative systematic review included four randomized trials of vitamin E supplementation to prevent or treat viral respiratory infections among elderly adults [20]. The evidence was mixed, and no meta-analysis was attempted.

Omega-3 Fatty Acids

Omega-3 long-chain polyunsaturated fatty acids (LC-PUFAs) have demonstrated effects in reducing inflammation and enhancing immune responses. Husson and coworkers' 2016 narrative systematic review of animal and human studies observed an *increased* risk of influenza infection and higher mortality in mice supplemented with omega-3 fatty acids but were unable to locate any randomized prevention or treatment trials in humans [21].

Flavonoids

Flavonoids are organic compounds with multiple phenol rings (polyphenolic); they are contained in many types of fruits and vegetables, as well as in wine, tea, and chocolate. They can also be found in popular herbal supplements, either as individual flavonoids like anthocyanidins, quercetin, and curcumin or as combinations of flavonoids. These compounds have demonstrated anti-inflammatory and anti-oxidant properties and have been shown to reduce viral replication in the laboratory. Somerville and coworkers' 2016 systematic review and meta-analysis included randomized trials of flavonoid supplements to prevent colds and other upper respiratory tract infections [22]. Six of the trials reporting on incidence of new infections, all with sample sizes below 200, showed a one-third reduced risk of infection during follow-up. Four of those trials also reported on total number of days sick with these infections, but no significant reduction was observed. Several of the included trials were funded by flavonoid manufacturers, raising the possibility of biased designs or analyses. Finally, Kow and colleagues' recent systematic review and meta-analysis of curcumin as treatment for COVID-19 included three small randomized trials from Iran and India and reported a large reduction in mortality risk [23]. Given the large number of persons taking flavonoids and other herbal supplements, additional, larger supplementation trials are needed.

Zinc

Two Cochrane reviews have analyzed randomized trials of daily zinc supplementation in relation to infection among children living in low- and middle-income countries. The 2014 review by Mayo-Wilson and colleagues included 80 randomized trials in over 200,000 children under 12 years of age [24]. The authors found no reduction in risk of death or malaria but a 13% reduction in risk of diarrheal disease. The 2016 Cochrane review by Lassi and coworkers restricted its analysis to children under 5 years and observed a statistically significant 21% reduction in risk of chest X-ray-confirmed pneumonia in children who received daily supplements [25]. In summary, zinc supplementation may reduce risks of diarrhea and pneumonia in children living in low- and middle-income countries with inadequate dietary zinc intake.

Among adults, the recent systematic review and meta-analysis by Abioye and colleagues included 5 prevention trials and 11 treatment trials in relation to acute respiratory infections, mostly from high-income countries [26]. The prevention trials showed no evidence of reduced risk of contracting new infections, but the 11 treatment trials demonstrated a nearly 50% reduction in duration of colds and other acute respiratory infections. The authors did not comment on the potential for bias due to funding of the included trials by zinc supplement manufacturers. Tabatabaeizadeh's recent systematic review and meta-analysis of zinc treatment of COVID-19 included three small randomized trials and two larger observational studies; the trials showed no reduction in mortality risk among those randomized to zinc treatment [27].

Probiotics

Probiotics are intended to promote a more favorable environment of microorganisms in the intestinal tract. They contain the "good" bacteria and/or yeast that may affect the microorganisms inhabiting the gastrointestinal tract, the so-called intestinal microbiome, and hence the risks of common infections caused by pathogenic (disease-causing) microbes. Some probiotic formulations contain single bacterial species, while others are mixtures of two or more species. They have been used successfully to prevent diarrhea caused by antibiotic treatment and to treat excessive crying in early infancy ("colic"). But the alteration in the microorganism environment of the gastrointestinal tract has also been reported to enhance systemic immunity, primarily by improving the function of white blood cells, which are responsible for ingesting and destroying bacteria and viruses, immune recognition, and antibody production.

For treatment of gastrointestinal infection (diarrhea of proven or suspected infectious origin), Collinson and coworkers' 2020 Cochrane review examined 82 randomized trials in over 12,000 participants, most of whom were children [28]. Probiotics did not significantly reduce the average duration of diarrhea, the proportion with duration ≥48 h or ≥14 days, or the risk of hospitalization. The authors found statistical evidence of publication bias, that is, under-representation of studies showing longer durations of symptoms in participants randomized to probiotic treatment. Saa and colleagues' 2018 systematic review, however, found no evidence that industry-funded trials were more likely to obtain beneficial effects of probiotic treatment than trials funded by non-industry sources [29].

For prevention of gastrointestinal infection, I was unable to find systematic reviews or individual randomized trials in adults, probably because such infections are usually mild and probably not worth the effort and cost of daily probiotics. Ahmad and colleagues' recent systematic review and meta-analysis, however, examined 15 randomized trials of probiotics in over 6000 infants and young children attending daycare centers [30]. Such centers are good settings to consider preventive treatment, because daycare attendees are at high risk of contracting gastrointestinal and respiratory infection from other infants and children. Attendees randomized to probiotics had a 26% lower risk of one or more gastrointestinal infections, but no significant difference in the total number of days with gastrointestinal symptoms or in number of days absent from daycare. Nine of the 15 trials were industry-funded, but the authors of the review did not compare trial results according to funding source.

Another approach to prevention is probiotic supplementation of infant formula, which has become increasingly frequent in recent years. Pastor-Villaescusa and coworkers' 2021 systematic review and meta-analysis found three randomized trials of formulas supplemented with *Lactobacillus fermentum*, the same "good" bacterium found in breast milk [31]. The overall results showed a halving of the rate of gastrointestinal infection in the supplemented group, but the trials were small, the trial reporting the largest effect was co-authored by an employee of the company that funded the trial (which may have led to a conflict of interest in its analysis or reporting), and duration or severity of episodes was not reported.

I was unable to locate any systematic reviews or individual randomized trials of probiotics used to treat respiratory infections. Probiotics have been tested, however, for their ability to prevent common colds and other acute upper respiratory tract infections in both children and adults. Zhao and coworkers' recent Cochrane review included 23 randomized prevention trials, most of which used a placebo control group [32]. The overall results indicated a 24% reduction in risk of one or more infections in the 16 trials reporting that outcome.

Summary

Both under- and over-nutrition can adversely affect health, and the benefits of a well-balanced diet are well established. Dietary supplements are used by a very large fraction of the population in high-income countries, especially by healthy persons consuming a good diet, who are least likely to benefit from the supplements. Vitamin A supplements provide modest protection against measles and gastrointestinal infection in preschool children living in low- or middle-income countries with a high prevalence of vitamin A deficiency but are unnecessary in fully vaccinated children in high-income settings. Vitamins C and D have very small effects in reducing the risk of contracting respiratory infections. Vitamin D supplements are ineffective in preventing COVID-19 infection but do reduce severe outcomes when used to treat infected adults. The evidence base is insufficient for vitamin E and omega-3 fatty acids. Zinc supplementation reduces the risk of both diarrhea and pneumonia in young children living in low- and middle-income countries. In adults in high-income settings, zinc supplementation does not reduce the risk of contracting respiratory infections but may substantially reduce the duration of symptoms among those infected.

Two of the most promising dietary supplements are flavonoids and probiotics. Flavonoids appear to lower the risk of contracting respiratory infections by about one-third but not the number of sick days due to such infections. Curcumin (a flavonoid contained in turmeric, the yellow spice used in curry and other foods) may help prevent death in adults infected with COVID-19, but larger trials are needed. The available evidence suggests that probiotics do not reduce the duration of diarrhea or the risk of hospitalization when used to treat gastrointestinal infection, although they may help prevent such infections in infants and young children attending daycare. This possible benefit may not be worth the cost and effort of getting young kids to take probiotics on a daily basis, however. Probiotics may help to reduce both the risk and duration of the common cold and other respiratory tract infections and are probably safe, but daily supplementation is not cheap, and it may be worth waiting for more and better trials before making the required investment.

References

1. Beisel WR. History of nutritional immunology: introduction and overview. J Nutr. 1992;122(3 Suppl):591–6.
2. Winick M, editor. Hunger disease: studies by the Jewish Physicians in Warsaw Ghetto, Current concepts in nutrition, vol. 7. New York: John Wiley & Sons; 1979.
3. Scrimshaw NS. Historical concepts of interactions, synergism and antagonism between nutrition and infection. J Nutr. 2003;133(1):316S–21S.
4. Wood S, Harrison SE, Judd N, Bellis MA, Hughes K, Jones A. The impact of behavioural risk factors on communicable diseases: a systematic review of reviews. BMC Public Health. 2021;21(1):2110.
5. Mishra S, Stierman B, Gahche JJ, Potischman N. Dietary supplement use among adults: United States, 2017–2018. NCHS Data Brief. 2021;399:1–8.
6. Gahche J, Bailey R, Burt V, Hughes J, Yetley E, Dwyer J, Picciano MF, McDowell M, Sempos C. Dietary supplement use among U.S. adults has increased since NHANES III (1988–1994). NCHS Data Brief. 2011;61:1–8.
7. 2017 CRN Consumer Survey on Dietary Supplements. http://www.nrnusa.org/survey.
8. Vatanparast H, Adolphe JL, Whiting SJ. Socio-economic status and vitamin/mineral supplement use in Canada. Health Rep. 2010;21(4):19–25.
9. Savikko N, Pitkälä KH, Laurila JV, Suominen MH, Tilvis RS, Kautiainen H, Strandberg TE. Secular trends in the use of vitamins, minerals and fish-oil products in two cohorts of community-dwelling older people in Helsinki—population-based surveys in 1999 and 2009. J Nutr Health Aging. 2014;18(2):150–4.

10. Lin JR, Lin YS, Kao MD, Yang YH, Pan WH. Use of supplements by Taiwanese adults aged 19–44 during 2005–2008. Asia Pac J Clin Nutr. 2011;20(2):319–26.
11. Skeie G, Braaten T, Hjartåker A, Lentjes M, Amiano P, Jakszyn P, Pala V, Palanca A, Niekerk EM, Verhagen H, Avloniti K, Psaltopoulou T, Niravong M, Touvier M, Nimptsch K, Haubrock J, Walker L, Spencer EA, Roswall N, Olsen A, Wallström P, Nilsson S, Casagrande C, Deharveng G, Hellström V, Boutron-Ruault MC, Tjønneland A, Joensen AM, Clavel-Chapelon F, Trichopoulou A, Martinez C, Rodríguez L, Frasca G, Sacerdote C, Peeters PH, Linseisen J, Schienkiewitz A, Welch AA, Manjer J, Ferrari P, Riboli E, Bingham S, Engeset D, Lund E, Slimani N. Use of dietary supplements in the European Prospective Investigation into Cancer and Nutrition calibration study. Eur J Clin Nutr. 2009;63(Suppl 4):S226–38.
12. Merino J, Joshi AD, Nguyen LH, Leeming ER, Mazidi M, Drew DA, Gibson R, Graham MS, Lo CH, Capdevila J, Murray B, Hu C, Selvachandran S, Hammers A, Bhupathiraju SN, Sharma SV, Sudre C, Astley CM, Chavarro JE, Kwon S, Ma W, Menni C, Willett WC, Ourselin S, Steves CJ, Wolf J, Franks PW, Spector TD, Berry S, Chan AT. Diet quality and risk and severity of COVID-19: a prospective cohort study. Gut. 2021;70(11):2096–104.
13. Imdad A, Mayo-Wilson E, Haykal MR, Regan A, Sidhu J, Smith A, Bhutta ZA. Vitamin A supplementation for preventing morbidity and mortality in children from six months to five years of age. Cochrane Database Syst Rev. 2022;3:CD008524.
14. Wu T, Ni J, Wei J. Vitamin A for non-measles pneumonia in children. Cochrane Database Syst Rev. 2005;3:CD003700.
15. Mathew JL. Vitamin A supplementation for prophylaxis or therapy in childhood pneumonia: a systematic review of randomized controlled trials. Indian Pediatr. 2010;47(3):255–61.
16. Jolliffe DA, Camargo CA Jr, Sluyter JD, Aglipay M, Aloia JF, Ganmaa D, Bergman P, Bischoff-Ferrari HA, Borzutzky A, Damsgaard CT, Dubnov-Raz G, Esposito S, Gilham C, Ginde AA, Golan-Tripto I, Goodall EC, Grant CC, Griffiths CJ, Hibbs AM, Janssens W, Khadilkar AV, Laaksi I, Lee MT, Loeb M, Maguire JL, Majak P, Mauger DT, Manaseki-Holland S, Murdoch DR, Nakashima A, Neale RE, Pham H, Rake C, Rees JR, Rosendahl J, Scragg R, Shah D, Shimizu Y, Simpson-Yap S, Trilok-Kumar G, Urashima M, Martineau AR. Vitamin D supplementation to prevent acute respiratory infections: a systematic review and meta-analysis of aggregate data from randomised controlled trials. Lancet Diabetes Endocrinol. 2021;9(5):276–92.
17. Hosseini B, El Abd A, Ducharme FM. Effects of vitamin D supplementation on COVID-19 related outcomes: a systematic review and meta-analysis. Nutrients. 2022;14(10):2134.
18. Pauling L. Vitamin C and the common cold. London: Bantam; 1970.
19. Hemilä H, Chalker E. Vitamin C for preventing and treating the common cold. Cochrane Database Syst Rev. 2013;1:CD000980.
20. Shokri-Mashhadi N, Kazemi M, Saadat S, Moradi S. Effects of select dietary supplements on the prevention and treatment of viral respiratory tract infections: a systematic review of randomized controlled trials. Expert Rev Respir Med. 2021;15(6):805–21.
21. Husson MO, Ley D, Portal C, Gottrand M, Hueso T, Desseyn JL, Gottrand F. Modulation of host defence against bacterial and viral infections by omega-3 polyunsaturated fatty acids. J Infect. 2016;73(6):523–35.
22. Somerville VS, Braakhuis AJ, Hopkins WG. Effect of flavonoids on upper respiratory tract infections and immune function: a systematic review and meta-analysis. Adv Nutr. 2016;7(3):488–97.
23. Kow CS, Ramachandram DS, Hasan SS. The effect of curcumin on the risk of mortality in patients with COVID-19: a systematic review and meta-analysis of randomized trials. Phytother Res. 2022;36(9):3365–8.
24. Mayo-Wilson E, Junior JA, Imdad A, Dean S, Chan XHS, Chan ES, Jaswal A, Bhutta ZA. Zinc supplementation for preventing mortality, morbidity, and growth failure in children aged 6 months to 12 years of age. Cochrane Database Syst Rev. 2014;5:CD009384.
25. Lassi ZS, Moin A, Bhutta ZA. Zinc supplementation for the prevention of pneumonia in children aged 2 months to 59 months. Cochrane Database Syst Rev. 2016;12:CD005978.

26. Abioye AI, Bromage S, Fawzi W. Effect of micronutrient supplements on influenza and other respiratory tract infections among adults: a systematic review and meta-analysis. BMJ Glob Health. 2021;6(1):e003176.
27. Tabatabaeizadeh SA. Zinc supplementation and COVID-19 mortality: a meta-analysis. Eur J Med Res. 2022;27(1):70.
28. Collinson S, Deans A, Padua-Zamora A, Gregorio GV, Li C, Dans LF, Allen SJ. Probiotics for treating acute infectious diarrhoea. Cochrane Database Syst Rev. 2020;12:CD003048.
29. Saa C, Bunout D, Hirsch S. Industry funding effect on positive results of probiotic use in the management of acute diarrhea: a systematized review. Eur J Gastroenterol Hepatol. 2019;31(3):289–302.
30. Ahmad HH, Peck B, Terry D. The influence of probiotics on gastrointestinal tract infections among children attending childcare: a systematic review and meta-analysis. J Appl Microbiol. 2022;132:1636–51.
31. Pastor-Villaescusa B, Blanco-Rojo R, Olivares M. Evaluation of the effect of *Limosilactobacillus fermentum* CECT5716 on gastrointestinal infections in infants: a systematic review and meta-analysis. Microorganisms. 2021;9(7):1412.
32. Zhao Y, Dong BR, Hao Q. Probiotics for preventing acute upper respiratory tract infections. Cochrane Database Syst Rev. 2022;8:CD006895.

Common Sense or Nonsense? Non-Drug Treatments for the Common Cold

5

Introduction

During the first 25 years of my academic career, I worked as a pediatric clinician in the Emergency Department of the Montreal Children's Hospital. As part of that work, I did encounter a few children with genuine emergencies. But most of the time, parents were using the Emergency Department as a "walk-in" clinic for their child's infections, minor accidents, and other non-urgent complaints. The majority of the infections I saw were simple upper respiratory tract infections: that is, common colds.

In the course of that work, I saw many hundreds, perhaps thousands, of children with colds. After I related my diagnosis ("Your child has a cold"), many of the parents asked what treatments they should use. From my training and my reading to keep up on recent research, I was convinced that no treatment they could provide would shorten the duration or reduce the severity of the cold.

The parents would usually ask my advice about what to feed or not feed their child, and about such measures as "getting plenty of rest and fluids," use of a room vaporizer or humidifier, and over-the-counter (non-prescription) cold medications. If the child had a fever or seemed to have a headache or other source of pain or discomfort, I would usually recommend children's acetaminophen (Tylenol). Otherwise, I would inform the parents that if they followed all the advice given and used all the measures that had been recommended in the past or used themselves when they had a cold, the child's illness would probably last about 7 days, whereas if they did none of those things, it would last a week. That information amused some of them, but it irritated others: how good a doctor was I if I couldn't recommend *anything*?

I this chapter, I will review several non-drug practices and remedies often recommended by well-meaning doctors, parents, spouses, other family members, and friends. These "common-sense" practices and remedies include bedrest, supplemental fluids (including chicken soup), humidifiers/vaporizers, and nasal irrigation.

Before summarizing the published scientific evidence bearing on the prevalence of use of these treatments and on their effectiveness, I will first trace their historical and cultural origins. When and where did they originate? Who first used and recommended them? What social and cultural factors led to their current popularity?

Historical Origins

Bed rest has been advocated for many medical conditions, including the common cold, since ancient times. Some illnesses leave their victim so weak that it is impossible for him or her to get out of bed. Perhaps because of this association between severe illness and the bed (that is, being bed-ridden), it became common for physicians in both ancient and modern times to *recommend* bed rest as a treatment. Hippocrates wrote that "In any movement of the body, whenever one begins to endure pain, it will be relieved by rest" [1]. He also specifically recommended bedrest for treating a bloody productive cough, which was often caused by tuberculosis. Bedrest became an increasingly common recommendation in the nineteenth century, when "rest cures" were prescribed for tuberculosis and many other illnesses.

Questions and objections related to this practice became more frequent in the twentieth century. Virginia Woolf, for example, poked fun at the rest cure in her 1925 novel, *Mrs. Dolloway*, and suggested at least one potential adverse effect: "You…order rest in bed; rest in solitude; silence and rest; rest without friends, without books, without messages; six months of rest; until a man who went in weighing seven stone six comes out weighing twelve." [A stone is a British measure of weight equivalent to 14 pounds, or 6.35 kg.] As emphasized by the famously feisty British pediatrician, RS Illingworth, "No one has ever explained to me why it should be expected that a child with, say, a sore throat or chickenpox…who would like to sit in a chair…should recover less rapidly than a child…sitting in bed" [2].

The historical origins of supplemental fluids are more obscure. As far as I can determine, they were not commonly prescribed by Hippocrates, Galen, and other ancient Greek physicians, although their use may have been originated in the perceived need to loosen phlegm, one of the four humors that served as the belief system underlying health and disease during that period. Their origins may also be related to the well-documented risk of dehydration that occurs in cholera and other diarrheal diseases. I don't ever recall seeing a dehydrated child with a cold or other respiratory infection during my 25 years of pediatric clinical practice, nor ever hearing a reasonable rationale for recommending "plenty of fluids" in children or adults.

The consumption of hot liquids probably had its origins over 2000 years ago in traditional Chinese medicine and the hot-cold theory of disease. Hot water and tea are beverages that, according to the theory, help combat the cold and restore the body's yin-yang balance and harmony. Maimonides, the 12-century AD Jewish theologian and physician, prescribed another type of hot liquid, chicken soup, to treat colds, leprosy, other infections, and even headaches [3]. Whether or not hot

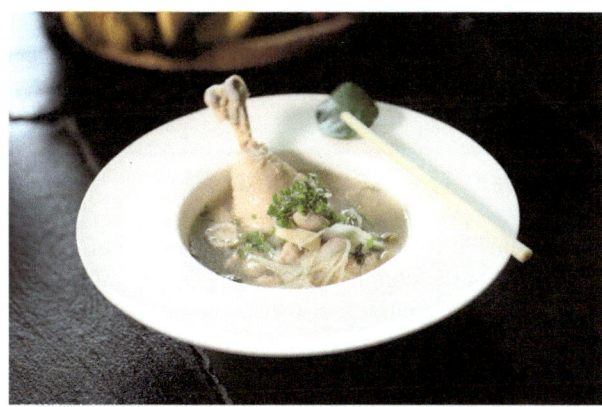

Fig. 5.1 Chicken soup: a modern version of a medieval treatment for the common cold

chicken soup is related to traditional Chinese medicine, or even to the hot-cold theory of disease, this so-called Jewish penicillin continues to this day to be advocated for colds and other minor infections (Fig. 5.1).

The history of humidifiers and vaporisers is also lost in the mists of time (pun intended). Their use may be related to the ancient Egyptian practice of placing plants or seeds on heated stones and congregating around those stones to smell the vapors. I have no idea where the idea emerged to use humidifiers or mist vaporizers to treat colds or other respiratory infections. The presumed rationale may have been to "loosen" phlegm and facilitate coughing it up.

The first mist vaporizers were patented in the 1920s, and I remember my mother using one in my bedroom when I was ill as a child growing up in the 1950s. During my pediatrics residency training in the 1970s, we frequently used mist in the hospital ward showers or cool mist created in tents placed over the bed to treat infants and toddlers with croup. Croup is a viral respiratory tract infection that affects the windpipe just below the larynx (voice box) and causes a barky, seal-like cough and difficulty inhaling (breathing in). In more recent years, that mist treatment has been shown to be ineffective and is now replaced by treatments of proven effectiveness like inhaled epinephrine and oral or inhaled cortisone-like medications called corticosteroids. Ordinary mist vaporizers and humidifiers continue to be sold and promoted by physicians and, of course, the manufacturers, "to moisten the respiratory passages" of the cold sufferer.

Nasal irrigation using a physiological salt (saline) solution administered into the nose through a plastic squeeze bottle or bulb has also become popular in recent years. It may be based on the ancient Hindu practice of Ayurveda (the science of life), which includes the practice of jala-neti: cleansing the nose with water. More recently, nasal irrigation is increasingly recommended by physicians faced with the ineffectiveness of most over-the-counter medications. Because the salt concentration in the irrigation solutions is similar to that found in the blood and therefore presumed to be safe, nasal saline irrigation has been promoted by manufacturers as a "natural" remedy to help "clear the nasal passages" of mucus. The manufacturers are not required to report how fast the mucus reaccumulates, nor any beneficial effect on discomfort, sleep, or the duration of cold symptoms.

Who Uses These Cold Remedies?

I was unable to locate a systematic review of current use of non-pharmaceutical remedies of the common cold or of factors affecting such use. I did, however, find two individual studies that shed some light on recent practices, one among U.S. parents, the other among European general practitioners (GPs).

A 1998 study reported on the use of home-based remedies for the common cold, based on interviewing a non-representative "convenience" sample of mothers of children attending one of three health care centers in Hartford, Connecticut, USA [4]. These clinical sites were chosen to provide a sufficient number of respondents among each of the four major ethnocultural groups living in the Hartford area: 85 non-Hispanic Whites, 68 African-Americans, 108 Puerto Ricans, and 20 Caribbean Blacks. The mothers were asked to list all the remedies they had used to treat their children when afflicted by a cold. Vaporizers or humidifiers were used by a large fraction of the non-Hispanic White mothers but not by those in the three other ethnic groups. Extra fluids were used by all four groups, but the type of fluid differed among them. Surprisingly to me, chicken soup was reported by all four groups, but by a higher proportion of the African-American mothers. Juices were reported only by non-Hispanic White and African-American mothers, while teas were reported by a high proportion of Caribbean Black mothers and a few African-American mothers, but not by mothers in the two other groups. The study mothers did not report using nasal irrigation and were not asked about bedrest or other physical activity restrictions.

Cultural influences are not limited to patients and their families, but also affect the recommendations given by practicing physicians. A 2014 survey of about 200 GPs in each of Norway and Poland was based on four brief vignettes, or clinical summaries, of adults with acute respiratory infections [5]. The investigators asked the clinicians about their recommendations on bed rest, staying indoors, and exercise for each case vignette. One of the vignettes was a 45-year-old woman with a common cold. Differences were striking between the two countries, with 87% of the Polish GPs recommending that the woman remain at home versus only 9% of the Norwegian GPs. Bedrest was recommended by 36% versus 1% and refraining from exercise by 69% versus 40%, respectively, of the Polish versus Norwegian GPs. Even when limited to those physicians recommending restrictions, the recommended duration of the restrictions was longer among the Polish GPs. Both groups of GPs were highly experienced, and the large differences in recommendations strongly suggest cultural influences on perceived severity of the infection, patients' expectations, or differences in the physicians' beliefs of their effectiveness, probably reflecting the beliefs of the physicians who trained them.

Key Evidence Points
- Published studies of the effectiveness of non-drug treatments of the common cold have generally been small and have lacked methodological rigor.
- Bedrest, supplemental fluids, use of humidifiers or vaporizers, or nasal irrigation are ineffective in reducing the severity or duration of cold symptoms.
- On a positive note, these treatments do not appear harmful, although young children may object to them, and parents may therefore struggle to administer them.
- The popularity of "common-sense" treatments is probably due to the wish to do *something*, and manufacturers' perennial eagerness to profit from that wish.

Detailed Review of the Scientific Evidence[1]

Because of the potential for bias due to confounding, reverse causality, and the placebo effect, I will rely heavily on systematic reviews of placebo-controlled randomized trials, and especially on Cochrane reviews. Randomized trials of non-drug treatments and advice cannot eliminate all sources of bias, however, since it is impossible to blind participants to their allocated treatment. People know whether or not they are advised to stay in bed, exercise, drink more fluids, use a vaporizer, or irrigate their nose, and their reporting of symptoms and responses to treatment are likely to be influenced by that knowledge.

Bedrest and Exercise

Allen and colleagues' 1999 systematic review of bedrest analyzed 24 trials in which bedrest was prescribed after medical procedures and 15 trials in patients with a variety of medical illnesses, but none of the latter included the common cold [6]. Another approach to analyzing the benefits and risks of bedrest is to evaluate the other end of the physical activity spectrum: exercise. I did not succeed in locating any randomized trials of exercise among patients with colds, but Grande and coworkers' recent Cochrane review and meta-analysis analyzed acute respiratory infections, including both common colds and lower respiratory infections like bronchitis and pneumonia, in 14 trials of exercise prescribed to healthy participants, all adults [7]. They reported on occurrence of infection, which reflects the effect of exercise on preventing infection, but also on the severity and duration of symptoms *among* participants with an infection. The latter might be a good proxy for the effect of exercise that *would* be observed if it were prescribed or advised as *treatment* of

---

[1] Readers who prefer to skip the Detailed Review should proceed to the Summary at the end of the chapter.

patients who already had an infection. No difference was observed in the six trials that reported on duration of symptoms among participants with respiratory infection. Only two trials reported on severity of symptoms among participants with infection, but the severity was significantly *lower* in the exercise group. Given the potential for biased reporting, however, this latter finding may not reflect a true beneficial effect of exercise. In any case, the evidence suggests no evidence of harm with exercise during colds and other respiratory infections.

Supplemental Fluids

Guppy and colleagues' 2011 Cochrane review found no randomized trials of advice to increase fluid intake in treating patients with colds or other respiratory infections [8]. One recent observational study from the UK provides some useful information on this topic. Eccles and Mallefet studied 55 adults with moderate or severe colds who were interviewed and examined and underwent blood and urine tests on two occasions: once during the acute illness and then again after they recovered 2 or 3 weeks later [9]. Although subjective reports indicated increased thirst at Visit 1 versus Visit 2, no differences were observed between the two visits in urine color or specific gravity (which reflects concentration) or numerous blood tests indicating degree of hydration. These results provide no evidence that colds cause dehydration. The increased thirst seen during the acute phase of colds almost certainly reflects the dry mouth and throat induced by mouth breathing caused by nasal congestion (stuffy nose).

Sakethoo and coworkers objectively measured the speed at which mucus moved inside the nose and resistance to airflow in the nose (reflecting degree of congestion) in 15 healthy adults who volunteered to come to a research laboratory for these measurements on six separate days [3]. At each those visits, they received one of the following liquids given in random order: hot water by sip or by straw, chicken soup by sip or by straw, cold water by sip, or sham (no liquid) by straw. The two objective measurements were made at baseline (before each liquid) and 5 and 30 min after drinking. The results showed that the none of the liquids affected nasal airflow, but sipping hot water or chicken soup significantly increased the speed of nasal mucus movement. The results are intriguing, but their relevance to treating colds is unclear. People with colds already complain of excess nasal mucus production, and increasing the speed of its flow seems unlikely to provide any relief of cold symptoms.

Rennard and coworkers tested the effect of chicken soup on the movement of white blood cells collected from healthy volunteers, that is, people without a cold, in a laboratory-based experiment [10]. The chicken soup slowed the movement of the cells, and a dose-response relationship was observed; that is, higher concentrations of soup slowed the white blood cell movement to a greater extent. Once again, the relevance of this effect for reducing (or even increasing) the severity or duration of the common cold is unclear.

Humidifiers and Vaporizers

Singh and colleagues' 2017 Cochrane review and meta-analysis analyzed six small, low-quality randomized trials of heated humidified air in 387 children and adults with colds [11]. The effect of the treatment on the severity was based on only two of the trials and differed depending on the choice of statistical method for analyzing the results: significantly lower symptom scores using the less conservative statistical method but no significant benefit using the more conservative statistical method. Two different trials reported no significant effect on subjective response to treatment, and a fifth trial in 20 volunteers experimentally infected with rhinovirus, the most common cause of the common cold, found no significant effect on rate of positive cultures from the nose between the two treatment groups. Given the subjective nature of self-reported symptoms, the authors of the review concluded that the humidification treatment was neither beneficial nor harmful but called for larger and more rigorous randomized trials.

Nasal Irrigation

A 2015 Cochrane review by King and coworkers analyzed three randomized trials in 544 children and two trials in 205 adults with colds [12]. Based on two trials reporting on duration of symptoms, no significant reduction was observed in the nasal irrigation group. One large trial in 401 children 6–10 years of age observed small but statistically significant reductions in symptom scores for nasal secretions and breathing through the nose in the irrigation group, but the subjective nature of these symptoms may well have been the result of non-blinding of the children and their parents. The authors concluded that larger trials are needed, with use of more objective outcome measures.

Summary

Bedrest has been recommended for common colds and many other illnesses since the time of the ancient Greeks. Consumption of hot liquids, including water and tea, can be traced to traditional Chinese medicine, and prescription of chicken soup to Maimonides. Humidifiers and vaporizers became popular in the twentieth century, and saline nasal irrigation, although a longstanding practice in ancient Hindu (Ayurvedic) medicine, has recently become a popular cold treatment in the West. Based on a few published studies, the use of these non-drug treatments by parents, as well as their recommended use by physicians, varies widely by geography and culture. Unfortunately, however, none has been demonstrated to reduce the severity or duration of cold symptoms.

Given the meager evidence for their effectiveness in treating the common cold, why have these measures been recommended and used by so many for so long? The biology of the human organism is complex, and it is not difficult to come up with physiological rationales to support these treatments and practices. Clearing the nasal passages, loosening phlegm, preventing dehydration, and allowing the immune system to fight the infection all sound reasonable, don't they? Common sense, many would (and do) say.

Published studies have generally been small and have lacked methodological rigor. In fairness, it is impossible to blind participants in randomized trials of these practices to the treatment group to which they are allocated, and self-reported symptoms are subjective and are likely to be biased by knowledge of the treatment received. On a positive note, the available evidence does not suggest that these treatments are harmful, although any parent who has attempted to irrigate the nose of a baby or toddler with a cold knows that the child is not very happy to receive it!

I suspect that the popularity of "common-sense" treatments is due primarily to the need to do *something*, and to manufacturers' perennial eagerness to profit from that need. Few people accept that *nothing* can be done to shorten the duration or lessen the severity of a cold. As I related at the beginning of this chapter, my 25 years of experience in treating children with colds taught me that many parents did not appreciate my nihilistic advice to do nothing and let nature take its course. But I was simply incapable of recommending measures that had no evidence to support them.

References

1. Hippocrates. The genuine works of Hippocrates. London: The Sydenham Society; 1849.
2. Illingworth RS. Restrictive practices in paediatrics. Acta Paediatr Scand. 1967;Suppl 172:84–92.
3. Saketkhoo K, Januszkiewicz A, Sackner MA. Effects of drinking hot water, cold water, and chicken soup on nasal mucus velocity and nasal airflow resistance. Chest. 1978;74(4):408–10.
4. Pachter LM, Sumner T, Fontan A, Sneed M, Bernstein BA. Home-based therapies for the common cold among European American and ethnic minority families: the interface between alternative/complementary and folk medicine. Arch Pediatr Adolesc Med. 1998;152(11):1083–8.
5. Halvorsen PA, Godycki-Cwirko M, Wennevold K, Melbye H. Would GPs advise patients with respiratory tract infections to refrain from exercise, stay indoors or stay in bed? Survey of GPs in Poland and Norway. Eur J Gen Pract. 2014;20(3):209–13.
6. Allen C, Glasziou P, Del Mar C. Bed rest: a potentially harmful treatment needing more careful evaluation. Lancet. 1999;354(9186):1229–33.
7. Grande AJ, Keogh J, Silva V, Scott AM. Exercise versus no exercise for the occurrence, severity, and duration of acute respiratory infections. Cochrane Database Syst Rev. 2020;4(4):CD010596.
8. Guppy MPB, Mickan SM, Del Mar CB, Thorning S, Rack A. Advising patients to increase fluid intake for treating acute respiratory infections. Cochrane Database Syst Rev. 2011;2:CD004419.
9. Eccles R, Mallefet P. Observational study of the effects of upper respiratory tract infection on hydration status. Multidiscip Respir Med. 2019;14:36.
10. Rennard BO, Ertl RF, Gossman GL, Robbins RA, Rennard SI. Chicken soup inhibits neutrophil chemotaxis in vitro. Chest. 2000;118(4):1150–7.
11. Singh M, Singh M, Jaiswal N, Chauhan A. Heated, humidified air for the common cold. Cochrane Database Syst Rev. 2017;8:CD001728.
12. King D, Mitchell B, Williams CP, Spurling GK. Saline nasal irrigation for acute upper respiratory tract infections. Cochrane Database Syst Rev. 2015;4:CD006821.

Part III

Skin and Eye Conditions

Duct (or Duck) Tape for Treating Warts: A Quack Remedy?

6

Introduction

Warts are raised bumps on the skin, most commonly occurring on the hands, fingers, feet, and toes. They can be single or grouped in a single location or scattered in different locations. Warts can be painful when they occur on the soles of the feet (plantar warts), but many never come to medical attention. Warts are caused by a virus called human papilloma virus (HPV), which includes over 100 genetic strains. HPV strains causing genital warts and cancer of the uterine cervix are different from those causing common warts on the hands and feet.

Most people develop warts at some time in the lives. They occur more frequently in children but also affect adults, including the elderly. One study of institutionalized children who were repeatedly examined over a 2-year period observed that about 20% of them were affected at any one time [1]. About two-thirds of the individual warts disappeared over the study period, but new ones occasionally appeared in other locations. It is not unusual for multiple warts to disappear simultaneously, suggesting that immunologic factors play a role in both the initial infection and eventual resolution.

A Brief History of Duct (or Duck) Tape

As reviewed by Woods, duct tape was originally called duck tape, because it contains a layer of *duck cloth*, which strengthens adhesive tape and, when coated with polyethylene plastic, makes it more water resistant and easier to peel off [2]. Duck cloth has nothing to do with ducks; it comes from *doek*, the Dutch and Afrikaans word for cloth. Duck tape was originally proposed by Vesta Stoudt, an employee in an ammunition packing factory during World War II. Ms. Stoudt had two sons in the Navy and wanted a better product for sealing ammunition cases.

M. S. Kramer, *Believe It or Not*, https://doi.org/10.1007/978-3-031-46022-7_6

Her factory bosses were not convinced by her idea, so she wrote directly to President Franklin Roosevelt, whose military officials convinced Johnson & Johnson to develop and manufacture the tape, which was originally olive green, like many other items of army equipment. It was used for many purposes other than sealing ammunition boxes, including repairs of tents, boots, and other military equipment.

After World War II, the color of duck tape changed from army green to silver and became popular outside of the military, including the household. One popular use was to seal and connect air conditioning and heating ducts. As a result, the common name changed from duck tape to duct tape. The tape often became brittle when heated, however, and occasionally caught fire, so it is no longer recommended for heating ducts. A final irony is that Duck tape has become a popular brand of duct tape, bringing the etymologic origins of the tape around full circle!

Who Uses or Recommends Duct Tape to Remove Warts?

What, you may well ask, does all this tape talk have to do with warts? Litt first reported successful treatment of warts near or under fingernails by wrapping ordinary adhesive tape (neither duck nor duct) around the affected finger for a week at a time for 4 successive weeks, with a 12-h "break" between applications [3]. The author claimed that other, untreated warts often resolved simultaneously. This publication is what is called a case series: a description of successfully treated cases of patients with warts. Unsuccessful cases were not reported, nor was a control treatment compared to the tape treatment. Twenty years later, a published letter from a family physician claimed an 80% success rate with this same treatment, but no cases were described in detail, and again, no control treatment was compared [4]. I was unable to find any published surveys of duct tape use by wart patients, parents, or physicians (Fig. 6.1).

Key Evidence Points
- Warts often disappear on their own, even entire groups of them.
- Salicylic acid (with or without lactic acid) applied directly to the wart significantly increases the rate of disappearance, as does freezing with liquid nitrogen.
- Duct tape (originally called duck tape) and other types of adhesive tape have no proven benefit over placebo or no treatment in the clearing of warts.

Fig. 6.1 Duct (or duck) tape for warts: does it work?

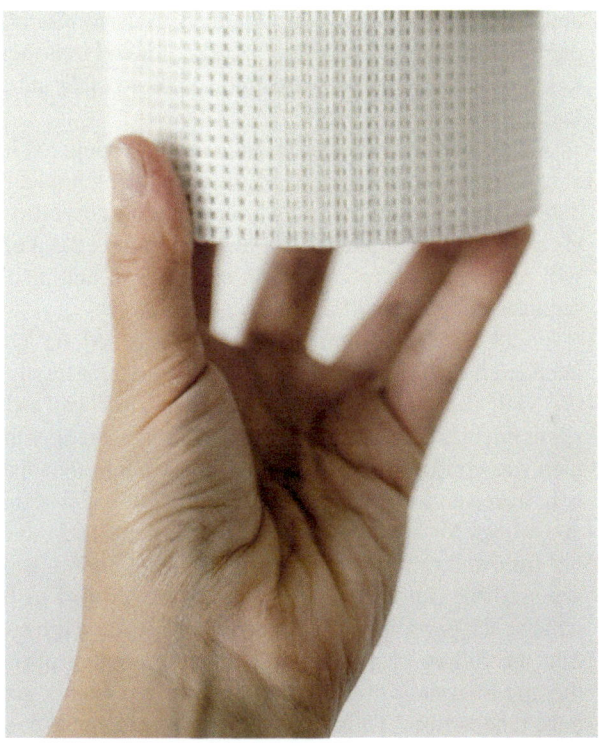

Detailed Review of the Evidence[1]

Based on Kwok and colleagues' 2012 Cochrane review of randomized trials of wart treatments [5], two commonly used topical treatments (products applied to the skin) have been shown to be effective and safe. One is a solution of salicylic acid, often combined with lactic acid, which can be bought over the counter, that is, without a prescription. It causes peeling and irritation and may work by stimulating the immune system to fight the virus. The solution is applied daily to one or more individual warts and leads to a 60% increase in cure rate over placebo or no treatment. The second common topical treatment is cryotherapy (freezing). It is the treatment preferred by dermatologists, who usually apply liquid nitrogen to the warts every 2–4 weeks.

Cryotherapy has a similar increase in cure rate as salicylic acid when compared to placebo or no treatment but is less convenient and, depending on the health care system, more expensive than salicylic acid. Four of the trials reviewed by Kwok and colleagues were head-to-head comparisons of cryotherapy and salicylic acid and observed similar cure rates in the two treatment groups. A recent systematic review

---

[1] Readers who prefer to skip the Detailed Review should proceed to the Summary at the end of the chapter.

and meta-analysis of 14 randomized trials by García-Oreja and colleagues compared cryotherapy to a variety of other topical treatments. The review was restricted to patients with plantar warts and found no clear superiority or inferiority of cryotherapy [6].

Kwok and coworkers' 2012 Cochrane review [5] included three randomized trials of duct tape treatment of warts: two in which duct tape was compared to placebo and one in which duct tape was compared to cryotherapy. Because randomized trials are the "gold standard" for evaluating the causal effects of medical treatments, I will review these three trials in some detail and also discuss two additional trials published since the 2012 Cochrane review.

Focht and coworkers' 2002 trial enrolled 61 children and adolescents who attended a single medical center with warts not involving the fingernails or toenails [7]. Half the children were randomized to receive daily occlusion with standard silver duct tape, which was removed for one night at the end of each week; this regimen was continued for up to 2 months or until disappearance of the wart. The other half were randomized to cryotherapy: 10 s of freezing with liquid nitrogen every 2–3 weeks for a maximum of six treatments. Of the 61 trial participants, ten were not followed up: a large fraction of those randomized. Physicians and nurses who assessed the outcome were meant to be blinded to (unaware of) the treatment to which each participant had been allocated when the children returned for follow-up. Yet, the follow-up procedure was not the same in the two groups: at every cryotherapy treatment in the group randomized to that group and every 4 weeks in the duct tape group. Thus the blinding would have been very difficult to maintain. Moreover, methods of outcome assessment at follow-up are not detailed. The reported rate of complete cure at 2 months was higher in the duct tape group than in the cryotherapy group (85% vs. 60%), although the difference was not statistically significant.

The second trial was carried out by de Haen and colleagues in 103 children 4–12 years of age who attended one of three primary schools in Maastricht, the Netherlands [8]. The children were randomized to transparent duct tape applied weekly (again, removed for one night per week) or a placebo corn pad: an adhesive doughnut-shaped pad placed over, but not covering, the wart one night per week. When children had multiple warts, the largest one was chosen for treatment. Treated warts were assessed at the child's school by a single blinded physician at 2, 4, and 6 weeks after initiating the treatment. No children were lost to follow-up. Cure rates in both groups treatment were much lower than in the above-mentioned Focht trial: 16% in the duct tape group and 6% in the placebo group, a statistically non-significant difference.

The third trial included in the Kwok Cochrane review also used a placebo treatment and was published in 2007 by Wenner and colleagues [9]. This trial recruited 90 adults with single or multiple warts from a single medical center; when multiple warts were present, the largest was chosen for treatment. Half the participants were randomized to receive the active treatment, pads of moleskin (a soft cloth) adherent pads with transparent duct tape added to the underside of the moleskin. The other half were randomized to the placebo treatment: look-alike moleskin pads without the added duct tape. The fact that the two treatments looked alike enabled both the participants and outcome assessors to remain blinded to which one was received. Participants were seen in follow-up after 1 and 2 months, although no details are provided on the number and types of outcome assessors. Ten of the 90 participants were lost to follow-up. Rates of cure at 2 months were virtually identical (21% and 22%) among those followed up in the two treatment groups.

Two relevant trials were published after, and therefore not included in, the 2012 Cochrane review. A 2020 trial by Abdel-Atif and coworkers enrolled 100 Egyptian adults with plantar warts, that is, warts on the sole of the foot [10]. The design was similar to that of the 2002 Focht trial in children [7], comparing duct tape occlusion (this time using conventional silver-colored duct tape) with cryotherapy. As in the Focht trial, duct tape was applied for 6 consecutive days per week, followed by removal for 1 day, then reapplied each week, for a total of 8 weeks or until the wart disappeared. The cryotherapy was given every 2–3 weeks for a maximum of four treatments. A complete response, or cure, was observed three times as frequently in the cryotherapy group (58%) as in the duct tape group (20%). The authors claim the participants were "randomly divided into two groups" but provide no details on the method of randomization. The fact that exactly 50 participants were assigned to each group, and that those who were non-compliant with their treatment (exactly six in each group!) were "replaced," indicates that this trial was neither designed nor analyzed as a bona fide randomized trial. In fact, consent for the trial was not obtained until the treatment had been completed!

Finally, another non-randomized trial from Korea published in 2013 enrolled 50 adults with warts to compare a cream containing 5% imiquimod, a drug that stimulates cellular immunity (not involving antibodies) versus a petrolatum (Vaseline) control [11]. The 25 participants in each group applied the cream or petrolatum once daily and at night covered it with a strip of standard silver duct tape, which was removed in the morning. The treatment was continued for up to 16 weeks or until disappearance of the wart, and participants returned for physician evaluation every 2 weeks. Five participants were lost to follow-up in each group. Since both treatments included duct tape application at night, that part of the treatment could not be compared in the two groups. Nonetheless, the treated wart disappeared in *none* of the 20 participants treated with petrolatum and duct tape versus 8 (40%) in those receiving imiquimod and duct tape. This result strongly supports the findings of Wenner, de Haen, and Abdel-Atif suggesting no benefit of duct tape.

Summary

Warts are very common, especially in young children, and are caused by infection with certain strains of the human papilloma virus (HPV). Warts can be uncomfortable or even painful, especially when they occur on the sole of the feet, but are usually only of cosmetic concern (appearance). Warts often disappear on their own, even entire groups of them. Salicylic acid (with or without lactic acid) applied directly to the wart significantly increases the rate of disappearance, as does freezing with liquid nitrogen. Duct tape (originally called duck tape) and other types of adhesive tape have no proven benefit over placebo or no treatment in the clearing of warts.

References

1. Massing AM, Epstein WL. Natural history of warts. A two-year study. Arch Dermatol. 1963;87:306–10.
2. Woods PM. Six historic facts about duct tape. Educational Now! (blog). 22 Sept 2019.
3. Litt JZ. Don't excise–exorcise. Treatment for subungual and periungual warts. Cutis. 1978;22(6):673–6.
4. Walbroehl G. Treating periungual warts with adhesive tape. Am Fam Physician. 1998;57(2):226.
5. Kwok CS, Gibbs S, Bennett C, Holland R, Abbott R. Topical treatments for cutaneous warts. Cochrane Database Syst Rev. 2012;2012(9):CD001781.
6. García-Oreja S, Álvaro-Afonso FJ, Tardáguila-García A, López-Moral M, García-Madrid M, Lázaro-Martínez JL. Efficacy of cryotherapy for plantar warts: a systematic review and meta-analysis. Dermatol Ther. 2022;35(6):e15480.
7. Focht DR 3rd, Spicer C, Fairchok MP. The efficacy of duct tape vs. cryotherapy in the treatment of verruca vulgaris (the common wart). Arch Pediatr Adolesc Med. 2002;156(10):971–4.
8. de Haen M, Spigt MG, van Uden CJ, van Neer P, Feron FJ, Knottnerus A. Efficacy of duct tape vs. placebo in the treatment of verruca vulgaris (warts) in primary school children. Arch Pediatr Adolesc Med. 2006;160(11):1121–5.
9. Wenner R, Askari SK, Cham PM, Kedrowski DA, Liu A, Warshaw EM. Duct tape for the treatment of common warts in adults: a double-blind randomized controlled trial. Arch Dermatol. 2007;143(3):309–13.
10. Abdel-Latif AA, El-Sherbiny AF, Omar AH. Silver duct tape occlusion in treatment of plantar warts in adults: is it effective? Dermatol Ther. 2020;33(3):e13342.
11. Kim SY, Jung SK, Lee SG, Yi SM, Kim JH, Kim IH. New alternative combination therapy for recalcitrant common warts: the efficacy of imiquimod 5% cream and duct tape combination therapy. Ann Dermatol. 2013;25(2):261–3.

Aloe Vera: Does It Work? A Burning Question

7

Introduction

When I was growing up in Miami, Florida, in the 50s and early 60s, we had an *Aloe vera* plant in our backyard. I remember the very sharp, pointy tips of its leaves (see Fig. 7.1). I also remember my parents breaking off a leaf from the plant near its base and squeezing a clear, gooey liquid directly on our skin whenever my brother or I burned ourselves or had a bad case of sunburn. The application of the cool, soothing goo was always accompanied by a promise that the burn would heal within a few days. Which it always did. Of course, as a kid I knew nothing about randomized trials or the post hoc fallacy (post hoc, *ergo propter hoc*, see Chap. 1). And like most kids, I assumed that my parents knew best.

Fast forward half a century, and my eldest son and his wife had their own aloe plant, which they bought because they were convinced from their own experience and "common knowledge" of the plant's wonderful properties. They told me how they had used it on multiple occasions to successfully treat their own and their kids' burns. Of course, now as an epidemiologist and professional skeptic, I pooh-poohed the idea but didn't attempt to disabuse them of their belief. After all, I was pretty sure it was harmless and would at least help sooth a crying child in need of consolation.

History

The name of the *Aloe vera* plant is derived from the Arabic word *alloeh*, meaning a bitter and shiny substance, and the Latin *vera* (true). Over 3000 years ago, the Egyptian queen Nefertiti used aloe leaf as a cosmetic, part of her beauty regime. A thousand years later, Alexander the Great was allegedly persuaded by Aristotle to capture the island of Socotra in the Indian Ocean, well known for its extensive growth of the plant, which he wanted to treat wounds among his soldiers. It was also

Fig. 7.1 The *Aloe vera* plant

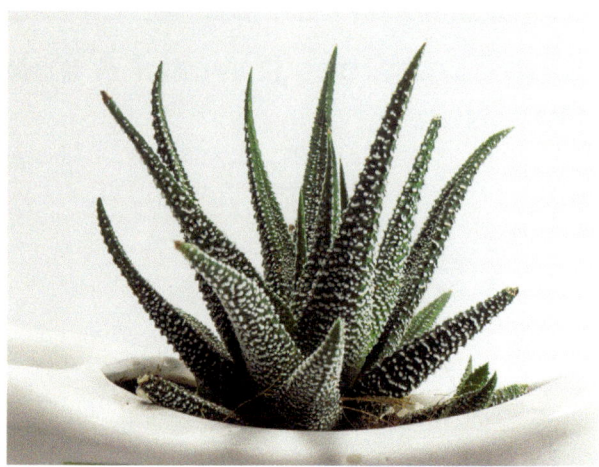

used for burns and other wounds in ancient India (where it remains part of Ayurveda, the science of life), by the Mayan Indians in Central America, and by sixteenth-century Spanish monks [1, 2]. Also in ancient times, aloe was taken internally as laxative but was gradually replaced by less toxic alternatives [1]. Aloe remains widely cultivated in North Africa, the Middle East, Mediterranean Europe, southern USA, Mexico, India, and China.

The aloe leaf gooey liquid contains a large number of chemicals [3]. Those chemicals include sugars and polysaccharides, which likely account for aloe's soothing and moisturizing effects. Compounds like aloesin, aloin, and emodin have antioxidant and anti-inflammatory effects, which might theoretically promote wound healing, while anthraquinones are probably responsible for the cathartic (laxative) effect when aloe is consumed orally. Since the 1950s, however, aloe has been used almost exclusively as a skin moisturizer and cosmetic and as a home-based "natural" remedy to treat thermal burns and sunburn and to promote wound healing. It is now sold commercially over the counter (without prescription) in a variety of gels and creams, which are easier to access for most people than buying and cultivating their own aloe plants.

How Are Burns Currently Treated?

I was able to find only two studies reporting on the prevalence of using *Aloe vera* as burn treatment. Alomar and coworkers administered questionnaires about parents' preferred burn treatments when they accompanied their child to the pediatric emergency departments of four major hospitals in Riyadh, Saudi Arabia [4]. The children came for a variety of ailments (not for burns). Just over 100 parents were surveyed at each of the hospitals (408 in total) about their first-choice treatment for treating a burn in their child, whether or not the child had been burned in the past. The highest-ranked treatment for the burn was application of cool or cold water, which was endorsed by 43% of the parents. *Aloe vera* was ranked in 11th position, endorsed by only 1%.

Bennett and colleagues compared children seen for burns in pediatric emergency departments in Cardiff, Wales, and Denver, Colorado over a 30-month period from 2015 to 2017 [5]. A total of 500 children were seen at each site. A substantial difference was observed in receipt of first aid before arrival: 90% in Cardiff versus 61% in Denver. Of those who received some first aid, children in Cardiff were more likely to have had their burns cooled with water: 82% versus 60%. Only a handful of children in either site had received topical application of *Aloe vera*, either alone or with other coverings or dressings.

Key Evidence Points
- Published randomized trials of *Aloe vera* treatment of burn wounds have been small and subject to bias due to non-blinding of participants and outcome observers.
- Nonetheless, those randomized trials (and systematic reviews of trials) suggest that applying creams or gels containing *Aloe vera* to burn wounds is at least as effective antibiotic creams and ointments in promoting healing and preventing infection.
- Placebo controls would be difficult to defend from an ethical standpoint, but laboratory studies in rats support the effectiveness of Aloe treatment.

Detailed Review of Scientific Evidence[1]

Randomized controlled trials (RCTs) are essential in evaluating the effectiveness of *Aloe vera*, either compared to a look-alike placebo product or to another treatment known to be effective, with blinding of the trial participants and of the observers who assess the outcome. The 2017 Cochrane review by Norman and coworkers analyzed five RCTs of *Aloe vera*, all involving comparisons with a topical antibiotic (applied to the burned skin, not taken orally) [6]. Using topical antibiotics or antiseptics is the standard of care for treating mild and moderate burns. No trials compared *Aloe vera* to no treatment or a placebo, which would be highly questionable from an ethical standpoint. The five trials were all relatively small, and although most participants were adults, some children were included. The burns were all mild or moderate (first- or second-degree). The two major outcomes assessed were time to healing and rate of infection of the burn wound, and non-blinding of participants and observers may have biased ascertainment of these outcomes. The three trials that reported on time to healing reported that the participants whose burns were treated with Aloe healed 1 week faster (2 vs. 3 weeks, on average) than those treated with topical antibiotics, but the small sample sizes of the trials and wide differences

---

[1] Readers who prefer to skip the Detailed Review should proceed to the Summary at the end of the chapter.

among them in time to healing (ranging from 11 to 31 days) led to the large average difference not achieving statistical significance. The three trials reporting on infection rates observed nearly identical risks of around 3.5% in that outcome.

Sharma and colleagues' recent non-Cochrane systematic review limited its analysis to burn wound healing in four RCTs treating second-degree burns (with blisters), comparing *Aloe vera* cream or gel versus a comparison cream [7]. The average time to complete wound healing was 4 days less in the Aloe group, although these results were highly heterogeneous and highly influenced by one low-quality trial that observed a 13-day shorter time to healing. The three other trials observed average differences of 1.5–3 days.

I found two additional RCTs not included in either systematic review, both published in 2022 [8, 9]. Both trials were small (34 and 30 participants) and both were from Iran, albeit from different cities (Tabriz and Kerman), with non-overlapping authors, and used different control antibiotic creams (silver sulfadiazine and nitrofurazone). Yet, these two trials used an identical, unusual design: all patients had burn on *both* sides of the body, and had both the *Aloe vera* and control treatments, randomized on the right- and left-sided burn wound. Although this is a rigorous design, neither trial apparently blinded either the participants or the observers who rated the wound healing, neither took the paired design into account in the statistical analysis, and two of the three outcomes studied in the Tabriz trial [8] (pain and itching) were subjective and self-reported. The Tabriz trial [8] reported differences favoring the Aloe treatment for the two subjective outcomes (especially itching), but the Kerman trial [9] found no differences between the Aloe and control results.

Overall, the RCT-based evidence suggests that the use of *Aloe vera* is not less effective than topical antibiotic creams or gels for treating burn wounds. Larger, more rigorous trials would be necessary to establish whether they are superior to antibiotics in accelerating healing. Because of the absence of RCTs comparing *Aloe vera* with placebo, I also searched evidence based on experimental burns in animals. Lin and colleagues reported significantly faster reduction in burn wound size among rats with experimentally induced burns treated with Aloe than controls treated with vehicle only, that is, with no active ingredient [10]. Finally, a recent experimental rat study compared topical application of *Aloe vera* with injection into the burn wound of mesenchymal stem cells obtained from rat bone marrow [11]. The rats receiving aloe had wound healing that was at least as fast and complete as those treated with stem cells.

Summary

Despite the thousands of years and wide geographic distribution of topical use of *Aloe vera* for burn treatment, limited evidence from Saudi Arabia, the USA, and U.K. suggest a very limited use. I was unable to find any descriptive studies of its use in Iran, but the large fraction of published randomized trials of Aloe strongly suggest its popularity in that country. As is true of many "natural" remedies, however, popularity does not necessarily mean efficacy. Many herbal and other natural remedies are popular but have absolutely no scientific evidence that they are effective, and some have even been shown to be harmful.

Based on the evidence from systematic reviews of randomized trials and several individual trials published since the systematic reviews, *Aloe vera* applied to burn wounds of mild and moderate severity (first- or second-degree) appears at least as effective as topical antibiotics in promoting healing and preventing infection. Studies using experimentally induced burns in rats comparing treatment with topical aloe to either a placebo control treatment or to injection with mesenchymal stem cells suggest that aloe may in fact be superior to those treatments. Since no human trials have compared Aloe to placebo, however, it is possible that neither Aloe nor topical antibiotics are effective. But given that antibiotics creams or ointments are the standard of care, parents and physicians who prefer a non-medicinal ("natural") remedy can feel confident that topical aloe treatment is at least as good antibiotic creams or ointments.

References

1. Manvitha K, Bidya B. Aloe vera: a wonder plant its history, cultivation and medicinal uses. J Pharmacogn Phytochem. 2014;2(5):85–8.
2. Roberts G. The magical and medicinal Aloe vera plant. Bloomspace. 21 Nov 2018.
3. Sánchez M, González-Burgos E, Iglesias I, Gómez-Serranillos MP. Pharmacological update properties of *Aloe vera* and its major active constituents. Molecules. 2020;25(6):1324.
4. Alomar M, Rouqi FA, Eldali A. Knowledge, attitude, and belief regarding burn first aid among caregivers attending pediatric emergency medicine departments. Burns. 2016;42(4):938–43.
5. Bennett CV, Maguire S, Nuttall D, Lindberg DM, Moulton S, Bajaj L, Kemp AM, Mullen S. First aid for children's burns in the US and UK: an urgent call to establish and promote international standards. Burns. 2019;45(2):440–9.
6. Norman G, Christie J, Liu Z, Westby MJ, Jefferies JM, Hudson T, Edwards J, Mohapatra DP, Hassan IA, Dumville JC. Antiseptics for burns. Cochrane Database Syst Rev. 2017;7:CD011821.
7. Sharma S, Alfonso AR, Gordon AJ, Kwong J, Lin LJ, Chiu ES. Second-degree burns and Aloe vera: a meta-analysis and systematic review. Adv Skin Wound Care. 2022;35(11):1–9.
8. Mahboub M, Aghazadeh Attari AM, Sheikhalipour Z, Mirza Aghazadeh Attari M, Davami B, Amidfar A, Lotfi M. A comparative study of the impacts of Aloe vera gel and silver sulfadiazine cream 1% on healing, itching and pain of burn wounds: a randomized clinical trial. J Caring Sci. 2022;11(3):132–8.
9. Sabaghzadeh Irani P, Ranjbar H, Varaei S, Bostani S, Akbari O, Askarymahani M. Comparison of the effectiveness of Aloe vera gel with 2% nitrofurazone ointment on the healing of superficial partial-thickness burns: a randomized clinical trial study. Nurs Pract Today. 2022;9(1):7–14.
10. Lin LX, Wang P, Wang YT, Huang Y, Jiang L, Wang XM. Aloe vera and vitis vinifera improve wound healing in an in vivo rat burn wound model. Mol Med Rep. 2016;13(2):1070–6.
11. Imbarak N, Abdel-Aziz HI, Farghaly LM, Hosny S. Effect of mesenchymal stem cells versus Aloe vera on healing of deep second-degree burn. Stem Cell Investig. 2021;8:12.

Diet and Acne: Should Teenagers Avoid Pizza and Chocolate?

8

Introduction

Common acne, or *acne vulgaris* in "medicalese" (Latin), affects nearly all teenagers of all races and socioeconomic conditions. The Ebers Papyrus, a compilation of ancient Egyptian writings from around 1550 BC, describes medical formulations for treating acne dating from the first dynasty (around 3400 BC) [1]. Although acne usually begins during puberty, it continues into the third decade of life in the majority of individuals and, in a substantial fraction, into the thirties and even the forties [2].

Acne is caused in part by the increased secretion of sebum, an oily secretion of the sebaceous glands that surround hair follicles on the face, neck, back, and chest. Sebum secretion begins in early puberty, as does the increased replication and turnover of the skin cells (keratinocytes) that line the ducts of the sebaceous glands. Levels of male hormones increase in early puberty in both sexes. Although the most potent of these hormones, testosterone, comes from the male testes, the ovaries and adrenal glands secrete masculinizing hormones of lower potency in girls.

These masculinizing hormones increase the production of sebum, which provides an excellent source of nutrition for a skin bacterium called *Propionibacterium acnes* and increases the shedding of keratinocytes, which can block the sebaceous gland ducts and hence the transit of sebum to the pores on the skin surface. The resulting increased pressure within the duct leads to leakage of the sebum outside of the sebaceous gland, causing irritation and inflammation of the surrounding skin, especially when combined with the acne bacterium. When the sebum remains within the gland and the duct, the sebum forms *open comedones*, called "blackheads," owing to the discoloration of the sebum reaching the skin surface from oxidation by the air. When the sebum and skin cells block the duct at or just under the pore, *closed comedones* (so-called whiteheads) are formed. When the increased pressure leads to the leakage of sebum and bacteria outside the duct, the resulting skin inflammation and infection leads to *papules* (red bumps) and *pustules* (in which the red areas have a tiny central cavity containing pus), which together are often referred to as *pimples*. When the leakage, inflammation, and infection become more severe, larger nodules and cysts can occur.

Studies comparing the occurrence and severity of acne in identical versus non-identical twins, and in family members versus unrelated individuals, have shown a very strong genetic contribution to acne causation. Environmental factors also contribute, however. They include psychological stress, application of oily cosmetics, and pressure from leaning the face onto one's hands or against mobile telephones. Many parents believe that poor hygiene is responsible, probably because they interpret the black color of open comedones as indicators of insufficient washing, but the evidence suggests that frequent washing is not beneficial for prevention or treatment [2].

Some parents also believe that teenagers' eating habits and preferences are to blame. To quote Isaac Asimov, the Russian-born biochemist and prolific science fiction writer, "The first law of dietetics seems to be: If it tastes good, it's bad for you" [3]. Of course, adolescence is a stage of life when most children emerge from parental control, at least to some degree, and express their new independence in what they eat, both inside and outside the home. Pizza, french fries and other oily foods, chocolate, and dairy products are the "usual suspects." In the next section, I will review the accumulated published evidence on these and other components of the diet, as well as dietary supplements. Given the potential for bias due to confounding factors related to differences in age, ethnicity, stress, and climate, I will prioritize systematic reviews of randomized trials of dietary interventions (Fig. 8.1).

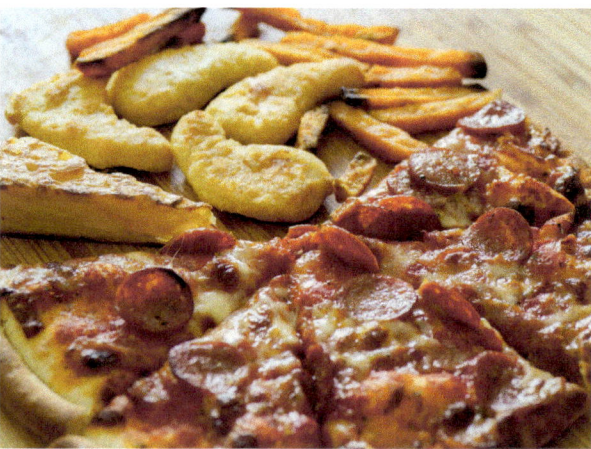

Fig. 8.1 Some of the oily foods commonly believed to cause or worsen acne

Current Beliefs About Diet and Acne

In a questionnaire-based survey of 500 students aged 14–17 years attending four randomly selected secondary schools in Podgorica, Montenegro, 82% and 73% responded that sweets and greasy food, respectively, would worsen acne [4]. The prevalence of these beliefs was nearly identical among respondents with and without acne. A similarly designed survey from Belgrade, Serbia, was based on 1452 students from six randomly selected schools but was limited to adolescents with current or past acne [5]. The percentages believing that sweets and greasy foods would worsen acne substantial but lower than those in the Montenegrin study: 40% and 27%, respectively, for sweets and greasy foods.

An acne questionnaire survey of 316 students attending four high schools in Athens, Greece, found that nearly two-thirds of them believed that diet could cause or worsen acne, with chocolate the most commonly reported offending food [6]. In a dermatology clinic-based survey of 49 adolescent and young adult acne patients from Houston, Texas, over 90% of them believed that diet could affect acne [7]. Over two-thirds believed that fried or greasy foods would worsen acne, and over half believed the same about chocolate. Finally, an Indian dermatology clinic-based survey of adolescent and young adult acne patients found that 85% of respondents believed that diet was a cause of acne, and the foods most commonly believed to worsen the disease were chocolate and fatty foods [8].

Key Evidence Points
- Acne is a skin disease originating in the sebaceous (oil) glands around the time of puberty that usually improves in the late teens or twenties.
- Its development and peak severity in adolescence may have led to suspicion about the causal role of teen dietary preferences like pizza, other oily foods, and chocolate.
- Beliefs about the causal role of these dietary preferences are highly prevalent among adolescents and young adults around the world.
- Most published evidence on the role of diet in the development and severity of acne is based on cross-sectional studies, which do not permit inference of a causal role.
- Randomized trials of chocolate intake do not suggest that chocolate consumption increases acne severity. No such trials have been published on pizza or oily foods.
- One small randomized trial of vitamin D supplementation reported a reduction in acne severity, a result that requires confirmation in future trials.
- Based on placebo-controlled randomized trials, zinc dietary supplements appear effective in reducing acne severity—as effective as oral antibiotics.

Detailed Review of Scientific Evidence[1]

Systematic reviews have been published on diet and dietary supplements suspected to affect (increase or decrease) the risk or severity of acne. These include the glycemic index of carbohydrates, dairy products, chocolate, long-chain polyunsaturated fatty acids (LCPUFAs), vitamins D and E, and zinc. I was unable to find systematic reviews on pizza or fried, greasy foods. Unfortunately, most of the systematic reviews are based on observational studies, rather than on randomized trials, at least partly owing to the paucity of published trials.

Glycemic Index

High-glycemic index carbohydrates include refined sugar, white bread, potatoes, pasta, and rice; they share the effect of a quick rise in the blood glucose (sugar) and insulin levels, thereby increasing the blood levels of insulin-like growth hormone, which is suspected to stimulate secretion of sebum and proliferate keratinocytes in sebaceous glands. Low-glycemic index carbohydrates include whole-grain breads, breakfast cereals, and citrus fruits. Cao and coworkers' 2015 Cochrane review included only two randomized trials of high- versus low-glycemic index carbohydrate diets in patients with acne. No significant difference was observed in number of acne lesions after 10–12 weeks of the diets when results of the two trials were combined (meta-analyzed) [9]. For some reason, Reynolds and colleagues' 2010 randomized trial in adolescent boys with acne was not included in the Cao systematic review [10]. After 8 weeks of the high- or low-glycemic diets in that trial, acne severity declined in *both* groups, with no significant difference in improvement between the two groups.

Chocolate

For chocolate, Dall'Oglio and colleagues' recent narrative systematic review of randomized trials of dietary interventions for acne was limited to trials published between 2009 and 2020 and did not include a meta-analysis [11]. It therefore excluded the trial of chocolate by Fulton and coworkers published in 1969, a well-designed crossover trial in which 65 adolescents with mild or moderate acne (lesions limited to comedones, papules, and pustules) were randomized to consume a daily chocolate bar for 4 weeks or a similar-tasting placebo bar containing no chocolate [12]. The placebo bar was necessary to blind the subjects, most of whom apparently believed that eating chocolate would worsen their acne. The real chocolate contained 10 times the usual chocolate content. After the initial 4-week treatment period, all participants had a 3-week washout period to eliminate any effect of the

---

[1] Readers who prefer to skip the Detailed Review should proceed to the Summary at the end of the chapter.

initial treatment, followed by another 4-week treatment period in which they consumed the opposite bar from the one they consumed in the initial period. No significant difference between the two treatment periods was observed in the proportions of participants who improved (reduction of at least 30% in the number of total lesions on one side of the face), worsened (increased by at least 30%), or remained unchanged (<30% change) after each period, nor in the quantity or biochemical composition of their sebum. My only criticism of this otherwise excellent trial is the apparent lack of blinding to treatment by the examining dermatologist, which should have been easy to implement.

The first of the two trials included in the Dall'Oglio review [11] was that of Caperton and colleagues, published in 2014 [13]. That trial was indeed double-blind but was very small (13 young men) and did not use a crossover design. Instead, the researchers combined varying quantities of gelatin and cocoa into capsules to create different concentrations of chocolate. The capsules were consumed as a "binge" at one sitting, and blinded clinical examinations were performed at baseline and at 4 and 7 days after the binge. Instead of comparing severity in groups receiving high versus low doses of chocolate, the authors based their primary analysis on overall changes in number of acne lesions in the *entire group* of 13 participants, regardless of chocolate intake; they observed a significant increase over baseline in acne lesions on both day 4 and day 7 of follow-up. Since most of the participants received some chocolate, the observers' expectations of an increase in acne lesions may well have biased their observations. The authors also observed modest correlations between chocolate "dose" and subsequent increase in lesions, but they did not report the statistical significance of those correlations. In any case, the response to a single dose of chocolate provides little useful evidence about the effect of frequent consumption.

The second trial included in the Dall'Oglio review [11] resembled the Fulton trial in its use of a crossover design. That trial recruited 54 college students, who were apparently not required to have current acne or even an acne history [14]. As in the Caperton trial, the intervention consisted of a single dose of a small (43 g, 1.5 ounces) Hershey's milk chocolate bar and was compared to a single consumption of 15 jellybeans. A 4-week washout period was provided between the two treatment periods, and a dermatologist blindly rated the number of acne lesions from photographs taken 48 h after the consumption of both products. The results showed a significant increase in acne lesions after the chocolate but not after the jellybeans. These results were apparently analyzed based on two independent groups, rather than as differences *within* the same participants during the two treatment periods, which would be the appropriate analysis for a crossover trial. Moreover, the participants were obviously not blinded to their treatments, and no mention is made of their beliefs about chocolate's effect on acne, which might well have led to stress about their appearance after ingesting the chocolate! When combined with the very low, single dose of chocolate studied, it is difficult to infer an adverse effect of the chocolate.

Vitamin D

Vitamin D has both anti-inflammatory and antioxidant properties. The 2021 systematic review and meta-analysis by Wang and coworkers focused on studies comparing blood vitamin D concentrations in participants with versus without acne, although the authors' objective does not distinguish between vitamin D as a prevention or treatment of acne [15]. Their meta-analysis found a significantly lower average concentration of 25-hydroxyvitamin D (the standard blood measurement for assessing vitamin D levels) in acne patients versus controls without acne. The included studies are labeled as case-control studies by the authors, but they were actually cross-sectional in design. Vitamin D levels were measured *after* the development of acne, and therefore exposure to the reported vitamin D levels did not correspond to a time *before* the acne occurred. Moreover, no mention is made of whether and how differences in confounding factors like age, sex, season, climate, psychological stress, and socioeconomic status were accounted for in the included studies. The reported differences cannot, therefore, be attributed to a causal effect of vitamin D on the risk or severity of acne.

The Wang review also cited two randomized *treatment* trials (rather than prevention trials) of vitamin supplementation in persons with acne, which the authors curiously dismiss as producing results that "cannot be used for research purposes" [15]. As readers of earlier chapters will know by now, randomized trials provide the strongest research evidence of causal effects, and I will therefore summarize the methods and results of the two treatment trials. Lim and coworkers' 2016 double-blind trial randomized 39 Korean patients with acne who had low blood levels of vitamin D to receive daily vitamin D supplements or placebo for 8 weeks, with photograph-based counts of acne lesions at baseline and after 2, 4, and 8 weeks of treatment [16]. No difference was observed between the two groups for comedones, but a significantly greater reduction in inflammatory lesions (papules, pustules, and nodules) was observed in those randomized to receive vitamin D supplements. A second double-blind, placebo-controlled trial by Ahmed Mohamed was published in 2021 [17]. One hundred acne patients were randomly assigned to receive vitamin D or placebo once daily for 3 months. The severity of acne was reduced in the vitamin D group at the end of follow-up versus the baseline assessment, but the authors did *not* compare changes in acne between the two treatment groups. I suspect the placebo group may have improved to the same degree!

Long-Chain Polyunsaturated Fatty Acids (LCPUFAs)

Omega-3 LCPUFAs are known to have anti-inflammatory properties, whereas omega-6 fatty acids have been reported to improve skin integrity. The previously-cited 2021 narrative systematic review by Dall'Oglio and coworkers [11] listed two small randomized controlled trials of LCPUFAs as treatment for established acne. Jung and colleagues randomized 45 Korean patients with mild or moderate acne to one of three treatment groups of 15 patients each for a period of 10 weeks: an omega-3 fatty acid group receiving a combination of eicosapentaenoic acid and docosahexaenoic acid; an omega-6 fatty acid group receiving gamma-linolenic acid; or no treatment [18]. No placebo was used for the control group. Both of the LCPUFA groups had improvements in acne severity, based on participants' subjective assessment, as well as on lesion counts made by two dermatologists from clinical photographs obtained at follow-up. The absence of a placebo group means that the participants knew whether or not they were receiving an active treatment and thus were not blinded. Nor is any mention made of blinding the clinical examiners. Despite the positive findings of the trial, therefore, it is impossible to infer a beneficial effect of either active treatment.

The other randomized trial in the Dall'Oglio review [11] focused on sunflower seeds, a good source of omega-6 linoleic acid. Mohebbipur and colleagues randomized 50 Iranian patients with mild or moderate acne who attended a dermatology clinic into two dietary groups, one of which was asked to stop eating sunflower seeds for 7 days, while the other group were each given a bag per day containing 25 g of sunflower seeds for the same period of time [19]. One dermatologist used two acne severity scales to examined the participants at baseline and after 14 days, that is, 7 days after completing the dietary intervention. That timing was based on the first author's previous experience in having observed an increase in severity 10–14 days after eating sunflower seeds. Neither the patients nor the examining dermatologist were blinded to the diet followed. The group consuming sunflower seeds had worsening acne over the 7-day follow-up, whereas the group who stopped eating the seeds had improved. Given the lack of blinding and the dermatologist's previous experience, a biased follow-up assessment of acne severity seems a far more likely explanation for the findings than an adverse effect of sunflower seeds!

Other Nutrients

Two other nutrients have been the subjected to systematic reviews: dairy products and vitamin E. Unfortunately, these reviews were restricted to observational studies, rather than randomized treatment or prevention trials. Systematic reviews and meta-analyses by Juhl and colleagues [20] and Aghasi and coworkers [21] were both based on 14 observational studies of associations between dairy intake and acne in nearly 80,000 children, adolescents, and young adults. The Juhl review [20] based its analyses on the association between any intake of milk, yogurt, or other dairy product (including cheese) and the presence of acne; the authors also analyzed associations based on weekly intake of milk. Analyses in the Aghasi review [21] were based on acne prevalence in the highest versus lowest categories of reported consumption. As with the above-mentioned systematic review of vitamin D, all studies included in both reviews of dairy intake were cross-sectional in design with respect to dairy intake and acne. Diets were compared among participants with and without acne at the time they reported their dairy intake, even though some of those studies had a prospective (follow-up) design for other study objectives. Moreover, the acne diagnosis was often self-reported by questionnaire, rather than diagnosed by clinicians.

The Juhl review [20] reported that any dairy intake was associated with a modest increase (25%) in reported acne; similar associations were observed for any milk, milks of different fat intakes, yogurt, and cheese. No clear gradient in risk was seen with increasing quantities of milk intake. In contrast, the Aghasi review [21] observed large increases in prevalence among participants in the highest versus lowest categories of total dairy and of milk of any fat content, but not with intakes of yogurt or cheese. Given the cross-sectional design of the studies reviewed, the frequently self-reported acne, and the potential for uncontrolled confounding, it is impossible to infer a causal effect of dairy consumption on the risk of developing acne from these two systematic reviews. Rigorous randomized trials would provide far stronger evidence for or against the role of milk and other dairy products in the development of acne (prevention) or in its severity (treatment) once it has developed.

Like vitamin D, vitamin E has both anti-inflammatory and antioxidant properties. Vitamin E is also a popular component of many cosmetic skin creams, but without any scientifically demonstrated benefits. Liu and coworkers' 2021 systematic review and meta-analysis included observational studies of the association between blood vitamin E levels and several inflammatory skin diseases, including acne [22]. As with several of the systematic reviews discussed in this section, the authors erroneously refer to their included studies as case-control studies, even though the actual design was cross-sectional, because the vitamin E levels compared were obtained after, rather than before, the diagnosis of their skin disease. For acne, the authors meta-analyzed three studies comparing blood vitamin E levels in 284 cases of acne and 186 controls without acne. A moderately lower (about one-third of a standard deviation) vitamin E level was observed in acne cases versus controls. Similar findings were observed for atopic eczema, psoriasis, and vitiligo (an immune disease leading to white spots without skin pigment), suggesting that confounding differences between cases and controls, especially in factors like age or ethnicity, are more likely to explain the observed differences than a causal effect of vitamin E intake on the development of acne.

Zinc

Zinc is an important nutrient contained in meat, shellfish, eggs, dairy products, eggs, beans and other legumes, nuts, and seeds. Zinc deficiency is rare in high-income countries but not among children in low-income countries, especially those with frequent or severe diarrhea. Zinc has proven anti-inflammatory properties. To my knowledge, it has not been used as a dietary supplement to prevent acne, but rather as an oral treatment for people with established acne. Dhaliwal and colleagues' 2020 narrative systematic review (without meta-analysis) found clear evidence of its effectiveness in randomized trials in which it was compared to placebo, but not when compared to oral antibiotics [23]. In one of the trials included in the review, the supplement contained lactoferrin (a milk-derived protein with antibacterial and anti-inflammatory properties) and vitamin E, as well as zinc [24]. Although the supplemented group had a significantly greater reduction in acne severity than the placebo group, it is impossible to identify which component was responsible for the difference.

Fatty or Oily Foods

As stated earlier, I was unable to find any systematic reviews concerning the association between consumption of pizza, french fries, or other fatty or oily foods and the development or severity of acne. One recent, large, cross-sectional web-based survey of French adults observed a strong association between consumption of fatty and sugary foods (surveyed as a combined category) and current acne, but the cross-sectional design, self-reported acne, and potential for uncontrolled confounding does not permit an inference of causality [25].

Summary

It is reasonable to ask whether foods favored by teenagers are responsible for the nearly universal occurrence of acne in adolescents. Hormonal changes at puberty clearly play a role in the high prevalence among adolescents, as do genetic factors; psychological stress, oily cosmetics, and facial pressure may also contribute in some cases. Gels and creams containing antibiotics and/or medications that loosen the keratinocyte cells that block sebaceous glands are highly effective in treating established acne, as are antibiotics taken by mouth. The published evidence does *not* support a causal role for chocolate, dairy products, or high-glycemic index carbohydrates, nor does it suggest a beneficial effect of omega-3 or omega-6 fatty acids. Blood vitamin E levels are lower in acne patients than in healthy controls, but the same is true for other skin diseases, and uncontrolled confounding better explains these findings than does a beneficial effect of vitamin E. The nutrient with the strongest evidence of benefit in treating established acne is zinc, and it appears to be as effective as oral antibiotics. For vitamin D, one small double-blind randomized trial suggests a beneficial effect on reducing severity. Additional larger trials of vitamin D supplementation are necessary before recommending its routine use by acne patients.

I was unable to find any systematic reviews or randomized trials concerning consumption of pizza, french fries, or other fatty or oily foods and acne. In other words, the evidence permits an answer concerning only one of the two foods I proposed in the chapter's title. Of course, it would be impossible to design a double-blind randomized trial of pizza or french fries!

References

1. Mahmood NF, Shipman AR. The age-old problem of acne. Int J Womens Dermatol. 2016;3(2):71–6.
2. Bhate K, Williams HC. Epidemiology of acne vulgaris. Br J Dermatol. 2013;168(3):474–85.
3. Wolf R, Matz H, Orion E. Acne and diet. Clin Dermatol. 2004;22(5):387–93.
4. Ražnatović Đurović M, Janković J, Đurović M, Spirić J, Janković S. Adolescents' beliefs and perceptions of acne vulgaris: a cross-sectional study in Montenegrin schoolchildren. PLoS One. 2021;16(6):e0253421.
5. Markovic M, Soldatovic I, Bjekic M, Sipetic-Grujicic S. Adolescents' self perceived acne-related beliefs: from myth to science. An Bras Dermatol. 2019;94(6):684–90.
6. Rigopoulos D, Gregoriou S, Ifandi A, Efstathiou G, Georgala S, Chalkias J, Katsambas A. Coping with acne: beliefs and perceptions in a sample of secondary school Greek pupils. J Eur Acad Dermatol Venereol. 2007;21(6):806–10.
7. Nguyen QG, Markus R, Katta R. Diet and acne: an exploratory survey study of patient beliefs. Dermatol Pract Concept. 2016;6(2):21–7.
8. Kaushik M, Gupta S, Mahendra A. Living with acne: belief and perception in a sample of Indian youths. Indian J Dermatol. 2017;62(5):491–7.
9. Cao H, Yang G, Wang Y, Liu JP, Smith CA, Luo H, Liu Y. Complementary therapies for acne vulgaris. Cochrane Database Syst Rev. 2015;1:CD009436.
10. Reynolds RC, Lee S, Choi JY, Atkinson FS, Stockmann KS, Petocz P, Brand-Miller JC. Effect of the glycemic index of carbohydrates on Acne vulgaris. Nutrients. 2010;2(10):1060–72.
11. Dall'Oglio F, Nasca MR, Fiorentini F, Micali G. Diet and acne: review of the evidence from 2009 to 2020. Int J Dermatol. 2021;60(6):672–85.
12. Fulton JE Jr, Plewig G, Kligman AM. Effect of chocolate on acne vulgaris. JAMA. 1969;210(11):2071–4.
13. Caperton C, Block S, Viera M, Keri J, Berman B. Double-blind, placebo-controlled study assessing the effect of chocolate consumption in subjects with a history of acne vulgaris. J Clin Aesthet Dermatol. 2014;7(5):19–23.
14. Delost GR, Delost ME, Lloyd J. The impact of chocolate consumption on acne vulgaris in college students: a randomized crossover study. J Am Acad Dermatol. 2016;75(1):220–2.
15. Wang M, Zhou Y, Yan Y. Vitamin D status and efficacy of vitamin D supplementation in acne patients: a systematic review and meta-analysis. J Cosmet Dermatol. 2021;20(12):3802–7.
16. Lim SK, Ha JM, Lee YH, Lee Y, Seo YJ, Kim CD, Lee JH, Im M. Comparison of vitamin D levels in patients with and without acne: a case-control study combined with a randomized controlled trial. PLoS One. 2016;11(8):e0161162.
17. Ahmed Mohamed A, Salah Ahmed EM, Abdel-Aziz RTA, Eldeeb Abdallah HH, El-Hanafi H, Hussein G, Abbassi MM, El Borolossy R. The impact of active vitamin D administration on the clinical outcomes of acne vulgaris. J Dermatolog Treat. 2021;32(7):756–61.
18. Jung JY, Kwon HH, Hong JS, Yoon JY, Park MS, Jang MY, Suh DH. Effect of dietary supplementation with omega-3 fatty acid and gamma-linolenic acid on acne vulgaris: a randomised, double-blind, controlled trial. Acta Derm Venereol. 2014;94(5):521–5.
19. Mohebbipour A, Sadeghi-Bazargani H, Mansouri M. Sunflower seed and acne vulgaris. Iran Red Crescent Med J. 2015;17(9):e16544.
20. Juhl CR, Bergholdt HKM, Miller IM, Jemec GBE, Kanters JK, Ellervik C. Dairy intake and acne vulgaris: a systematic review and meta-analysis of 78,529 children, adolescents, and young adults. Nutrients. 2018;10(8):1049.
21. Aghasi M, Golzarand M, Shab-Bidar S, Aminianfar A, Omidian M, Taheri F. Dairy intake and acne development: a meta-analysis of observational studies. Clin Nutr. 2019;38(3):1067–75.
22. Liu X, Yang G, Luo M, Lan Q, Shi X, Deng H, Wang N, Xu X, Zhang C. Serum vitamin E levels and chronic inflammatory skin diseases: a systematic review and meta-analysis. PLoS One. 2021;16(12):e0261259.

23. Dhaliwal S, Nguyen M, Vaughn AR, Notay M, Chambers CJ, Sivamani RK. Effects of zinc supplementation on inflammatory skin diseases: a systematic review of the clinical evidence. Am J Clin Dermatol. 2020;21(1):21–39.
24. Chan H, Chan G, Santos J, Dee K, Co JK. A randomized, double-blind, placebo-controlled trial to determine the efficacy and safety of lactoferrin with vitamin E and zinc as an oral therapy for mild to moderate acne vulgaris. Int J Dermatol. 2017;56(6):686–90.
25. Penso L, Touvier M, Deschasaux M, Szabo de Edelenyi F, Hercberg S, Ezzedine K, Sbidian E. Association between adult acne and dietary behaviors: findings from the NutriNet-Santé prospective cohort study. JAMA Dermatol. 2020;156(8):854–62.

I Can See Clearly Now: Do Glasses Make You More Nearsighted?

9

Introduction

Nearsightedness (*myopia* in "medicalese") is a visual impairment whereby distant objects appear blurry, whereas nearby objects are seen clearly. It is caused by the eye's focusing the optical image in front of the retina, rather than directly on it. The retina is the back wall of the eye and contains photoreceptor cells that convert the optical signal to a nerve impulse. The usual reason for the frontward focus is a front-to-back elongation of the eyeball, although changes in the curvature of the cornea (the layer of cells covering the lens and iris) can also be a cause. Most myopia begins at early school age and progresses at least until late adolescence. One recent long-term prospective study from Australia, however, documented new-onset myopia and progression in the degree of myopia into the third decade of life [1].

The degree of myopia is usually measured in terms of negative diopters, which denotes the amount of correction required to achieve normal vision. A correction of −0.50 diopters (or a larger negative number) is a common threshold to define myopia and the need for treatment, with values of −6.00 diopters (or a larger negative number) denoting severe myopia. If left untreated, myopia can lead to severe eye problems like macular (retinal) degeneration, retinal detachment, glaucoma (high pressure in the eyeball, with consequent damage to the nerve conveying visual signals to the brain), and cataract (lens opacity). Untreated myopia is a major global health problem, leading to an annual estimated loss of 250 billion U.S. dollars in 2015 [2].

Nearsightedness was recognized by Aristotle around 350 BC, although the Greek physician Galen first used the word *myopia* to refer to nearsightedness in the second century AD. The Roman emperor Nero was nearsighted and was said to have watched gladiator fights through a concave emerald! [3] The earliest glasses appeared around the end of the thirteenth century, when they were introduced by the Franciscan friar Roger Bacon. Rafael's 1517 portrait of Pope Leo X showed the pontiff with a concave glass: a lens curved inwards that sharpens (unblurs) the image of distant objects. However, it was the early seventeenth-century astronomer Johannes Kepler, himself myopic, who first demonstrated that myopia was caused by the forward displacement of the focused image. Kepler also demonstrated that myopia could be corrected by a concave lens. Twenty years later, the Dutch physician Klempius demonstrated that the erroneous focal point was due to an axial (front-to-back) elongation of the eyeball.

Studies comparing prevalence of myopia in identical and non-identical twins, as well as family studies not involving twins, demonstrate a strong genetic effect on risk. If both of your parents are myopic, the chances of your escaping the condition are slim. Many genes have been demonstrated to increase the risk of myopia, but even taken together, those genes account for only a small fraction of all cases. The evidence thus suggests that many genes are involved, most causing only small increases in risk.

Genes are not the entire story, however, since myopia incidence has been increasing for decades, especially in urban areas of the world. Genes do not change that fast in human populations, and the increase must therefore be due to environmental factors. One important environmental risk factor is near work, that is, activities that require focus on nearby objects such as reading and use of video games and other screen devices [4]. A recent umbrella review (that is, a review of systematic reviews), mostly based on prospective observational studies, found that children who spent more time outdoors had a significantly lower risk of developing myopia [5]. Randomized trials from Taiwan and China have confirmed that spending more time outdoors on school days can reduce the risk, probably owing to greater exposure to sunlight [6, 7]. These environmental factors not only affect the risk of developing myopia in the first place, but also the rate of progression of myopia once it develops [8]. As confirmation of these effects, a systematic review of observational studies observed an increased rate of progression of myopia among children during the COVID-19 lockdown, when most children were learning remotely (online) and spending less time outdoors [9].

Ethnic and Geographic Differences and Temporal Trends

Holden and colleagues' systematic review and meta-analysis included 145 studies with 2.1 million participants across the globe [10]. The authors estimated that 1.4 billion people (23% of the world's population) were affected by some degree of myopia, figures they predicted would rise to 4.8 billion and 50% by the year 2050. Temporal increases have been substantial since the year 2000. Marked geographic differences were noted in the systematic review, with the highest rates observed in high-income countries in East and Southeast Asian regions (50% in 2020); 40% in North America and Western Europe; 30% in Latin America, South Asia, the Caribbean, the Middle East, and Eastern Europe; and <10% in most of Africa and Oceania. In 2000, the prevalence was highest among people 10–39 years of age, but prevalence is predicted to flatten out at older ages by 2050, as the recent increases at earlier ages will lead to higher future prevalence at older ages (Fig. 9.1).

Fig. 9.1 Myopia affects half the population in East and Southeast Asia

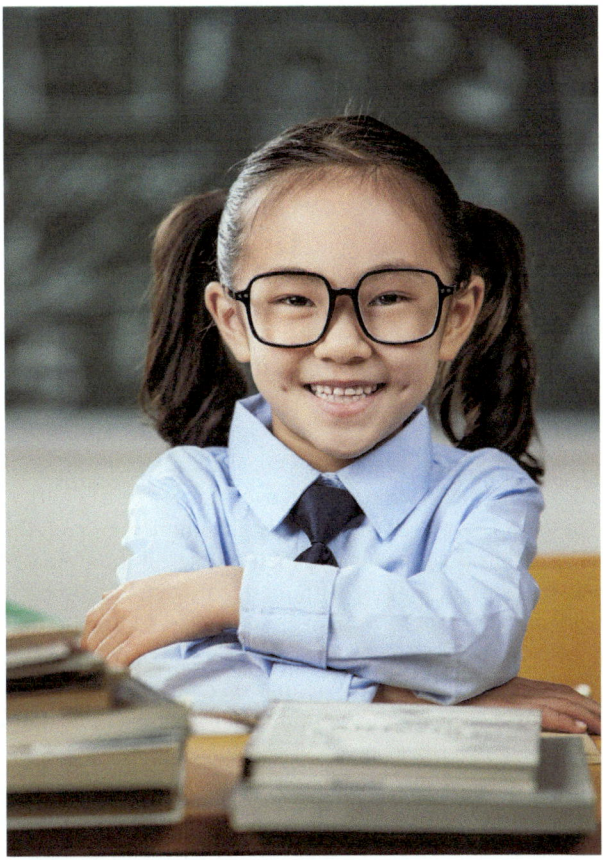

Differences in prevalence among countries may be at least partly due to differences in ethnicity. Ethnic differences are better studied by comparing prevalence among ethnic groups *within* the same multi-ethnic countries. Kleinstein and colleagues recruited a non-representative sample of children in grades 1–8 in four U.S. communities [11]. The authors compared the prevalence of myopia in four ethnic groups: non-Hispanic Whites, Blacks, Hispanics (mostly Mexican-Americans), and Asians. These samples were not necessarily representative of state or national populations but had similar distributions of sex and age among the four ethnic groups. Myopia prevalence was highest among Asians, intermediate in Hispanics, and lowest (and similar) in Whites and Blacks.

The National Health and Nutrition Examination Survey is a cross-sectional survey carried out regularly (now annually) on a representative sample of the child and adult population in the United States. This survey was mentioned in Chap. 4 when discussing temporal trends in the use of dietary supplements. Vitale and coworkers compared the prevalence of myopia in the right eye by age and sex in 1971–72 with the prevalence in 1999–2004, based on over 8000 Black and White participants from age 12 to 54 years, using the same eye examination techniques in the two periods [12]. Overall, the prevalence was higher in Whites than in Blacks, and in females than in males, at all ages. The prevalence increased from 25% to 42% overall, with large increases observed in all age groups, both races, both sexes, and for all degrees of myopia severity.

Current Beliefs About Wearing Glasses

In one Nigerian study, a survey questionnaire was administered to a random sample of 500 undergraduate students 18–30 years of age attending the University of Benin [13]. Only half of those surveyed said they would wear spectacles if prescribed by their doctor, and nearly two-thirds believed they were harmful to the eyes. Two-thirds had never had a test of vision, 60% thought that glasses are meant for old people, and 57% feared they would be mocked or teased for wearing them. In the southern Mexican state of Oaxaca, a random sample of 5–18 year-old school children who had been provided eyeglasses free of charge were examined unannounced in their schools 18 months after having been given their glasses [14]. Only 13% of the children were wearing their glasses at the time of the examination, and another 34% had their glasses with them but were not wearing them. Children with myopia documented at the time of the "surprise" examination were of course significantly more likely to be wearing their glasses, but so were younger children and those from rural areas. A random sample of children and adults living in Tehran, Iran were recruited door-to-door and invited to a clinic interview and eye examination [15]. Of those qualifying as needing spectacles (most of whom were myopic), one-third did not wear glasses. The risk of "unmet need" (needing, but not wearing, spectacles) was significantly higher in older participants and those with lesser education.

Two school-based studies of random samples of rural Chinese children were carried out by the same group of investigators. The first examined 1892 adolescents 13–17 years of age in Xichang [16]. Half of the children had refractive errors (most were myopic) that would benefit from glasses, but only 40% of those children owned spectacles. Among the 580 children who owned spectacles, 18% did not wear them at school. Among the 476 children who wore spectacles at school, 25% had prescriptions that grossly under-corrected their visual defect. Girls were significantly more likely to be wearing their spectacles than boys. Among children who would benefit from spectacles but did not wear them, 17% believed spectacles would weaken their eyes, but nearly 80% said that their families would be willing to pay for them.

The second study from these authors was based on focus groups (small discussion groups led by a facilitator) of randomly selected myopic students 14–18 years of age, parents, and teachers from three schools (one high school and two junior high schools) in the rural Chaoshan region of southern China [17]. Separate focus groups were held for the students, parents, and teachers at each of the three schools to better understand barriers to wearing glasses. All three groups of participants believed that wearing glasses should be delayed, because they might hasten the progression of the myopia. Parents cited inconvenience ("too busy with work"), rather than expense, as the major reason for not purchasing glasses for their children. Teachers cited students' concern about their appearance and lack of concern about their vision as the major barriers.

In contrast to the above studies in low- and middle-income countries, a population-based sample of 2353 12-year-old children from Sydney, Australia were examined in their schools [18]. Only 19% of the children wore spectacles for myopia or other refractive eye problems, and only 8% of them had under-corrected prescriptions. Only eight children (0.3%) had an unmet need for glasses.

Key Evidence Points
- Myopia is caused by elongation of the eyeball from front to back. It usually starts in childhood and progresses during adolescence and even into early adulthood.
- Myopia has been increasing in frequency across the world, owing to increases in screen use, reading, and other near work and reduction in time spent outdoors.
- Contrary to some beliefs, failure to correct or under-correction of myopia hastens its progression.
- Multifocal soft contact lenses or spectacles slow progression of myopia.
- Orthokeratology (ortho-K), which uses rigid scleral lenses worn at night to change the shape of the cornea, has an even larger effect on slowing progression of myopia than multifocal lenses.
- A novel treatment with repeated low-level red light shows promise for slowing progression of myopia, but large, placebo-controlled randomized trials with prolonged follow-up are necessary to confirm its effectiveness.
- Atropine drops applied at night have the largest effect on slowing myopia progression, and the magnitude of effect increases with concentration of the drug. Unfortunately, however, high concentrations ($\geq$0.5%) also cause blurry vision and should be avoided.

Detailed Review of Scientific Evidence: What Slows Progression of Myopia?[1]

As seen in the previous section, many children and adults believe that wearing glasses will weaken their eyes, that is, hasten the progression of their myopia. I suspect that belief is an extension of the "Use it or lose it" concept that applies to muscles, but myopia is **not** related to weak eye muscles. As explained at the beginning of this chapter, it is the front-to-back (axial) elongation of the eyeball that

---

[1] Readers who prefer to skip the Detailed Review should proceed to the Summary at the end of the chapter.

causes myopia. The main known causes of the elongation are genetic predisposition, near work, and insufficient time outdoors.

How do we know that the common belief that glasses hasten myopia progression is incorrect? In fairness, I am unaware of any randomized trials in children or adults in which myopic individuals have been randomized either to wear corrective concave lens glasses or to "placebo" glasses (clear glass without concavity or convexity), or even to no glasses. Ong and colleagues carried out a small observational 3-year follow-up study in 43 children from the onset of their myopia [19]. Four groups were compared: (1) full-time spectacle wearers; (2) children who wore them for distance vision only; (3) children who switched from distance-only to full-time wear; and (4) non-wearers. The non-wearers had twice the progression as the full-time wearers over the 3-year follow-up, but the small sample size prevented even this large difference from achieving statistical significance. Moreover, the absence of randomization raises the potential of confounding differences among the studied groups.

In the remainder of this evidence review, I will restrict my discussion to randomized trials, based on the 2023 Cochrane review by Lawrenson and coworkers [20]. These authors analyzed 64 randomized trials in over 11,000 children 18 years or younger. The treatments compared included spectacles, contact lenses, and eye drops containing atropine or other active medications, as well as their combinations, in children. Follow-up periods varied across trials, but most were 1 or 2 years, and the control treatments were either placebos (for medicated eye drops) or single-focus spectacles or contact lenses.

Children randomized to wear under-correcting spectacles had a slightly increased rate of myopia progression over 1 year of follow-up (differences of −0.15 diopters in refractive error and +0.05 mm in axial length) versus those randomized to fully-correcting spectacles. In other words, contrary to the common "Use it or lose it" belief, the under-corrected group had a greater progression of their myopia, although the observed differences were of borderline statistical significance. Differences after 2 years of follow-up were negligible.

Other randomized trials compared multifocal soft contact lenses with standard, single-vision soft contact lenses for correcting distance vision. The multifocal lenses incorporate different lens curvatures at different distances. Children randomized to soft contact lenses with multifocal lenses had slower progression than those randomized to single-vision lenses (differences of 0.26 diopters in refractive error at 1 year and 0.30 diopters at 2 years; −0.11 mm in axial length at 1 year and −0.15 mm at 2 years). Differences only about half of those just cited were observed in trials comparing multifocal (progressive) versus single-vision spectacles, rather than soft contact lenses. Newly-designed progressive spectacles improve central vision but provide a deliberate myopic de-focus for peripheral vision to counteract the hyperopic de-focus of single-vision spectacles. Randomized trials of these spectacles have shown improvements at 1 and 2 years that were greater than those achieved with multifocal soft contact lenses.

Specialty contact lenses have also been studied in several randomized trials. Rigid, gas-permeable contact lenses (which land on the sclera, the white part of the eye outside the colored iris) did not slow progression of myopia compared to standard soft contact lenses, which are applied to the cornea, the transparent layer of cells lying over the pupil and iris. On the other hand, orthokeratology (often abbreviated as ortho-K) uses rigid scleral lenses worn only at night to reshape the cornea and thereby affect its refractive properties to help focus light on, rather than in front of, the retina. Since ortho-K flattens the cornea at night, no substantial refractive error is detectable the following day. Therefore, the effect on myopia progression is measurable only by comparing changes in axial length in treatment versus control groups. In seven trials analyzed in the systematic review [20], ortho-K substantially slowed myopia progression compared to single-vision soft contact lenses, with a −0.19-mm difference in axial elongation over 1 year of follow-up, and a −0.28-mm difference in the two trials reporting 2-year follow-up.

The most effective treatment for slowing progression of myopia in the systematic review [20] was the use of eye drops containing atropine or similar-acting medications, usually a single drop applied at night. The concentration of atropine studied has varied 100-fold, from 0.01% to 1%. Higher concentrations are more likely to cause blurred vision at near distances, owing to the drug's ability to partially paralyze the ciliary muscle, which controls the shape of the eye's lens. Differences favoring high-dose (≥0.5%) atropine drops versus placebo drops were 0.90 and 1.26 diopters in refractive error at 1 and 2 years, respectively, and −0.33 and −0.47 mm, respectively, for axial elongation. Improvements in trials of low-dose (<0.1%) atropine were about one-third as large as those observed with high-dose atropine, whereas the two trials of intermediate-dose atropine (0.1% to <0.5%) unsurprisingly observed improvements that were smaller than those seen with high-dose atropine, but larger than those using a low dose. It is not known *how* atropine drops work to slow myopia progression. The atropine is believed to lead to biochemical changes in the retina, but the exact mechanism is unknown. Tsai and coworkers' recent systematic review and meta-analysis suggests that the combination of ortho-K and low-dose atropine appears particularly effective in slowing myopia progression [21].

A novel treatment for myopia is the use of repeated low-level red light (RLRL) shined into the eye for 3 min, twice per day. Tang and colleagues' recent systematic review and meta-analysis analyzed eight small studies of RLRL in myopic children, mostly randomized trials, but also including several observational studies [22]. Follow-up times were short, but impressive reductions in myopia progression were observed between the RLRL and control groups. The mechanism by which RLRL achieves its beneficial effect is unknown. Larger, placebo-controlled randomized trials with longer follow-ups are required to situate this treatment among the effective treatment options currently available.

Summary

Myopia (nearsightedness) has been recognized since antiquity. It is very common, affecting many school-age children, adolescents, and adults across the world, especially among Asians. The prevalence of myopia has been increasing world-wide, probably attributable to changes in lifestyle involving more reading and screen time and less time spent outdoors. Nonetheless, many children and adults are reluctant to wear glasses or contact lenses, especially in less developed areas of the world, at least partly owing to the belief that they will "weaken" the eyes and thereby hasten the progression of myopia.

The belief that wearing glasses will hasten progression of myopia is not supported by rigorous scientific evidence. In fact, the data from one small observational study of no treatment and the systematic Cochrane review of randomized trials of under-correction suggest that failure to correct or even under-correction may *hasten*, rather than slow, myopic progression. Treatments proven to slow progression include progressive spectacles and multifocal soft contact lenses, orthokeratology, repeated low-level red light, and (especially) atropine eye drops. The latter are used at low concentrations, because they carry increased risks of blurred near vision when used at higher concentrations.

References

1. Lee SS, Lingham G, Sanfilippo PG, Hammond CJ, Saw SM, Guggenheim JA, Yazar S, Mackey DA. Incidence and progression of myopia in early adulthood. JAMA Ophthalmol. 2022;140(2):162–9.
2. Naidoo KS, Fricke TR, Frick KD, Jong M, Naduvilath TJ, Resnikoff S, Sankaridurg P. Potential lost productivity resulting from the global burden of myopia: systematic review, meta-analysis, and modeling. Ophthalmology. 2019;126(3):338–46.
3. de Jong PTVM. Myopia: its historical contexts. Br J Ophthalmol. 2018;102(8):1021–7.
4. Dutheil F, Oueslati T, Delamarre L, Castanon J, Maurin C, Chiambaretta F, Baker JS, Ugbolue UC, Zak M, Lakbar I, Pereira B, Navel V. Myopia and near work: a systematic review and meta-analysis. Int J Environ Res Public Health. 2023;20(1):875.
5. Dhakal R, Shah R, Huntjens B, Verkicharla PK, Lawrenson JG. Time spent outdoors as an intervention for myopia prevention and control in children: an overview of systematic reviews. Ophthalmic Physiol Opt. 2022;42(3):545–58.
6. Wu PC, Tsai CL, Wu HL, Yang YH, Kuo HK. Outdoor activity during class recess reduces myopia onset and progression in school children. Ophthalmology. 2013;120(5):1080–5.
7. He M, Xiang F, Zeng Y, Mai J, Chen Q, Zhang J, Smith W, Rose K, Morgan IG. Effect of time spent outdoors at school on the development of myopia among children in China: a randomized clinical trial. JAMA. 2015;314(11):1142–8.
8. Pärssinen O, Kauppinen M, Viljanen A. The progression of myopia from its onset at age 8–12 to adulthood and the influence of heredity and external factors on myopic progression: a 23-year follow-up study. Acta Ophthalmol. 2014;92(8):730–9.
9. Cortés-Albornoz MC, Ramírez-Guerrero S, Rojas-Carabali W, de-la-Torre A, Talero-Gutiérrez C. Effects of remote learning during the COVID-19 lockdown on children's visual health: a systematic review. BMJ Open. 2022;12(8):e062388.

10. Holden BA, Fricke TR, Wilson DA, Jong M, Naidoo KS, Sankaridurg P, Wong TY, Naduvilath TJ, Resnikoff S. Global prevalence of myopia and high myopia and temporal trends from 2000 through 2050. Ophthalmology. 2016;123(5):1036–42.

11. Kleinstein RN, Jones LA, Hullett S, Kwon S, Lee RJ, Friedman NE, Manny RE, Mutti DO, Yu JA, Zadnik K, Collaborative Longitudinal Evaluation of Ethnicity and Refractive Error Study Group. Refractive error and ethnicity in children. Arch Ophthalmol. 2003;121(8):1141–7.

12. Vitale S, Sperduto RD, Ferris FL 3rd. Increased prevalence of myopia in the United States between 1971–1972 and 1999–2004. Arch Ophthalmol. 2009;127(12):1632–9.

13. Ebeigbe JA, Kio F, Okafor LI. Attitude and beliefs of Nigerian undergraduates to spectacle wear. Ghana Med J. 2013;47(2):70–3.

14. Castanon Holguin AM, Congdon N, Patel N, Ratcliffe A, Esteso P, Toledo Flores S, Gilbert D, Pereyra Rito MA, Munoz B. Factors associated with spectacle-wear compliance in school-aged Mexican children. Invest Ophthalmol Vis Sci. 2006;47(3):925–8.

15. Fotouhi A, Hashemi H, Raissi B, Mohammad K. Uncorrected refractive errors and spectacle utilisation rate in Tehran: the unmet need. Br J Ophthalmol. 2006;90(5):534–7.

16. Congdon N, Zheng M, Sharma A, Choi K, Song Y, Zhang M, Wang M, Zhou Z, Li L, Liu X, Liu X, Lam DS. Prevalence and determinants of spectacle nonwear among rural Chinese secondary schoolchildren: the Xichang pediatric refractive error study report 3. Arch Ophthalmol. 2008;126(12):1717–23.

17. Li L, Lam J, Lu Y, Ye Y, Lam DS, Gao Y, Sharma A, Zhang M, Griffiths S, Congdon N. Attitudes of students, parents, and teachers toward glasses use in rural China. Arch Ophthalmol. 2010;128(6):759–65.

18. Robaei D, Kifley A, Rose KA, Mitchell P. Refractive error and patterns of spectacle use in 12-year-old Australian children. Ophthalmology. 2006;113(9):1567–73.

19. Ong E, Grice K, Held R, Thorn F, Gwiazda J. Effects of spectacle intervention on the progression of myopia in children. Optom Vis Sci. 1999;76(6):363–9.

20. Lawrenson JG, Shah R, Huntjens B, Downie LE, Virgili G, Dhakal R, Verkicharla PK, Li D, Mavi S, Kernohan A, Li T, Walline JJ. Interventions for myopia control in children: a living systematic review and network meta-analysis. Cochrane Database Syst Rev. 2023;2:CD014758.

21. Tsai HR, Wang JH, Huang HK, Chen TL, Chen PW, Chiu CJ. Efficacy of atropine, orthokeratology, and combined atropine with orthokeratology for childhood myopia: a systematic review and network meta-analysis. J Formos Med Assoc. 2022;121(12):2490–500.

22. Tang J, Liao Y, Yan N, Dereje SB, Wang J, Luo Y, Wang Y, Zhou W, Wang X, Wang W. Efficacy of repeated low-level red-light therapy for slowing the progression of childhood myopia: a systematic review and meta-analysis. Am J Ophthalmol. 2023;252:153–63.

Eye Strain and Headache: A Change in Viewpoint

10

Introduction

In both children and adults, headaches are common symptoms that range in severity from mild to debilitatingly severe. They can occur alone or with infections or other illnesses. And they can vary in characteristics like one-sided versus generalized or pounding versus constant; in location such as the front, back, or side of the head; and in accompanying symptoms like nausea, blurry vision, or dizziness. With some migraine headaches, they can be preceded by a so-called aura with flashing lights, strange sounds, or a sense of impending doom. Parents or adult patients often fear the worst (brain cancer), but that diagnosis is almost always accompanied by convulsions, double vision, limb or facial weakness, limp, vomiting, or sleepiness.

When I was doing my residency (clinical specialty training) in pediatrics half a century ago, I saw many children complaining of headache. Rarely, the headache was severe enough to result in an Emergency Department visit. Sometimes, the child's regular pediatrician would refer the child to see a pediatric neurologist in a subspecialty clinic that I and other pediatric residents would rotate through. But more commonly, the child's parents would make an appointment in the pediatric outpatient clinic.

I was taught, both by senior pediatricians and pediatric neurologists, that the two most frequent types of headaches were tension headaches and migraines, and to enquire about symptoms that were "typically" observed in one type versus the other. (I was never clear as to why this distinction was so important, since the treatments were generally similar, at least initially.) But I was also taught that "eye strain" was not a cause of headache; rather, it was a lazy diagnosis that encouraged referral to optometrists or ophthalmologists, rather than trying to undercover the child's underlying psychological or physiological problems. Since my pediatric training, and especially after training as an epidemiologist and professional skeptic, I never doubted the "lazy diagnosis" characterization of eye strain as an explanation for headaches in adults or children.

That is, not until I recently started developing headaches myself after working on my laptop for several hours straight. When my optometrist daughter Elise suggested eye strain as a possible explanation, I of course would have none of it. Elise told me that the biological explanation was still uncertain but assured me that she had had numerous patients whose headaches resolved after prescription of corrective lenses.

Always the skeptic, I had my doubts but tried a few rounds of de-challenge and re-challenge: stopping my computer work for half an hour or so when I felt a headache coming on, without taking acetaminophen or other pain killer, then restarting when the headache resolved. After multiple successful de-challenges after stopping and relapses after re-challenge, my skepticism began to recede. Of course, I was not "blinded" to these de-challenges and re-challenges, so I could not rule a placebo effect.

My skepticism receded further after Elise's examination of my eyes, when she noted no change in my mild myopia (nearsightedness) and even milder presbyopia (blurry vision for small print at reading distance), but detected a substantial increase in astigmatism, or distortion of the optical image, especially at the middle distances typical for computer use. Astigmatism is caused by an asymmetrical change in curvature of the lens or of the cornea, the clear surface that covers the front of the eyeball. With new glasses to correct for the astigmatism, the headaches improved. Of course, I could not refrain from re-challenging my eyes with computer work without the glasses, with inevitable relapses, to lessen the likelihood of a placebo response!

A Brief History

As reviewed in the previous chapter, myopia was first identified by the ancient Greeks, but it was not until the seventeenth century that the optical defect was understood and that corrective spectacles (eyeglasses) were commonly worn. The "discovery" of eye strain had to wait another two centuries, however. Nineteenth century ophthalmologists observed a range of symptoms in patients with a range of visual defects, including refractive errors in focusing light, such as myopia, presbyopia, hyperopia (farsightedness), and astigmatism [1, 2]. The symptoms included pain in the front of the eye, headache, dizziness, and even general fatigue. During the same period, the American neurologist Silas Weir Mitchell "legitimized" eye strain as a cause of headache [3].

Since Greek and Latin were the chosen languages for medicine in those days (or perhaps because "eye strain" was too easily understood by the general public!), the ophthalmologists came up with the Greek-based term *asthenopia*, which literally means weak vision [4]. In the absence of evidence that refractive error or dry eye denotes "weakness," I will avoid that term. Treatments for eye strain in the late nineteenth century included atropine eye drops and corrective spectacles.

Why Should Refractive Errors Cause Headache?

In the remainder of this chapter, I will concentrate my discussion of symptoms on headache. I started the chapter by discussing what I was taught and practiced in treating children with headache—not children with refractive errors or other visual problems. Part of my unwillingness to attribute headache to refractive errors was based on what I was taught by faculty in both pediatrics and neurology. Another part was (and still is) my skeptical inclination. But a third part remains: despite a fair bit of reading on the subject while writing this chapter, I still find the "explanations" for headache weak and unconvincing.

The best explanation I can find relates to the ciliary muscle, the muscle that con- trols the curvature of the lens, which needs to change when looking at nearby objects versus when looking at distant ones. This change is called *accommodation*. Without it, we would need to change lenses whenever we regarded objects at differing distances, much as we change the focus of binoculars. That is why many people with myopia who develop presbyopia (inability to focus on nearby objects like words in books or newspapers) in middle or older age require bifocal or progressive lenses to see clearly at varying distances.

But why should overuse of the ciliary muscle cause a headache? Just because that muscle is in the head? So are all the extraocular muscles that control movement of the eyeball, whose malfunction leads to double vision. Why do so few people with double vision have headaches? The tongue is also in the head, but people who talk excessively are more likely to give *other* people headaches than complain of headaches themselves! I admit that the brain is a complex and poorly understood organ, but I have yet to read or hear a convincing biological explanation for how overuse of the ciliary muscle leads to headache.

The good news, however, is that understanding the mechanism is not a requirement for evaluating the cause-and-effect relationship between refractive errors and headache, nor the efficacy of treatments. Later in this chapter, I will review the scientific evidence bearing on the strength of these causal relationships.

Current Beliefs About and Prevalence of Eye Strain Headaches

I was unable to locate any systematic reviews, or even population-based surveys, on beliefs about eye strain. The published literature is quite plentiful, however, on its prevalence. In recent decades, eye strain has been increasingly reported in connection with computer use in adults. This link is now enshrined by the name *computer vision syndrome*, or CVS. Some ophthalmologists prefer the term *digital eye strain* (DES), in order to encompass digital devices other than computers, such as smartphones, hand-held video games, and electronic readers (Fig. 10.1).

Strong evidence supporting an increase in eye strain with computer work comes from Chu and colleagues' crossover trial in 30 young adults [5]. Wearing their usual spectacles or contact lenses, the subjects read aloud the identical text for 20 min at two sessions separated by at least 24 h: one session from a computer screen and one

Fig. 10.1 Headaches and other potential symptoms of eye strain have become increasingly common among workers and students who spend hours every day facing a computer screen. This phenomenon has given rise to the synonymous terms of digital eye strain (DES) and computer vision syndrome (CVS)

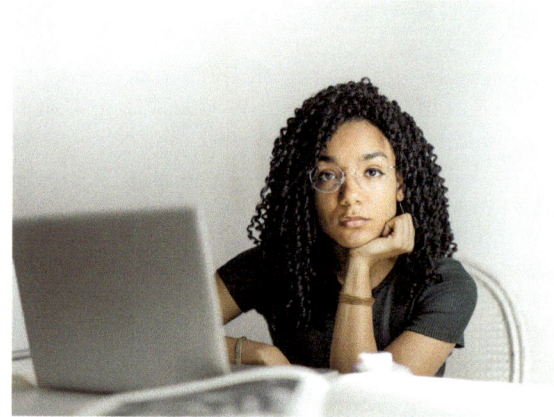

session from a hard copy, at an identical distance of 50 cm and with identical font, contrast, and lighting. After each reading, the subjects completed a written questionnaire rating each of ten symptoms (including headache) related to eye strain. The order of the two testing conditions was unfortunately not randomized but was alternated among subjects. A statistically significantly higher score was observed for the average score across all ten symptoms, but not separately for headache, when reading from the computer screen versus the hard copy. These results strongly suggest something specific about reading from a computer screen that leads to more eye strain symptoms than the same amount of time spent reading from a printed page.

In high-income countries, use of digital devices is now nearly universal among older children and young adults and has increased markedly even among the elderly [6]. Narrative reviews by Rosenfield [7] and Sheppard and Wolffsohn [6] cite surveys of office computer users in Australia, Mexico, India, and the U.S., all of which documented a very high prevalence of one or more symptoms of eye strain. The prevalence was generally higher in women than in men and increased with increased number of hours per day in front of a computer screen. With respect to headache in particular, a survey of over 500 office workers in New York City found that 22% of respondents reported headache to occur at least half of their time working on a computer [8].

Among children, a population-based cross-sectional survey was carried out in 1741 6-year-old children attending 34 primary schools in Sydney, Australia [9]. The children underwent comprehensive eye examinations, and their parents completed a detailed questionnaire regarding visual symptoms. One-eighth of the studied children had one or more symptoms of eye strain: blurred vision, sore eyes, double vision, or headaches. Only 3% of the children reported headaches. Most (82%) children with eye strain symptoms had normal eye examinations. Refractive errors were slightly more common among those with eye strain symptoms than among those without (15% vs. 10%), but 85% of children with symptoms had no refractive errors.

Finally, a recent narrative systematic review of 21 studies in children reported an increase in computer and other screen time attributed to the change to remote learning during the COVID-19 pandemic, with concomitant increases in refractive errors, eye strain, and headache [10]. Few of the studies included in the review followed the same children over time, however, and the effects of reduced time spent outdoors and increased reading and other near work could not be separated from those of increased screen time.

Key Evidence Points
- Use of computers and other screen devices has increased worldwide at all ages, especially with remote work and learning during the COVID-19 pandemic.
- Eye strain symptoms are more frequent when reading from a computer screen than from a printed page, even with identical distance, font size, contrast, and lighting.
- Prolonged screen time is associated with symptoms of eye strain, including blurred vision, eye discomfort, and headache.
- Refractive errors, and especially astigmatism, increase the symptoms of eye strain, including headache, although the underlying biological mechanisms are unknown.
- Progressive lenses with a focus at computer distance reduce eye strain symptoms, but blue light-filtering lenses do not.

Detailed Review of Scientific Evidence[1]

Do Refractive Errors Cause Eye Strain and Headache?

A recent narrative systematic review by Mataftsi and colleagues included 10 studies of digital eye strain (DES) in children and adults <40 years of age (that is, before the onset of presbyopia) but concentrated on screen time, rather than refractive errors [11]. The two observational studies that reported on daily screen time observed a statistically significant positive association between number of hours per day and DES symptom scores. Lanca and Saw's systematic review and meta-analysis did not observe a clear positive association in prevalence or incidence of myopia in children with increased screen time [12], but the authors' interest was in screen time as a cause of new cases of myopia or myopia progression—not myopia as a cause of DES. A more recent systematic review by Wang and coworkers restricted its included studies to smartphone use in children and young adults [13]. Most of the studies included in that review were cross-sectional in design, but no significant association was observed between smartphone use and myopia.

---

[1] Readers who prefer to skip the Detailed Review should proceed to the Summary at the end of the chapter.

In the remainder of this section, I will review the best individual studies I was able to find on the etiologic role of refractive errors in causing DES, and especially headache. As reviewed in Chap. 9, myopia, or nearsightedness, is a common refractive error usually due to an axial (front-to-back) elongation of the eyeball. Nearsighted people, however, do not usually have difficulty reading books or using computers or cellphones but have blurry vision when focusing on more distant objects. This may explain why published studies of the causal role of refractive errors have concentrated on astigmatism, rather than myopia.

In an excellent small experimental study by Sheedy and colleagues [14], 20 young adult students and staff at The Ohio State University with normal (20/20) vision were each asked to read text from printed sheets placed on a document holder placed 40 cm (16 in) from the eyes after being subjected to eight different optical stressors designed to cause eye strain. The eight stressors were astigmatism, strong magnifying glasses, upward gaze, dry eyes (lids kept open), lens flipper (reading sentences with lenses that alternated between slightly convex and slightly concave), small font, glare, and flickering light. The order of the stressors was randomized, and each was applied for up to 15 min each or until the subject complained of "barely tolerable" discomfort. After each stressor, the subjects rated nine eye strain symptoms on a scale from 0 to 100 and then had a 5-min rest before the next stressor was applied.

Based on a statistical technique called factor analysis, the symptoms clustered into two factors: an external symptom factor and an internal symptom factor. The external factor cluster comprised eye burning, tearing, irritation, and dryness, which is probably attributable to drying of the eye surface. This factor was strongly associated with holding the eyelids open, upward gaze, glare, small font, and flickering. The internal factor cluster comprised headache, eye ache, strain, double vision, and blur—that is, symptoms that are probably attributable to problems with accommodation and/or convergence (having both eyes move inward to see close objects). The internal factor was strongly associated with magnifying glasses, lens flipper, and small font stressors. These results suggest that internal symptoms are more likely to be caused by refraction errors, such as astigmatism or presbyopia, whereas external symptoms are probably caused by dry eye due to insufficient blinking. With respect specifically to headache, symptom scores did not vary much among the eight optical stressors, except that scores were much lower for keeping the eyelids open, suggesting that dry eye is not a cause of headache. Despite the experimental design of this study, its results might not be applicable to DES, because the testing was based on printed documents, rather than read off a computer screen.

Wiggins and coworkers published two excellent but small experimental studies in the early 1990s evaluating the role of astigmatism in causing eye strain [15, 16]. Both studies used a randomized, double-blind crossover design in which subjects read for 25 min from a computer screen. The first study recruited seven optometry students at the University of Alabama at Birmingham (UAB) School of Optometry and one student's spouse [15]. One pair of spectacles contained lenses that created astigmatism, while the other pair contained very weak (placebo control) lenses.

Both pairs of spectacles were applied over each subject's best-corrected prescription. The subjects completed an interview-based symptom rating of blur, visual discomfort, and eye strain after each 25-min session. Visual discomfort and eye strain, but not blur, were higher when using the astigmatism-inducing lenses, although the differences were of borderline statistical significance. All but one of the eight subjects preferred the control lenses.

The second study recruited 12 contact lens-wearing patients with some residual (uncorrected) astigmatism who attended the clinic at the UAB School of Optometry [16]. Unlike the first study, the experimental spectacles in this study corrected the residual astigmatism, while the weak placebo control spectacles did not. Both spectacles were used over each subject's usual contact lenses. The second study also differed by combining the symptoms into a single visual discomfort scale that included both blur and eye strain. Visual discomfort was significantly higher with the control (no correction) than with the experimental (corrective) spectacles, and all but 1 of the 12 subjects preferred the corrective glasses. In summary, neither study specifically inquired about headache, but the results of both show a causal effect of astigmatism on visual discomfort.

A more recent study by Rosenfield and coworkers [17] used a similar crossover design to the studies of Wiggins and colleagues [15, 16] and provides further evidence of astigmatism as a cause of eye strain. Twelve young adults were asked to read lines of text containing unrelated words from a computer screen for a 10-min period under four conditions: (1) using their usual spectacles or contact lenses; (2) placing an additional lens over their usual correction to induce mild astigmatism; (3) as in condition 2, but with doubling of the astigmatism; and (4) a repeat of condition 1. All sessions were separated by at least 24 h, and a written questionnaire was completed after each, with the subject requested to rate each of ten eye strain symptoms on a 0–10 scale. Two important methodologic differences from the Wiggins trials are worth underlining, however. The order of conditions was varied among subjects, but not randomized, and the absence of placebo spectacles made it impossible to "blind" the subjects to the condition imposed for each session, except perhaps for comparing conditions 2 and 3. The results showed statistically significantly higher symptom scores during the high-astigmatism lens condition (condition 3) than for the control conditions (1 and 4) for eye strain, eye discomfort, blurred vision, and "tired eyes," but not for dry eyes or headache.

The specific association of refractive errors with headache was addressed in an observational case-control study of 25 patients with migraine headaches and 25 age- and sex-matched controls, who were friends of the migraine patients but who did not themselves suffer from headaches [18]. Cases and controls underwent a detailed visual examination, with the order of patient versus "friend" control randomized and the examiner blind to the case versus control status of the person examined. The major finding was a significantly higher degree of astigmatism in the cases than in the controls, despite no difference in visual acuity, suggesting astigmatism as an important cause of migraine headaches. The pertinence of these findings to headache caused by DES is uncertain.

Does Correction of Refractive Errors Reduce Eye Strain and Headache?

The title of this section may suggest the same issue addressed in the previous section: that is, the causal effect of refractive errors on eye strain and headache. Although both sections address causal relationships, the previous section reviewed studies about whether refractive errors occurring naturally or induced experimentally produce eye strain symptoms, and especially headache. That is important, but probably not as important as whether people who already have headache or other symptoms of eye strain experience a reduction in their symptoms after treatment of their refractive errors.

The evidence in this section is all based on randomized or quasi-randomized trials. I have relied heavily on the 2018 Cochrane review by Heus and colleagues [19]. That review includes eight small trials among frequent computer users; six of the eight trials were restricted to presbyopic participants. One of those trials studied monofocal (also called single-vision) glasses with a focus at computer distance compared with progressive lenses that included a computer-distance focus; that trial observed reduced headache in the progressive lens group over a 12-month follow-up period. Two other trials compared progressive computer glasses with the conventional progressive lenses often used by presbyopic persons, which presumably do not do as good a job of ensuring a sharp image at computer distance. Those trials observed a short-term reduction in overall DES symptoms in the group randomized to the progressive computer glasses. Unfortunately, these trials cannot address the question of whether *any* computer-distance spectacles reduce headache and other eye strain symptoms compared to no spectacles.

Finally, Singh and colleagues' recent non-Cochrane systematic review and meta-analysis included three randomized trials comparing conventional spectacles for myopia to spectacles that selectively filtered out (blocked) blue light [20]. Visual fatigue (DES) symptoms were not significantly reduced by the blue-filter spectacles; headache was not reported separately.

Summary

The frequent and prolonged use of computers has increased in most parts of the world, especially with remote work and schooling during the COVID-19 pandemic. Eye strain symptoms are more frequent when reading from a computer screen than from a printed page, even with identical distance, font size, contrast, and lighting. Prolonged screen time is associated with symptoms of eye strain, including blurred vision, eye discomfort, and headache. These associations have led to the increased recognition of digital eye strain (DES), also known as computer vision syndrome (CVS).

Astigmatism experimentally induced by special lenses increases visual discomfort, albeit not headache. Migraine patients have more astigmatism, however, than controls not suffering from headaches, although the pertinence of this association to DES-induced headaches remains unclear. Randomized trials in frequent computer users with eye strain symptoms have compared treatment with progressive lenses incorporating a computer-distance focus with single-vision computer spectacles or with conventional progressive lenses and observed modest reductions in headache and other symptoms of visual discomfort with the progressive computer lenses. Other randomized trials have shown no benefit in DES symptoms with blue light-blocking lenses.

I still don't understand the biological mechanisms involved, but the evidence I have reviewed in this chapter has changed my "viewpoint." Eye strain due to heavy computer use does indeed seem to be a cause of headache.

References

1. Rider W. Headache from eye-strain. Am J Dent Sci. 1889;22(11):481–93.
2. De Schweinitz GE. Some ophthalmic observations based on experience during the past fifty years. Arch Ophthalmol. 1935;14(6):879–89.
3. Tomsak RL. Ophthalmologic aspects of headache. Med Clin North Am. 1991;75(3):693–706.
4. Cross FR. Asthenopia and ocular headache. Bristol Med Chir J (1883). 1893;11(40):73–84.
5. Chu C, Rosenfield M, Portello JK, Benzoni JA, Collier JD. A comparison of symptoms after viewing text on a computer screen and hardcopy. Ophthalmic Physiol Opt. 2011;31(1):29–32.
6. Sheppard AL, Wolffsohn JS. Digital eye strain: prevalence, measurement and amelioration. BMJ Open Ophthalmol. 2018;3(1):e000146.
7. Rosenfield M. Computer vision syndrome: a review of ocular causes and potential treatments. Ophthalmic Physiol Opt. 2011;31(5):502–15.
8. Portello JK, Rosenfield M, Bababekova Y, Estrada JM, Leon A. Computer-related visual symptoms in office workers. Ophthalmic Physiol Opt. 2012;32(5):375–82.
9. Ip JM, Robaei D, Rochtchina E, Mitchell P. Prevalence of eye disorders in young children with eyestrain complaints. Am J Ophthalmol. 2006;142(3):495–7.
10. Cortés-Albornoz MC, Ramírez-Guerrero S, Rojas-Carabali W, de-la-Torre A, Talero-Gutiérrez C. Effects of remote learning during the COVID-19 lockdown on children's visual health: a systematic review. BMJ Open. 2022;12(8):e062388.
11. Mataftsi A, Seliniotaki AK, Moutzouri S, Prousali E, Darusman KR, Adio AO, Haidich AB, Nischal KK. Digital eye strain in young screen users: a systematic review. Prev Med. 2023;170:107493.
12. Lanca C, Saw SM. The association between digital screen time and myopia: a systematic review. Ophthalmic Physiol Opt. 2020;40(2):216–29.
13. Wang J, Li M, Zhu D, Cao Y. Smartphone overuse and visual impairment in children and young adults: systematic review and meta-analysis. J Med Internet Res. 2020;22(12):e21923.
14. Sheedy JE, Hayes JN, Engle J. Is all asthenopia the same? Optom Vis Sci. 2003;80(11):732–9.
15. Wiggins NP, Daum KM. Visual discomfort and astigmatic refractive errors in VDT use. J Am Optom Assoc. 1991;62(9):680–4.
16. Wiggins NP, Daum KM, Snyder CA. Effects of residual astigmatism in contact lens wear on visual discomfort in VDT use. J Am Optom Assoc. 1992;63(3):177–81.
17. Rosenfield M, Hue JE, Huang RR, Bababekova Y. The effects of induced oblique astigmatism on symptoms and reading performance while viewing a computer screen. Ophthalmic Physiol Opt. 2012;32(2):142–8.
18. Harle DE, Evans BJ. The correlation between migraine headache and refractive errors. Optom Vis Sci. 2006;83(2):82–7.

19. Heus P, Verbeek JH, Tikka C. Optical correction of refractive error for preventing and treating eye symptoms in computer users. Cochrane Database Syst Rev. 2018;4:CD009877.
20. Singh S, McGuinness MB, Anderson AJ, Downie LE. Interventions for the management of computer vision syndrome: a systematic review and meta-analysis. Ophthalmology. 2022;129(10):1192–215.

Part IV

Foods and Beverages

The Benefits of Intermittent Fasting: Detox or Redux?

11

Introduction

Our hunter-gatherer ancestors ate when and what they could, usually only once or twice per day, occasionally going 24 h or longer without a meal. Moreover, hunting, fishing, and gathering all required substantial energy expenditure, while success was far from guaranteed. Obesity and other modern-day chronic diseases were rare. Undernutrition, and even frank starvation, were far more common, and average life expectancy was less than half of what it is today. Intermittent fasting in those days was not a lifestyle choice, but an unavoidable and unhealthy fact of life.

Eating three or more meals per day did not become common about until about 12,000 years ago, with the agricultural revolution of farming and the raising of domestic animals during what is called the Neolithic period (New Stone Age). These changes in the organization of human communities obviated the need for hunting and gathering but nonetheless required manual labor and high energy expenditure. The absence of long periods between meals may have reduced selection for genetic mutations (changes in DNA) that help maintain blood sugar and muscle mass during fasts.

The metabolic challenge has now become how to avoid excessive food intake, obesity, and their later adverse effects: type 2 diabetes, coronary heart disease, and high blood pressure. Over the last several decades, obesity rates have skyrocketed all over the world, and life expectancy in some countries may actually decline, despite general improvements in socioeconomic conditions and health care. Although the epidemic of obesity began in high-income countries, it has more recently affected low- and middle-income countries as well [1]. The wide availability, attractive taste, and low cost of high-calorie processed foods (so-called "junk foods") puts them within reach of nearly the entire world's population. Many low- and middle-income countries have now entered what has been referred to as the epidemiologic transition: the co-existence of stunting (short stature) and other indicators of undernutrition alongside obesity and overnutrition within the same country, region, or community. In fact, the two extremes can co-exist even within the

M. S. Kramer, *Believe It or Not*, https://doi.org/10.1007/978-3-031-46022-7_11

same person! An adult who was undernourished and stunted as an infant and toddler may become obese as an older child or adult.

Obesity rates vary widely by race, culture, socioeconomic status, and family history. In high-income countries, the poor tend to be more obese than the rich. Diet and physical activity are heavily influenced by culture and family eating habits. In some countries or regions, high-calorie junk foods are cheaper than fruits and vegetables and thus affordable even for poor families. A Big Mac at McDonald's contains about 550 calories—about 20–25% of the total daily calories needed by an average adult. A Big Mac takes only 5 min to eat, but burning off those 550 calories requires at least an hour or two of high-intensity physical activity!

Voluntary Fasting: A Brief History

It seems unlikely that our hunter-gatherer ancestors fasted voluntarily, and even Neolithic farmers may not have had sufficient food to encourage such a practice. But voluntary fasting later became an important aspect of religions in diverse regions of the world, including Hinduism, Judaism, Buddhism, Christianity, Islam, and Indigenous religions in both North and South America [2, 3]. It was believed that fasting helped prepare the mind to approach God in prayer and to receive divine revelations. Buddha, Christ, and Mohammed all preached the value of fasting for "purifying" the spirit and for healing the body [4].

The ancient Greeks believed that voluntary fasting improved cognition. Hippocrates, the fifth century B.C. "father" of medicine whose oath is still taken by modern medical graduates, was convinced of its ability to treat a variety of illnesses: "To eat when you are sick is to feed your illness." The idea that fasting could help the healing process continued well into the nineteenth century A.D. EH Dewey, a prominent American physician, pioneered what he called therapeutic fasting and advocated a "No Breakfast Plan." In his book, presumptuously entitled *The True Science of Living*, he wrote that all diseases were caused by "habitual eating in excess of the supply of gastric juices" [5].

The modern belief in the medical benefits of fasting appears to be based on the notion of *detoxification*, a periodic "cleansing" of the body that is intended to remove accumulated "toxins" that its proponents believe are contained in foods, either as natural components of those foods or as contaminants in the environment or from modern food processing. The liver and kidney are the body's organs tasked with either metabolizing (the liver) or excreting (the kidney) such toxins. Unfortunately, modern claims of "detox" fasts have not clearly identified the toxins that fasting is alleged to help eliminate. Another current attraction of intermittent fasting is based on the diet of hunter-gatherers. Because our ancestors were often lucky to get one or two meals per day, their apparent freedom from obesity and chronic cardiometabolic diseases like diabetes and high blood pressure (but, curiously, not their drastically reduced life span!) has been credited to their diet, at least in part. I call this return to our hunter-gatherer roots as a "redux" diet in the title of the chapter (Fig. 11.1).

Fig. 11.1 Beliefs about the health benefits of fasting have a long and colorful history

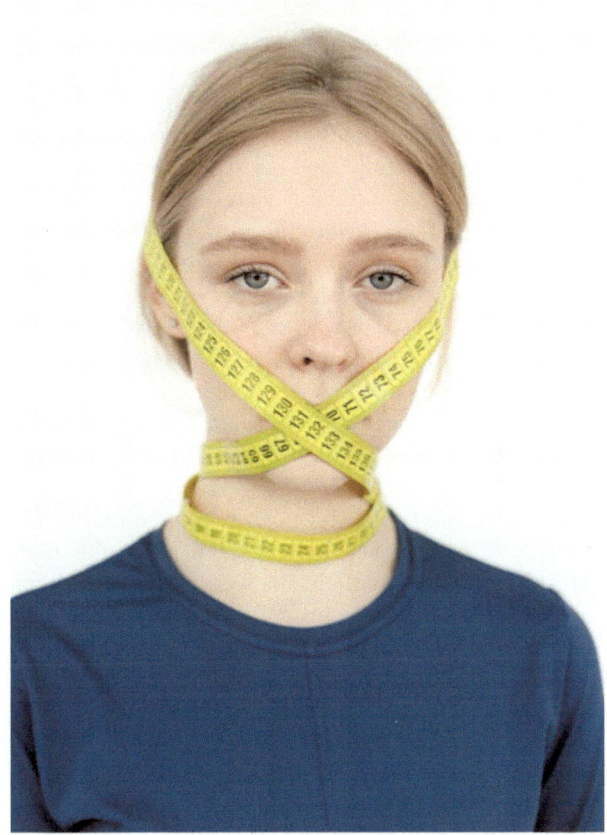

Current Beliefs and Practices About Intermittent Fasting

I was unable to find any systematic reviews of current beliefs and practices concerning intermittent fasting. In fact, even descriptive surveys about voluntary fasting (as opposed to fasting for religious reasons) appear to be few and far between. The only population-based survey I located was from the International Food Information Council, a food industry-funded consortium of food companies that has carried out a yearly web-based survey since 2006 among U.S. adults, using a sample that is statistically weighted to be representative of the adult U.S. population with respect to age, sex, race/ethnicity, education, and region. In the Council's 2022 survey, 10% of participants reported following an intermittent fasting diet [6], an identical proportion to that reported in 2018, the first year in which participants were asked about this diet.

Weinstock and Mazzeo surveyed 463 undergraduate women from a public university in Virginia, U.S.A. [7], of whom 8.4% reported following an intermittent fasting diet. Participants were also presented with five one-paragraph fictional vignettes, each describing a distinct dietary pattern, including one for intermitting fasting and one for a standard American diet. The vignette of a woman following the intermittent fasting diet was perceived significantly more negatively by the survey participants than the woman who was not dieting.

An online cross-sectional survey from the University of Bristol (UK) recruited participants (90% women) from a database of students and staff and by advertising on a Facebook dieting page [8]. Those who either were currently fasting intermittently, or previously did but were no longer doing so, were asked to complete a questionnaire. Over 90% of the participants had followed the 5:2 diet, that is, 5 days of ad lib (unrestricted) diets and two non-consecutive days of restriction to 500 (women) or 600 (men) calories per day each week. The remainder followed other fasting regimens, such as every other day. The former fasters were more likely to believe that eating three meals per day is healthy and to have eaten breakfast on fasting days. Despite the cross-sectional design, the authors attributed the fact that former fasters no longer adhered to the fasting diet to their beliefs about the value of breakfast and three meals per day, rather than their wish to justify why they had stopped fasting!

Brisebois and colleagues carried out an online diet and nutrition survey among over 2500 practitioners of CrossFit, a popular high-intensity exercise program. Most of the survey participants were from the U.S. and were recruited by distributing flyers at CrossFit gyms [9]. Sixty percent of respondents reported following a specific diet; intermittent fasting was practiced by 7.7% overall, but the proportion was higher among men (11.1%) than women (4.6%).

Finally, Alnasser and Almutain reported an online survey of 514 Saudi adults who fasted intermittently outside of Ramadan [10]. The participants were recruited through social media sites such as Twitter, WhatsApp, and Telegram. The majority had been voluntarily fasting for 3 months or less. Over 40% followed the same 16:8 pattern of fasting (16 h of fasting, 8 h of unrestricted eating per day) as during Ramadan. The most frequent reason for the diet was desire to lose weight, followed by other health reasons or religious reasons.

Key Evidence Points
- Our hunter-gatherer ancestors were probably lucky to eat once or twice a day and may have been obligated to skip meals entirely on some days.
- The agricultural revolution (farming and livestock) 12,000 years ago obviated the need for prolonged fasting but required heavy physical activity; the foods consumed were modest in calories, and sedentary activity was uncommon.
- The recent availability of high-calorie, low-cost processed food and reduction in physical activity have led to a world-wide epidemic of obesity, diabetes, and heart disease.
- More recently, so-called detox diets involving intermittent fasting have been promoted as ways to help rid the body of alleged toxins from the environment or food processing.

- No scientifically sound studies have identified those toxins, nor demonstrated their increased elimination relative to normal liver and kidney function.
- Intermittent fasting diets are followed by about 10% of adults in the few populations in which it has been studied, mostly as a weight control measure but also for other health or religious reasons.
- Randomized trials have found similar reductions in weight, body fat, and blood pressure and similar metabolic function with intermittent fasting versus continuous calorie restriction.
- All-day fasts, such as during the Jewish Day of Atonement (Yom Kippur), can increase the risks of going into labor and of preterm birth in pregnant women, but the dawn-to-dusk fast during the month of Ramadan appears safe for both the mother and baby.

Detailed Review of Scientific Evidence[1]

Caloric restriction increases the lifespan of rodents, to a greater degree in rats than in mice [11]. The evidence from monkeys is less convincing. In humans, complete fasting leads to metabolic breakdown of fat, which increases circulating ketone bodies after 8–12 h, a condition known as ketosis. Less extreme caloric restriction over a longer time period leads to modest weight loss but substantial reductions in insulin levels and improved insulin sensitivity, that is, an enhanced insulin effect of moving glucose from the blood into fat, muscle, and liver cells. It remains unclear, however, whether these metabolic benefits are due to a reduction in daily energy (calorie) intake or to the *pattern* of that reduction, that is, the degree to which total food intake is concentrated into one or two large meals every day, 1 day out of every two, the more popular 5 days of ad lib eating and 2 days of fasting each week, fasting from sunrise to sunset (as in the Muslim month-long fast of Ramadan), or reduced evenly across multiple meals and snacks every day.

Allaf and colleagues' 2021 Cochrane review analyzed 11 randomized trials in adults comparing intermittent fasting (very low caloric intake) to continuous restriction with a higher calorie intake over treatment periods of 3 weeks to 6 months [12]. Most of the participants in these trials were overweight or obese. No statistically significant differences were observed in body weight, waist circumference, blood pressure, or cholesterol or blood sugar levels, but it was not possible to ensure that the degree of overall caloric restriction was equivalent in the two groups. To put a positive spin on these results, intermittent fasting can be used as an effective alternative to continuous caloric restriction for those who wish (or need) to lose weight. In other words, some dieters may prefer intermittent fasting, while "letting go" with

---

[1] Readers who prefer to skip the Detailed Review should proceed to the Summary at the end of the chapter.

normal caloric intake between fasting periods, to non-stop but milder caloric restriction.

Vitale and Kim's systematic review was restricted to randomized trials in obese adults with type 2 diabetes; three of the trials compared intermittent fasting to continuous caloric restriction [13]. As in the trials reviewed by Allaf and colleagues [12], the trials were unable to ensure equivalent long-term caloric intake in the two dietary regimens. No significant differences were observed in changes in weight, percent body fat, or measures of blood sugar or longer-term diabetes control. The same positive spin can be put on these results for type 2 diabetics who prefer intermittent bouts of more severe "deprivation" to relentless but milder restriction.

Sadeghian and co-workers' 2021 narrative systematic review of intermittent fasting during chemotherapy for cancer included studies in experimental animals, human cells, and humans with various forms of cancer who were receiving chemotherapy [14]. None of the human studies were randomized trials, and it is therefore difficult to draw cause-and-effect inferences. Nonetheless, the descriptive summaries suggest that intermittent fasting while receiving chemotherapy may reduce nausea and vomiting, at the possible expense of increased fatigue and hunger. No solid evidence is available on effects of intermittent fasting on tumor progression, relapse, or survival.

Caloric restriction during critical care in the intensive care unit has been studied with respect to survival, duration of mechanical ventilation (on a breathing machine), and length of hospital stay. Perman and co-workers' 2018 Cochrane review included 15 randomized trials of caloric restriction (either by mouth or by intravenous nutrition) [15]. Most of the included trials did not achieve a substantial reduction in caloric intake versus the control group, however, and thus it is unsurprising that no differences in outcomes were observed in the two treatment arms.

Fasting during pregnancy is generally discouraged. In fact, pregnant Muslim women are not required to fast between dawn and dusk during the month of Ramadan, but many do fast for at least part of the month. Glazier and colleagues' 2018 systematic review and meta-analysis of 22 observational studies including over 3000 pregnant women found no increased risk of preterm birth (delivery before 37 completed weeks) or reduction in average birth weight (reflecting slower growth of the fetus) among those who fasted [16]. The only difference observed was a lower average placental weight in the fasting group, which was observed in only a single (but large) study. Jewish fasts for Yom Kippur (Day of Atonement) are complete fasts lasting 25 h and are followed by most religious Jews, even many pregnant ones. I was unable to find a systematic review of studies bearing on the effects of all-day fasting during pregnancy. Two single-center observational studies, however, observed increased births on the day *following* Yom Kippur [17, 18], while one single-center observational study over a 23-year period observed a doubling of the risk of delivering preterm *on* the day of the fast but did not analyze the risk on the day following the fast [19].

Finally, Singata and colleagues' 2013 Cochrane review assessed five randomized trials of food restriction in pregnant women during labor [20]. No differences were observed in risk of cesarean delivery, instrumental (forceps or vacuum) vaginal delivery, duration of labor, type of pain relief received, or the condition of the baby at delivery in the restricted group compared to the group randomized to eat what they wished.

Summary

The current popularity of intermittent fasting may reflect the romantic notion of returning to the eating patterns of our hunter-gatherer ancestors, which I have referred to as "redux" fasting. Our ancestors had no choice about how often or even how much they ate; many were undernourished, and the average lifespan was much shorter than it is today. "Detox" fasting is a modern notion that has no scientific basis either in identifying the toxins that it claims to remove or in evidence of health benefits. Intermittent fasting may be a preferable weight loss diet to long-term calorie restriction, however, for some people who are overweight or have type 2 diabetes.

Science cannot address whether fasting for religious reasons enriches the religious experience, but complete fasting for 24 h during pregnancy, such as during the Jewish Day of Atonement (Yom Kippur), can increase the likelihood of going into labor and of preterm birth. The dawn-to-dusk Ramadan fast, however, does not carry any risks to the pregnant mother or her baby.

References

1. NCD Risk Factor Collaboration (NCD-RisC). Worldwide trends in body-mass index, underweight, overweight, and obesity from 1975 to 2016: a pooled analysis of 2416 population-based measurement studies in 128.9 million children, adolescents, and adults. Lancet. 2017;390(10113):2627–42.
2. Kerndt PR, Naughton JL, Driscoll CE, Loxterkamp DA. Fasting: the history, pathophysiology and complications. West J Med. 1982;137(5):379–99.
3. Arbesmann R. Fasting and prophecy in pagan and Christian antiquity. Traditio. 1949–51;7:1–71.
4. Britannica, The Editors of Encyclopaedia. Fasting. Encyclopedia Britannica. https://www.britannica.com/topic/fasting. Accessed 21 Apr 2023.
5. Dewey EH. The true science of living. Norwich, CT: Henry Bill Publishing Co.; 1895.
6. International Food Information Council. 2022 Food and Health Survey. 18 May 2022. https://foodinsight.org/2022-food-and-health-survey.
7. Weinstock M, Mazzeo SE. College students' perceptions of individuals following popular diets and individuals with Orthorexia Nervosa. Eat Behav. 2022;47:101671.
8. Potter C, Griggs RL, Brunstrom JM, Rogers PJ. Breaking the fast: meal patterns and beliefs about healthy eating style are associated with adherence to intermittent fasting diets. Appetite. 2019;133:32–9.
9. Brisebois M, Kramer S, Lindsay KG, Wu CT, Kamla J. Dietary practices and supplement use among CrossFit® participants. J Int Soc Sports Nutr. 2022;19(1):316–35.
10. Alnasser A, Almutairi M. Considering intermittent fasting among Saudis: insights into practices. BMC Public Health. 2022;22(1):592.
11. de Cabo R, Mattson MP. Effects of intermittent fasting on health, aging, and disease. N Engl J Med. 2019;381(26):2541–51. https://doi.org/10.1056/NEJMra1905136. Erratum in: N Engl J Med 2020;382(3):298.

12. Allaf M, Elghazaly H, Mohamed OG, Fareen MFK, Zaman S, Salmasi AM, Tsilidis K, Dehghan A. Intermittent fasting for the prevention of cardiovascular disease. Cochrane Database Syst Rev. 2021;1(1):CD013496.
13. Vitale R, Kim Y. The effects of intermittent fasting on glycemic control and body composition in adults with obesity and type 2 diabetes: a systematic review. Metab Syndr Relat Disord. 2020;18(10):450–61.
14. Sadeghian M, Rahmani S, Khalesi S, Hejazi E. A review of fasting effects on the response of cancer to chemotherapy. Clin Nutr. 2021;40(4):1669–81.
15. Perman MI, Ciapponi A, Franco JV, Loudet C, Crivelli A, Garrote V, Perman G. Prescribed hypocaloric nutrition support for critically-ill adults. Cochrane Database Syst Rev. 2018;6(6):CD007867.
16. Glazier JD, Hayes DJL, Hussain S, D'Souza SW, Whitcombe J, Heazell AEP, Ashton N. The effect of Ramadan fasting during pregnancy on perinatal outcomes: a systematic review and meta-analysis. BMC Pregnancy Childbirth. 2018;18(1):421.
17. Kaplan M, Eidelman AI, Aboulafia Y. Fasting and the precipitation of labor: the Yom Kippur effect. JAMA. 1983;250(10):1317–8.
18. Lurie S, Baider C, Boaz M, Sulema V, Golan A, Sadan O. Fasting does not precipitate onset of labour. J Obstet Gynaecol. 2010;30(1):35–7.
19. Shalit N, Shalit R, Sheiner E. The effect of a 25-hour fast during the day of atonement on preterm delivery. J Matern Fetal Neonatal Med. 2015;28(12):1410–3.
20. Singata M, Tranmer J, Gyte GM. Restricting oral fluid and food intake during labour. Cochrane Database Syst Rev. 2013;2013(8):CD003930.

Preventing or Treating a Hangover: Dilution or Delusion?

12

Introduction

I have rarely had a hangover from excessive alcohol intake since my university days. At that age and in those times (late 1960s), the main *purpose* of drinking alcohol was to get drunk: publicly and socially, preferably with friends who acted equally silly while under the influence. I certainly can't remember enjoying the taste of the wine, spirits, or even the beer that I consumed. In those days, the legal age for drinking was 21 years, an age I did not attain until after graduating university. Obtaining alcohol illegally and getting drunk with friends was a double pleasure at that age and a badge of honor. But the inevitable price to pay for that pleasure and honor always awaited me the next morning: the hangover, characterized by a splitting headache, an inability to think straight, fatigue, nausea, and a mouth so dry that no amount of coffee, orange juice, or water would relieve my thirst.

I can't remember which of my brilliant university buddies who shared my drunken revels or their aftermath was the first to "explain" to me that my hangover symptoms were due to alcohol-induced dehydration. Although I studied biology as an undergraduate student and knew a fair bit about the biochemistry of metabolic pathways and the physiology of fresh- and saltwater fish, I knew next to nothing about medicine until I attended medical school. I certainly didn't know enough to doubt my friends' dehydration explanation for my hangover symptoms. I tried drinking large amounts of water to relieve my dry mouth, but the benefit lasted only several seconds and had no effect on my headache or cognitive difficulties. The headache reproducibly improved somewhat with aspirin or acetaminophen (Tylenol), and the other symptoms dissipated over time and were usually better by evening.

Even during medical school and specialty training in pediatrics residency, I never attended a lecture that discussed the physiological mechanisms of hangover, nor the effects of additional water consumption to prevent or treat it. I learned that alcohol has a diuretic effect, that is, it increases urine output. But so does caffeine. Yet, coffee and tea don't usually cause dehydration, let alone a hangover!

One of the many things I learned when researching the literature for this chapter was a new "medicalese" word for hangover: *veisalgia*, but I have never heard or encountered this word during my clinical training or practice. "Hangover" is both well-known and verbally descriptive, and I will use it throughout the rest of this chapter.

More than half a century has passed since my university days and first experiences of hangover, but the biological mechanisms underlying the phenomenon remain poorly understood [1]. Elevated levels of several inflammatory hormones, including prostaglandins and cytokines (the latter produced by white blood cells) have been documented during hangovers [2, 3], but they are also elevated in many other conditions that do not closely resemble hangovers. They may therefore merely reflect the body's reaction to the metabolic stress caused by high-alcohol consumption. The elevated prostaglandins and cytokines may explain why non-steroidal anti-inflammatory drugs (NSAIDs) like ibuprofen and aspirin relieve some of the discomfort of hangovers. But these drugs are also good pain relievers and have not proven superior to acetaminophen (Tylenol) for treating hangover, to my knowledge. The non-alcohol components (called congeners) of alcoholic beverages may also play a role, since dark hard liquors like whiskeys and brandies seem to have a higher potential to cause hangovers than do vodka, gin, or white wine, even for the same total alcohol intake [4].

Gunn and colleagues' systematic review and meta-analysis of hangover effects on cognitive function observed substantial deficits of about half a standard deviation in short-term memory, sustained attention, and psychomotor speed (reaction time) [5]. (Standard deviation units are used to pool results across studies reporting different measurement scales.) As previously noted for the biological mechanisms underlying the development of hangover, the nature of the neurological (brain) dysfunction underlying the transient cognitive deficits is unclear.

Historical and Cultural Overview

Residues of fermentation have been found in pottery jars in Northern China, suggesting alcohol consumption by humans for at least 8–9000 years [6]. Beer was brewed in ancient Egypt, and over 20 beer recipes have been found on Sumerian clay tablets. Evidence of wine production from Georgia (the country) can be dated to 6000 BC, but the ancient Greeks and Romans may have been the first to plant vineyards. In fact, both had a god of wine: Dionysus in Greece and Bacchus in Rome.

It is probably safe to assume that hangovers have as long a history as alcohol consumption. They are well described in the Ayurveda, the ancient Hindu system of medicine [7]. Some of the older remedies for hangovers are particularly colorful [1, 8]. The ancient Assyrians consumed a mixture of ground bird beaks and myrrh, while the Romans preferred raw owl eggs or fried canary. European doctors in the Middle Ages recommended raw eel and bitter almonds. The "prairie oyster," an unappetizing mixture of raw egg yolk, Worcestershire and Tabasco sauces, salt, and pepper, was introduced at the 1878 Paris World Exposition. In 1938, Ritz-Carlton

Fig. 12.1 The stinkbug, eaten as a remedy for hangovers by two ethnic groups in South Africa

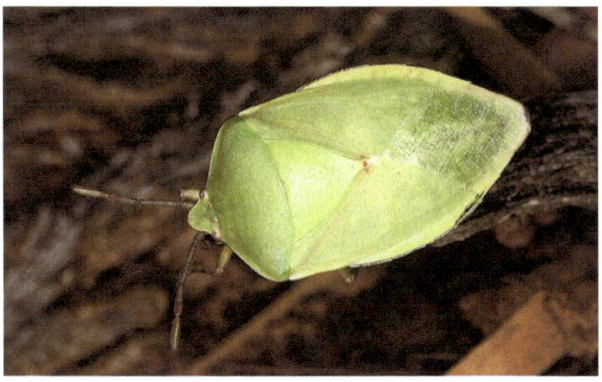

hotels offered a combination of Coca-Cola and milk as a hangover remedy. A well-known but equally dubious treatment is the so-called hair of the dog, that is, consuming alcohol to combat hangover symptoms. My own favorite, however, is stinkbugs (see Fig. 12.1 below), a common remedy still consumed by two ethnic groups in northeastern South Africa [9].

Current Beliefs and Practices

I was unable to find a systematic review or individual surveys of beliefs about why hangovers occur or practices to prevent or treat them, but I will summarize several studies of their frequency of occurrence. In one representative home-based interview survey of 1041 adults in western New York State, 86% of the participants reported at least occasional alcohol consumption in the previous year [10]. Among the drinkers, 35% reported having had at least one hangover during the year: 42% among men and 27% among women. A published survey of 127 undergraduate students attending the University of Missouri was based on electronic diaries over a 14-day period [11]. Forty percent reported at least one hangover during that period. Nearly half of the episodes of alcohol consumption were followed by a hangover, with a higher rate in girls than in boys and, unsurprisingly, among those consuming more drinks.

In a series of three randomized, placebo-controlled crossover trials in 54 Swedish merchant mariners (one trial) and 118 students from the Boston area (two trials), participants consumed sufficient alcohol to produce intoxication in the form of high-alcohol beer, bourbon, or vodka (the latter two mixed with caffeine-free cola) or alcohol-free beer or cola [12]. After consuming the alcohol, 76% of the participants reported a hangover at 7 AM the next morning versus 3% after consuming placebo. Neither sex, age, nor type of alcohol (beer, bourbon, or vodka) influenced the risk of hangover. The largest population survey I found included 36,000 men and women and observed 50–100% higher rates of hangover symptoms and of severe hangovers in women than in men, which were not explained by differences in quantity or type of alcohol consumed [13]. The inconsistencies noted by sex in the above-cited studies are likely to reflect differences in self-reporting, rather in occurrence. Women in some countries or cultures may under-report the true occurrence, whereas some men may consider hangovers as a "badge of courage." I found no studies investigating differences in risk of hangover by region or ethnic origin.

Some people seem resistant to hangovers. Based on a narrative systematic review of population surveys and experimental studies of alcohol administration, Howland and coworkers observed that nearly one-quarter of the participants in both types of studies did not experience hangovers even after heavy drinking bouts [14].

Hangovers are responsible for a substantial adverse economic impact. In their 2000 narrative systematic review, Wiese and colleagues reported huge losses in wages and productivity due to hangovers in the UK, Canada, the U.S., Australia, and New Zealand, estimated as $2000 per worker in 1998 [15]. That figure would of course be much higher in 2022. These losses are due to increased absenteeism, impaired job performance, and reduced productivity. Conversely, the high demand for hangover remedies can be economic stimulants. In South Korea alone, beverages, pills, and jellies marketed for hangover "cures" is an industry that generates over $200 million annually [1]. Whether the latter funds are well spent is another question, of course. In the next section, I will review the scientific evidence on whether such remedies are effective.

Key Evidence Points
- Humans have consumed alcohol for at least 8–9000 years.
- Headache, fatigue, nausea, and cognitive dysfunction are common hangover symptoms that occur the morning after consuming a large dose (binge) of alcohol.
- About 75% of persons who drink enough alcohol to get drunk develop a hangover, but the underlying biological mechanisms are incompletely understood.
- Hangovers have substantial adverse economic consequences, including absenteeism, impaired job performance, and reduced productivity.
- Many hangover remedies have been tested in randomized trials, including foods and beverages, dietary supplements, and medications.
- Most of the published trials have aimed to prevent, rather than treat, a hangover and have been small and of poor methodologic quality; attempted replication of results has been rare.
- None of the randomized trials has studied the effect of additional fluid consumption, but one intervention study found no association between alcohol dose consumed or severity of hangover symptoms and body water content.
- In the absence of strong evidence for beneficial remedies, the best way to prevent a hangover is to avoid binge drinking.
- Although not specifically tested in randomized trials for treatment of hangover symptoms, acetaminophen (Tylenol) and ibuprofen (Advil) are both probably effective in treating the headache that commonly occurs with a hangover.

What Works? Detailed Review of Scientific Evidence[1]

I was able to locate two systematic reviews of randomized trials of remedies to prevent a hangover or to treat its symptoms once it develops: an older one by Pittler and colleagues [16] and a recent one by Roberts and coworkers [17]. The Pittler review included only eight trials; yet, it included three trials not included in the more recent Roberts review. The treatments studied in the assembled trials are so different from one another that pooling their results in a meta-analysis is not appropriate.

Before summarizing the results of the trials included in the two systematic reviews, however, let me first consider the treatment of greatest interest to me: added water intake, or hydration therapy, which is not among the studied treatments in either review. Hydration therapy has become quite aggressive, including intravenous saline, that is, an infusion of water containing a similar concentration of salt (sodium and chlorine) as that in the blood, along with vitamins and minerals. Hydration therapy for hangover symptoms has become particularly popular treatments in "sin cities" like Las Vegas and New Orleans [18]. Unfortunately, the growing popularity of hydration therapy is not based on scientific evidence of its efficacy.

As far as I can tell, no one has carried out a randomized trial of hydration therapy, either as prevention or treatment of hangover, given either orally (drinking) or intravenously. But Lieb and Schmitt's 2020 trial compared three beverages given both 45 min before and immediately after ad lib consumption of wine or beer [19]. No significant association was observed in any of the groups between body water content (a measure of hydration) and either the dose of alcohol consumed during the 4-h evening alcohol drinking period or the severity of hangover symptoms the following morning.

Table 12.1 lists the treatments studied in randomized trials, including those analyzed in the systematic reviews by Pittler and colleagues [16] and Roberts and coworkers [17], as well as three trials not included in those reviews [19–21]. The references cited for each treatment studied are those of the review(s), plus the three individual trials not included in either review.

Surprisingly to me, three of the eight trials analyzed in the earlier review were not included in the recent review, but one of them [22] tested treatments for their effects on alcohol withdrawal symptoms in alcoholic patients admitted to hospital, not patients with hangovers, and should probably have been excluded (as it was from the recent review). The same could be said for an unpublished trial obtained from the manufacturer of the γ-linolenic acid product shown in the table [23]. Two of the pre-2005 trials included in Roberts's recent review [17] were not included in Pittler's 2005 review [16], and the three trials not included in either review were published in 1991, 2018, and 2020. These disparities underline that despite the superiority of systematic reviews to conventional (non-systematic) reviews discussed in Chap. 2, keyword searches and study selection, even within multiple databases, are not exact sciences!

---

[1] Readers who prefer to skip the Detailed Review should proceed to the Summary at the end of the chapter.

Table 12.1 Preventive and therapeutic interventions for hangover studied in randomized trials

A. Foods and beverages
   1. Glucose and fructose solutions [16]
   2. Juice from *Angelica keiskei*, green grape, and pear [20]
B. Dietary supplements
   1. *Cynara scolymus* (artichoke) extract [16, 17]
   2. *Opuntia ficus-indica* (prickly pear) extract [16, 17]
   3. γ-linolenic acid (omega-6 fatty acid) [16]
   4. Pyritinol (vitamin B_6) [17]
   5. Yeast extract + vitamins [16, 17]
   6. L-ornithine [17]
   7. *Acanthapanax senticosus* extract [17]
   8. *Hovenia dulcis* extract [17]
   9. Clove bud extract [17]
  10. *Phyllanthus amarus* extract [17]
  11. L-cysteine + vitamins (2 trials) [17]
  12. Probiotics [17]
  13. Curcumin [17]
  14. Multiple vitamins and minerals [19]
  15. Multiple vitamins, minerals, and plant extracts [19]
  16. Liv.52 (Ayurvedic herbal mixture) [21]
C. Medications
   1. Tolfenamic acid (non-steroidal anti-inflammatory drug, or NSAID) [16, 17]
   2. Propanolol (blocker of adrenaline used in heart disease and high blood pressure) [16, 17]
   3. Chlormethiazole (sedative used to treat alcohol withdrawal syndrome) [17]
   4. Naproxen (NSAID) + fexofenadine (a non-sedating antihistamine) [17]
   5. Loxoprofen (NSAID) [17]
   6. N-acetylcysteine (used to treat acetaminophen [Tylenol] overdose) [17]

None of the trials is large; most had a few dozen participants, and only two trials included more than 100 participants. Many of the trials used a crossover design, however, in which each participant consumed both the active treatment and the placebo (or other comparator) after an appropriate "washout period" to allow any effects of the first treatment to dissipate before administering the second. That design improves statistical power to detect a true effect of the active treatment, if one exists, because any non-treatment factors that affect the severity of hangover symptoms should remain constant within the same participant.

One of the trials in the 2005 Pittler review [16] by Ylikahri and colleagues [24] compared the effects of drinking glucose and fructose solutions to those of water when given either preventively (during the same evening period when alcohol was administered) or therapeutically (the next morning). (The Ylikahri trial is the second trial mentioned above that was included in the Pittler review [16] but not the more recent Roberts review [17].) The chlormethiazole trial [25] used the treatment both preventively (on the evening before) and therapeutically (the morning after) to all participants. The only trial in either of the systematic reviews that studied a treatment solely for its therapeutic effect, that is, to treat "morning-after" symptoms of hangover, was the trial of loxoprofen by Hara and coworkers [26]. I am disappointed to report that stinkbugs have not been evaluated in the published trials.

It is curious to me that most of the treatments used in these trials aimed to prevent a hangover, rather than treat one. Benjamin Franklin's famous dictum that "an ounce of prevention is worth a pound of cure" is certainly valid for smallpox, polio, COVID-19, cancer, and heart disease. But not so valid, perhaps, for a headache or even a full-blown hangover. I suspect that investigators have focused on prevention, rather than cure, at least partly because a preventive treatment can be (and was, in most trials) given before, with, or right after a standardized quantity of alcohol, often in a laboratory setting or hospital, rather than asking, without supervision, the participant to take a therapeutic treatment at home if and when they experience hangover symptoms the morning after the alcohol binge.

The most interesting aspect of Table 12.1 for me, however, is the large number of different types treatments studied in the trials, combined with the fact that only **one** of them was studied in more than a single trial (although a few had some overlapping components). This aspect prevented both published systematic reviews from including a meta-analysis. Most importantly, however, the abundance of different treatments suggests that few if any are likely to be effective. If they were, I presume that investigators would stop looking for new ones!

So, which of these many treatments yielded beneficial effects? From the two systematic reviews, the trials of several preventive treatments reported significant reductions in hangover symptoms: one for the NSAID tolfenamic acid, one for vitamin B_6, one for γ-linolenic acid, one of the two trials of L-cysteine plus vitamins, and one each for several of the herbal dietary supplements, including clove extract, *Hovenia dulcis*, red ginseng, and Korean pear juice. The Roberts systematic review [17] commented on the low quality of the trials published to date, with the major methodologic problems being insufficient details about the randomization procedure, failure to analyze all randomized participants, and difficulties in blinding the participants because of taste differences between herbal and placebo beverages. Among the three trials not reported in either of the systematic reviews [19–21], the one of the Ayurvedic herbal mixture (Liv.52) [21] reported no statistically significant benefit, one reported benefits at 6 h after alcohol consumption (too soon to be labeled a hangover) [20], and the third reported beneficial effects of a mixture of herbs and vitamins [19]. Surprisingly, the only trial of a therapeutic treatment (loxoprofen) given solely after the occurrence of hangover symptoms did not observe significant relief, despite its NSAID nature and its efficacy in reducing inflammation and synthesis of prostaglandins [26].

Summary

Hangover is a common occurrence in all countries and ethnic groups in which large amounts of alcohol are consumed over a short period of time, that is, "a binge." Nearly one-quarter of bingers seem resistant to hangovers, although the biological and/or psychological mechanisms underlying such resistance are unknown. Hangovers have often been attributed to dehydration, but what little evidence is available lends no support to that attribution. Moreover, no randomized trials have tested "dilution" (drinking additional water) as either a preventive treatment to prevent hangovers or as therapy to relieve hangover symptoms after they occur. So, the belief in the dehydration theory and "dilution" treatment may well be a delusion!

Among other treatments tested in randomized trials, almost all have been preventive in nature. The sheer number and variety of these treatments suggests an absence of clear benefit, and the fact that only one of them (L-cysteine plus vitamins) has been tested in more than one trial (two trials, one of which reported benefit) indicates the need for replication in new and larger trials of those treatments that show some promise. Some of the treatments with reported benefits are herbal supplements, but it is unclear why some seem to work and others do not. The potential for publication bias is very strong in this area, because negative results are less likely to be submitted for publication and less likely to be published if they are submitted.

Since hangover symptoms are not life-threatening and often dissipate after several hours, it is difficult to recommend routine treatment to prevent hangovers. Of course, an unequivocally effective preventive measure is to avoid bingeing altogether! But even in the absence of supportive evidence of randomized trials of therapeutic hangover treatments, the proven efficacy of acetaminophen (Tylenol) and NSAIDs like ibuprofen (Advil) in relief of headache suggests that waiting until a hangover occurs and then using one of these over-the-counter medications is a sensible approach.

References

1. Wikipedia contributors. Hangover. Wikipedia, The Free Encyclopedia. 20 Feb 2022, 19:31 UTC. https://en.wikipedia.org/w/index.php?title=Hangover&oldid=1073049734.
2. Parantainen J. Prostaglandins in alcohol intolerance and hangover. Drug Alcohol Depend. 1983;11(3–4):239–48.
3. Penning R, van Nuland M, Fliervoet LA, Olivier B, Verster JC. The pathology of alcohol hangover. Curr Drug Abuse Rev. 2010;3(2):68–75.
4. Damrau F, Goldberg AH. Adsorption of whisky congeners by activated charcoal. Chemical and clinical studies related to hangover. Southwest Med. 1971;52(9):179–82.
5. Gunn C, Mackus M, Griffin C, Munafò MR, Adams S. A systematic review of the next-day effects of heavy alcohol consumption on cognitive performance. Addiction. 2018;113(12):2182–93.
6. American Addiction Centers. The history of alcohol throughout the world. 29 Nov 2021. https://recovery.org.
7. Ravi Varma LA. Alcoholism in Ayurveda. Q J Stud Alcohol. 1950;11(2):484–91.
8. Suddath C. A brief history of hangover cures. Time. 2009;173(1):19.
9. Dzerefos CM, Witkowski ET, Toms R. Comparative ethnoentomology of edible stinkbugs in southern Africa and sustainable management considerations. J Ethnobiol Ethnomed. 2013;9:20.
10. Smith CM, Barnes GM. Signs and symptoms of hangover: prevalence and relationship to alcohol use in a general adult population. Drug Alcohol Depend. 1983;11(3–4):249–69.
11. Piasecki TM, Slutske WS, Wood PK, Hunt-Carter EE. Frequency and correlates of diary-measured hangoverlike experiences in a college sample. Psychol Addict Behav. 2010;24(1):163–9.
12. Howland J, Rohsenow DJ, Allensworth-Davies D, Greece J, Almeida A, Minsky SJ, Arnedt JT, Hermos J. The incidence and severity of hangover the morning after moderate alcohol intoxication. Addiction. 2008;103(5):758–65.

13. Tolstrup JS, Curtis T, Petersen CB, Eriksen L, Grønbaek M. Forekomsten af tømmermaend blandt danske kvinder og maend [the occurrence of hangovers among Danish men and women]. Ugeskr Laeger. 2008;170(51):4226–9.
14. Howland J, Rohsenow DJ, Edwards EM. Are some drinkers resistant to hangover? A literature review. Curr Drug Abuse Rev. 2008;1(1):42–6.
15. Wiese JG, Shlipak MG, Browner WS. The alcohol hangover. Ann Intern Med. 2000;132(11):897–902.
16. Pittler MH, Verster JC, Ernst E. Interventions for preventing or treating alcohol hangover: systematic review of randomised controlled trials. BMJ. 2005;331(7531):1515–8.
17. Roberts E, Smith R, Hotopf M, Drummond C. The efficacy and tolerability of pharmacologically active interventions for alcohol-induced hangover symptomatology: a systematic review of the evidence from randomised placebo-controlled trials. Addiction. 2022;117(8):2157–67.
18. Chan LN, Seres DS, Malone A, Holcombe B, Guenter P, Plogsted S, Teitelbaum DH. Hangover and hydration therapy in the time of intravenous drug shortages: an ethical dilemma and a safety concern. JPEN J Parenter Enteral Nutr. 2014;38(8):921–3.
19. Lieb B, Schmitt P. Randomised double-blind placebo-controlled intervention study on the nutritional efficacy of a food for special medical purposes (FSMP) and a dietary supplement in reducing the symptoms of veisalgia. BMJ Nutr Prev Health. 2020;3(1):31–9.
20. Kim MJ, Lim SW, Kim JH, Choe DJ, Kim JI, Kang MJ. Effect of mixed fruit and vegetable juice on alcohol hangovers in healthy adults. Prev Nutr Food Sci. 2018;23(1):1–7.
21. Chauhan BL, Kulkarni RD. Alcohol hangover and Liv.52. Eur J Clin Pharmacol. 1991;40(2):187–8.
22. Muhonen T, Jokelainen K, Hook-Nikanne J, Methuen T, Salaspuro M. Tropisetron and hangover. Addict Biol. 1997;2(4):461–2.
23. Moesgaard S, Hansen NV. GLA effectively reduces hangovers. Pharma Nord Research (unpublished report from manufacturer).
24. Ylikahri RH, Leino T, Huttunen MO, Pösö AR, Eriksson CJ, Nikkilä. Effects of fructose and glucose on ethanol-induced metabolic changes and on the intensity of alcohol intoxication and hangover. Eur J Clin Investig. 1976;6(1):93–102.
25. Myrsten AL, Rydberg U, Ideström CM, Lamble R. Alcohol intoxication and hangover: modification of hangover by chlormethiazole. Psychopharmacology. 1980;69(2):117–25.
26. Hara M, Hayashi K, Kitamura T, Honda M, Tamaki M. A nationwide randomized, double-blind, placebo-controlled Physicians' trial of loxoprofen for the treatment of fatigue, headache, and nausea after hangovers. Alcohol. 2020;84:21–5.

"Natural" Remedies to Improve Sleep: Perchance a Dream?

13

Introduction

Anyone who has had insomnia can attest to the frustration and adverse effects on productivity, mood, and quality of life caused by insufficient sleep. As with so many things, Shakespeare may have said it best (*Henry IV*, Part 2*)*:

> "O sleep, O gentle sleep,
>> Nature's soft nurse, how have I frightened thee,
>> That thou no more will weigh my eyelids down,
>> And steep my senses in forgetfulness?"

King Henry's speech above concludes with the often-cited line, "Uneasy lies the head that wears a crown," suggesting that a king cannot afford the luxury of a full night's sleep. Plato and other ancients considered excessive sleep as wasted time that could be more productively spent in creative or commercial activity [1].

Insomnia can be defined as dissatisfaction with the amount and/or quality of sleep [2]. As reviewed in the next section, insomnia is a very common complaint. It is therefore not surprising that remedies for preventing or combating insomnia are numerous and varied. They include sleep hygiene (recommendations to reduce caffeine intake, increase exercise, and adopt regular bedtimes); prescribed medications; over-the-counter drugs like antihistamines or melatonin that require no prescription; acupuncture and massage therapy; herbal teas and dietary supplements; warm milk at bedtime; and psychological interventions such as relaxation exercises, meditation, and cognitive behavioral therapy. The prescription medications most frequently used are benzodiazepines or the similarly-acting, so-called Z-drugs. These medications are highly effective but often cause daytime drowsiness and can lead to higher dose requirements and to troublesome withdrawal symptoms when they are stopped or reduced in dosage. Antihistamines and melatonin are less effective than prescription medications, and antihistamines can cause dry mouth and other side effects. The psychological interventions are also less effective than prescription medications but far safer. In this chapter, I focus on teas, herbal and other dietary supplements, warm milk, aroma therapy, and other so-called natural remedies that have been used for hundreds or even thousands of years.

Current Beliefs and Practices

I was unable to find a systematic review of the prevalence of insomnia or of its treatment, so I will cite individual studies. Insomnia is characterized by one or more of the following: difficulty falling asleep, waking up during the night and being unable to fall back asleep, early morning awakening, or feeling unrefreshed after sleeping. About 30% of adults self-report one or more of these sleep problems, although the prevalence falls to 10% if adverse daytime consequences are included in the definition [3]. The prevalence is consistently higher in women than in men, and rises with age in both sexes, especially in women after the menopause.

In an international collaborative study based on interviews of representative samples from seven high-income countries comprising over 10,000 participants, self-reported sleep problems in the previous year were reported by 56% in the U.S., 31% in Western Europe, and 23% in Japan [4]. Based on data from the National Health and Nutrition Surveys in a representative sample of around 4000 adults from the U.S., Blacks were more likely than Whites to report requiring over 30 min to fall asleep, as were respondents who had not graduated university, while respondents born in Mexico were less likely to report this problem than those born in the U.S. [5] Significant increases in prevalence of insomnia over time have been reported from the U.K. [6], U.S. [7], and Finland [8].

In a representative sample of over 30,000 U.S. adults participating in the 2002 National Health Interview Survey, 17.4% reported insomnia within the previous year, 4.5% of whom reported some form of alternative medicine treatment [9]. In a representative postal survey of nearly 1000 adults in the province of Quebec, 18.5% reported using "natural products" to improve sleep in the preceding year; the most common product (by far) was chamomile tea, followed by herbal and other compounds sold in tablet form [10]. In a questionnaire survey of 176 elderly persons visiting outpatient clinics or pharmacies in the province of Ontario, 3% reported using herbal products (including teas) to improve sleep [11]. Finally, in a population-based survey of nearly 3000 Canadian adults, 20% had sought professional help for insomnia within the previous 6 months, 15% had used prescribed medications for sleep, 7% had used over-the-counter (non-prescription) medications, and 12% had used natural products [12].

In two published surveys of general practitioners, one from the UK [13] and the other from Australia [14], the management strategies assessed included sleep hygiene measures, prescription medications, relaxation techniques, and psychological interventions. To my surprise, neither survey enquired about natural products. I suspect that most general practitioners assume that patients consult their physicians only after failing to succeed with natural products and over-the-counter medications.

Key Evidence Points
- Insomnia is a common complaint among adults; the prevalence rises with age, and is higher in women, especially after the menopause.
- Placebo-controlled randomized trials are essential for evaluating all insomnia treatments, especially because sleep quantity and quality are often self-reported.
- Valerian, chamomile, kava, oolong, passionflower, rosemary, saffron, crocetin, theanine, and Montmorency tart cherries have been studied as teas and/or capsule extracts in high-quality trials and found *not* to be effective in treating insomnia.
- Trials of other herbal teas and extracts, including those popular in traditional Chinese medicine, have not used placebo controls, which invalidates their reported large beneficial effects on self-reported sleep quantity or quality.
- Similar problems with the design and reporting of randomized trials of aroma therapy invalidate their large reported benefits.
- Ashwagandha root is a longstanding natural remedy used in Ayurvedic (ancient Hindu) medicine that shows promise, based on several well-designed but small randomized trials in India.
- Fermented milk has been studied in one rigorous randomized trial but found to be ineffective in treating insomnia.
- Single randomized trials of magnesium and vitamin D have been of insufficient quality to draw any conclusions about their effectiveness.

Detailed Review of Scientific Evidence: Do "Natural" Remedies Work?[1]

Given the strong potential for bias due to confounding and reverse causality in observational studies, and to a placebo effect in non-blinded studies, randomized, placebo-controlled, double-blind trials are essential in evaluating such treatments. Unfortunately, randomized trials testing the effectiveness of natural remedies have been fewer, smaller, and less rigorous than those used to test medications and psychological interventions. I will focus on eight systematic reviews (with meta-analyses) of such trials: two of valerian (a plant whose roots are used to make a tea) [15, 16]; one that included trials of several herbal teas, including valerian, chamomile, oolong, wuling, and kava [17]; three of traditional Chinese herbal extracts [18–20]; one of Ashwagandha root extract [21]; and one of aroma therapy [22].

Other interventions have not been systematically reviewed, to my knowledge; I shall therefore discuss individual randomized trials of warm milk, fermented milk,

---

[1] Readers who prefer to skip the Detailed Review should proceed to the Summary at the end of the chapter.

passionflower tea, mixed herbal teas, tart cherry juice, rosemary, saffron, vitamin D, and magnesium. I will limit my evidence review to healthy adults but exclude those with depression, anxiety disorder, or diabetes or other chronic diseases. I will include trials that measured sleep outcomes using questionnaires, including nightly sleep diaries, or more objective measures obtained from actigraphs (electronic movement-detection devices, usually worn on the wrist at night) or electroencephalograms (EEGs).

Herbal Teas and Extracts

Valerian is a plant whose root has been ground into extracts sold as capsules or teas. It has been used for millenia to treat insomnia and is the most common herbal product tested in randomized trials. It is included in three of the above-cited systematic reviews, which came to similar conclusions about its efficacy: no significant improvement in quantitative measures such as sleep latency (time required to fall asleep) or overall sleep quality score, but an increase in subjective dichotomous assessment (yes or no) of improved sleep. The meta-analysis by Bent and colleagues [15], however, found strong statistical evidence of publication bias for the latter outcome: small trials with no or small effects appeared to be missing from the published trials.

Chamomile is a flowering plant whose flowers have been consumed for at least 5000 years as a tea to improve sleep; it is also available as an extract in tablet form. It is probably used even more frequently than valerian but, for some reason, has been far less frequently evaluated in randomized trials. As reviewed in the

Fig. 13.1 Chamomile tea, a frequently used "natural" remedy for insomnia

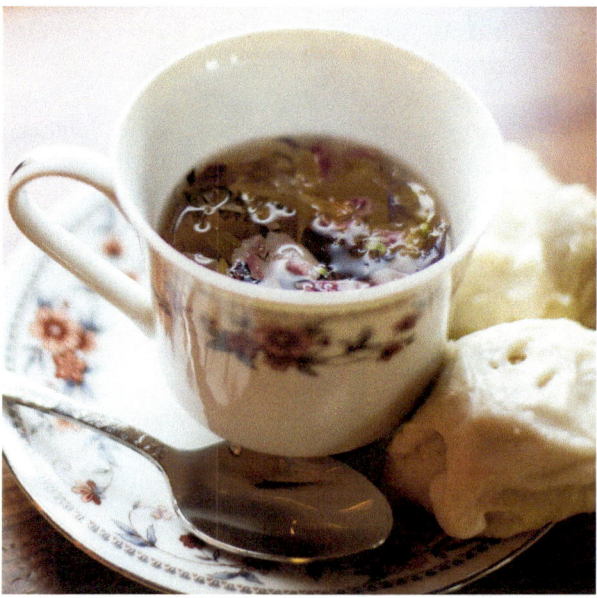

above-cited meta-analysis by Leach and Page [17], one small placebo-controlled, double-blind U.S. trial of chamomile extract found no significant improvement in sleep with chamomile extract. An Iranian placebo-controlled trial published after that meta-analysis did find a greater improvement in participants who received chamomile extract [23], but the authors provided no information about how participants were randomized and used a single-blind design in which researchers who measured the sleep outcomes were not blinded to the treatment received (Fig. 13.1).

Like valerian and chamomile, kava roots and oolong leaves are used to make other popular herbal teas that are believed to improve sleep. Each of these two herbs has been studied in one randomized trial (in capsule form, rather than as tea infusions, which facilitates placebo treatment and blinding), and both trials are included in Leach and Page's systematic review and meta-analysis [17]. Neither herb had significant beneficial effects on insomnia or sleep quality.

Wuling capsule is a Chinese patent medicine derived from a fungus and used for decades to treat insomnia. Zhou and colleagues' systematic review and meta-analysis included 19 randomized trials and observed a large and statistically significant improvement in sleep quality [18]. Sleep quality was based exclusively on the Pittsburgh Sleep Quality Index (questionnaire), however, and the only trial to use a placebo control found absolutely no effect.

Shumian capsule is a traditional Chinese patent medicine that includes several herb and animal components and is commonly used in China to treat insomnia. Wang and coworkers' 2021 systematic review and meta-analysis included nine randomized trials, all of which compared Shumian capsule to benzodiazepenes [19]. Outcomes were subjective "cure" and the score on the Pittsburgh Sleep Questionnaire, both of which slightly favored Shumian capsule. Adverse effects were far more common in the control (benzodiazepine) group. The absence of a placebo group and consequent impossibility of blinding the outcome assessments, however, make these results highly suspect.

Guizhi gancao longgu muli is an extract of herbs and oyster shell, a longstanding natural sleep remedy in traditional Chinese medicine. Chen and coworkers' recent systematic review and meta-analysis includes 15 randomized trials in which Guizhi extract was compared to "Western" medicine prescription treatment with benzodiazepines [20]. Three of the 15 trials included acupuncture along with Guizhi extract, and nine used the self-reported Pittsburgh Sleep Quality Index to compare outcomes. All 15 trials were assessed by the authors as having an "unclear risk" of measurement bias, which substantially understates the enormous potential risk due to non-blinding, since none of the trials used placebo controls. This bias completely undermines the meta-analysis's findings of improved sleep and reduced side effects in the experimental group!

Ashwagandha root is an ancient herbal remedy for insomnia from the Ayurveda alternative medicine system that is closely aligned with Hinduism. Cheah and coworkers systematically reviewed and meta-analyzed five small, randomized placebo-controlled trials of Ashwagandha extract, all of which were conducted in India [21]. The authors observed statistically significant beneficial effects on both questionnaire-based sleep quality and actigraphy-based measures of sleep duration.

The effects were large (approximately one standard deviation) for the subjective, questionnaire-based outcomes but more moderate (about half a standard deviation) for the actigraphy-based sleep durations. (Standard deviation units were used to account for different measurement scales reported in the trials.) These favorable results require confirmation in larger trials and in other settings.

Passionflower is a climbing vine with light-purple flowers that is another popular insomnia treatment in many parts of the world and is consumed as a tea but also sold as herbal extract tablets. In a placebo-controlled crossover trial comparing a tea from bags containing passionflower leaves, flowers, and seeds with tea made from bags containing parsley, 41 healthy young adults were treated with each tea consumed an hour before bedtime for 1 week [24]. The order of the two treatments was balanced, but apparently not randomized. A 1-week washout period between the two treatment periods was included to eliminate carry-over effects. No significant differences between the two teas were observed in total sleep time, sleep latency (time required to fall asleep), or number of awakenings during the night, either based on sleep diaries or on electroencephalographic (EEG) recordings in the ten participants who volunteered to undergo such recordings.

A small randomized trial of a traditional East Asian multi-herb tea compared 20 young adult Korean insomniacs randomized to twice-daily tea consumption for 4 weeks to 20 randomized to a waiting list and observed a significant improvement in the tea group following the treatment period and 4 weeks after completing the treatment [25]. But, of course, the absence of a placebo treatment, and therefore of blinding, makes it impossible to attribute the improvement to the tea.

Black and green tea leaves contain caffeine, a known stimulant that can interfere with sleep. L-theanine is an amino acid found in most tea leaves that has been reported to reduce anxiety. In a small placebo-controlled crossover trial, 20 young Japanese men consumed either 200 mg tablets containing L-theanine or placebo 1 h before bedtime for three consecutive nights, with a 1-day washout period between the two treatments [26]. Sleep duration was not significantly increased by L-theanine when assessed by questionnaire. In the ten men who complied with wrist-worn actigraphy monitors worn at night, total sleep time was unaffected despite a significantly reduced time awake after sleep onset while on the L-theanine treatment.

Rosemary is a common herb used in cooking. A single randomized trial from Iran compared the effects of its extract in capsule form versus placebo capsules in healthy university students and found no significant benefits on sleep latency or duration [27].

I was able to find four placebo-controlled randomized trials of saffron extract or its presumed active carotenoid ingredient, crocetin, in adult insomniacs but no systematic review or meta-analysis. Saffron is an expensive herb used to add a yellow color and a subtle floral flavor to cooked foods but has also been reported to relieve anxiety and depression. The two saffron extract trials are both recent: one from Australia [28], the other from Belgium [29]. The Australian trial sleep outcomes were based on questionnaires only, whereas the Belgian trial used questionnaires and a wrist-worn actigraph. Both trials focused their results on within-group changes, which showed improvements in several measures of sleep quantity and quality in both the saffron and placebo groups, with very few and very small differences *between* the two treatment groups.

The two crocetin trials were very similar and had overlapping authors. Both used a randomized, placebo-controlled crossover design in Japanese adults with mild insomnia and measured both objective (actigraphy [30] or EEG [31]) and questionnaire-based sleep outcomes [30, 31]. As with the two saffron trials, between-group differences in objectively measured sleep outcomes were small, and most were statistically non-significant between the crocetin and placebo treatments. The only exception was a difference of 1.6 awakening episodes per night at follow-up after the crocetin treatment in the Kuratsune trial [30], mostly due to an unexplained *increase* of 1.1 awakenings after the placebo treatment. In summary, neither saffron nor crocetin appears to be a very promising treatment for insomnia.

Montmorency tart cherries contain a high concentration of melatonin, a hormone produced by the pineal gland in the brain whose secretion rises at night and contributes to night-time sleepiness. Two small randomized, placebo-controlled crossover trials have compared twice-daily consumption of tart cherry juice versus a look-alike placebo juice [32, 33]. In crossover trials, each participant receives both treatments, the order of which should be randomized, with a washout period between the two to eliminate any carry-over effects. The first trial recruited seniors with chronic insomnia and observed no effect on sleep latency (the time required to fall asleep) or total sleep duration but a small reduction in awake time after sleep onset [32]. The second trial recruited healthy young adults and observed no significant differences in any of the three sleep diary measures, despite an increase in urinary melatonin levels after consuming the tart cherry juice [33]. Objective actigraphy measures obtained by an electrical movement monitor attached at night, however, suggested a higher total sleep time after the tart cherry juice among those participants who complied with the monitor.

Milk

I was unable to find any randomized trial of bedtime milk, whether cold or heated, as a preventive or remedial treatment for insomnia. One published trial, however, investigated the effect of 100 g per day of skim milk fermented with *Lactobacillus helveticus* in 29 healthy seniors living in Osaka, Japan [34]. Fermented milk contains bioactive peptides (small protein-like compounds) that the authors hypothesized might improve sleep. The trial used a randomized, placebo-controlled crossover design in which participants took both the fermented milk and a look-alike acidified (to mimic the sour taste) milk any time during the day for 3 weeks, with a 3-week washout period between the two treatments. Participants were requested to refrain from consuming any other milk or fermented products (yogurt, cheese) during the study. Wrist actigraph-based sleep outcomes showed no significant differences between the two treatments in sleep latency, wake time after sleep onset, or number of awakenings.

Dietary Supplements

Magnesium is known to affect ion channels and transmission of nerve signals in the brain, but its effects on sleep are largely unknown. In a randomized trial of supplementation with 250 mg magnesium versus placebo twice per day for 8 weeks in 43 Iranian adults 60–75 years of age, participants completed sleep diary questionnaires before and after the treatment period [35]. No details are provided about the randomization process or the placebo treatment. "Sleep time" (not defined) was significantly increased in the magnesium group versus the placebo group, but not total sleep time or awake time after sleep onset. Sleep latency was significantly reduced in the magnesium group. Curiously, mean sleep times were identical before and after the placebo treatment. Clearly, any beneficial effect of magnesium supplementation on insomnia requires confirmation in future randomized trials.

I was able to find one randomized trial evaluating the effect of vitamin D supplementation on insomnia [36]. The trial has several major methodologic shortcomings, primary among which is the fact that the original trial recruited 306 middle-aged Iranian adults with abdominal obesity, of whom 289 completed the trial and only 29 of whom reported insomnia symptoms at baseline (before treatment) and were included in the published report. In other words, the report is based on a post hoc decision to test a subgroup of the overall trial sample that was apparently not justified in the original trial protocol. The 29 participants were divided into the four treatment groups: low-fat milk with and without nano-capsules of vitamin D and low-fat yoghurt with and without the vitamin D for a 10-week supplementation period. The authors do not indicate the number of participants in each of the four treatment groups. Moreover, insomnia was assessed by questionnaire only, and the data shown in the two tables of the published article contradict one another. Finally, the analysis was based on before-and-after differences within treatment groups, rather than *between* groups. The authors claim that participants randomized to supplemented milk, but not those randomized to the supplemented yogurt, had a significant improvement in their insomnia. Given the above-noted problems, however, that claim is difficult to accept.

Aroma Therapy

Aroma therapy is a branch of complementary and alternative medicine based on inhaling odors from oils extracted from plants. Stone jars and vials probably used to contain these oils have been found in ancient Egyptian tombs. The oils are called "essential oils," but not because they are "essential" for health in the same way as essential amino acids or fatty acids. That is, not because they are required for physiological functions, cannot be synthesized by the body, and therefore must be consumed in the diet or in dietary supplements. Instead, essential oils are "essential" only in the semantic sense implied by the smell ("essence") of the oil. The fragrant oils comprise hundreds of organic compounds, most of which are fat-soluble, which explains their oil-like appearance and consistency.

Essential oils have been used for a variety of purposes to improve health, but they are not regulated by agencies that license and approve medications. It will therefore not surprise readers of this book to learn that few of their alleged benefits have been evaluated in placebo-controlled randomized trials. Since the oils are plant-based, they are "natural" and thus generally regarded as safe (GRAS). Although some essential oils can irritate the skin, they are not meant to be ingested or injected and therefore should not pose health risks if inhaled.

Some inhaled oils are used primarily to improve sleep; the most popular is lavender. A recent systematic review and meta-analysis by Cheong and colleagues included 34 randomized trials of aroma therapy for insomnia, most from Korea and most evaluating a single aroma (usually lavender) but some combining two or three aromas [22]. The trial outcomes were based primarily on self-reported questionnaires, with only one trial incorporating actigraphy. Because of the variety of outcome measures used, effect sizes were combined and pooled using standard deviation-like units. The pooled result for the primary outcome was a very substantial improvement in sleep outcomes of nearly two-thirds of a standard deviation. But the systematic review *fails to even mention* the treatments used in the control groups. In evaluating the trials' potential for bias, it seems clear that few of the trials described procedures to ensure blinding of participants, investigators, and outcome assessors. As discussed above, the absence of a placebo aroma control treatment completely invalidates the "positive" results of aroma therapy inferred by the authors of the systematic review.

Summary

Insomnia is a common complaint among adults. The prevalence rises with age and is higher in women, especially after the menopause. Potent and effective drugs are available to treat insomnia, but most prescription drugs are habit-forming and associated with morning grogginess or other side effects. Psychological treatments have been well studied and shown to have modest benefits. Many "natural" therapies have also been used to promote healthy sleep or treat insomnia. These include herbal teas and extracts, dietary supplements, and aroma therapy, but rigorous placebo-controlled randomized trials have been rare and have generally yielded little or no evidence of efficacy. Ashwagandha root has shown promise in five small, well-designed trials from India, but larger trials from other settings are necessary to confirm these findings. I was surprised that warm milk, one of the most popular natural treatments, has not been studied in randomized trials. It should be, although finding a good placebo will be a challenge!

References

1. Whitehead K, Beaumont M. Insomnia: a cultural history. Lancet. 2018;391(10138):2408–9.
2. Saddichha S. Diagnosis and treatment of chronic insomnia. Ann Indian Acad Neurol. 2010;13(2):94–102.

3. Roth T. Insomnia: definition, prevalence, etiology, and consequences. J Clin Sleep Med. 2007;3(5 Suppl):S7–10.
4. Léger D, Poursain B, Neubauer D, Uchiyama M. An international survey of sleeping problems in the general population. Curr Med Res Opin. 2008;24(1):307–17.
5. Grandner MA, Petrov ME, Rattanaumpawan P, Jackson N, Platt A, Patel NP. Sleep symptoms, race/ethnicity, and socioeconomic position. J Clin Sleep Med. 2013;9(9):897–905.
6. Calem M, Bisla J, Begum A, Dewey M, Bebbington PE, Brugha T, Cooper C, Jenkins R, Lindesay J, McManus S, Meltzer H, Spiers N, Weich S, Stewart R. Increased prevalence of insomnia and changes in hypnotics use in England over 15 years: analysis of the 1993, 2000, and 2007 National Psychiatric Morbidity Surveys. Sleep. 2012;35(3):377–84.
7. Ford ES, Cunningham TJ, Giles WH, Croft JB. Trends in insomnia and excessive daytime sleepiness among U.S. adults from 2002 to 2012. Sleep Med. 2015;16(3):372–8.
8. Kronholm E, Partonen T, Härmä M, Hublin C, Lallukka T, Peltonen M, Laatikainen T. Prevalence of insomnia-related symptoms continues to increase in the Finnish working-age population. J Sleep Res. 2016;25(4):454–7.
9. Pearson NJ, Johnson LL, Nahin RL. Insomnia, trouble sleeping, and complementary and alternative medicine: analysis of the 2002 national health interview survey data. Arch Intern Med. 2006;166(16):1775–82.
10. Sánchez-Ortuño MM, Bélanger L, Ivers H, LeBlanc M, Morin CM. The use of natural products for sleep: a common practice? Sleep Med. 2009;10(9):982–7.
11. Sproule BA, Busto UE, Buckle C, Herrmann N, Bowles S. The use of non-prescription sleep products in the elderly. Int J Geriatr Psychiatry. 1999;14(10):851–7.
12. Cheung JMY, Jarrin DC, Beaulieu-Bonneau S, Ivers H, Morin G, Morin CM. Patterns of concomitant prescription, over-the-counter and natural sleep aid use over a 12-month period: a population based study. Sleep. 2021;44(11):zsab141.
13. Everitt H, McDermott L, Leydon G, Yules H, Baldwin D, Little P. GPs' management strategies for patients with insomnia: a survey and qualitative interview study. Br J Gen Pract. 2014;64(619):e112–9.
14. Miller CB, Valenti L, Harrison CM, Bartlett DJ, Glozier N, Cross NE, Grunstein RR, Britt HC, Marshall NS. Time trends in the family physician management of insomnia: the Australian experience (2000–2015). J Clin Sleep Med. 2017;13(6):785–90.
15. Bent S, Padula A, Moore D, Patterson M, Mehling W. Valerian for sleep: a systematic review and meta-analysis. Am J Med. 2006;119(12):1005–12.
16. Fernández-San-Martín MI, Masa-Font R, Palacios-Soler L, Sancho-Gómez P, Calbó-Caldentey C, Flores-Mateo G. Effectiveness of valerian on insomnia: a meta-analysis of randomized placebo-controlled trials. Sleep Med. 2010;11(6):505–11.
17. Leach MJ, Page AT. Herbal medicine for insomnia: a systematic review and meta-analysis. Sleep Med Rev. 2015;24:1–12.
18. Zhou H, Zhao Y, Peng W, Han W, Wang D, Wang Z, Ren X, Pan G, Lin Q, Wang X. Efficacy and safety of Wuling capsule for insomnia disorder: a systematic review and meta-analysis of randomized controlled trials. Sleep Med. 2022;93:1–14.
19. Wang C, Yang Y, Ding X, Li J, Zhou X, Teng J, Qi X. Efficacy and safety of Shumian capsules in treating insomnia: a systematic review and meta-analysis. Medicine (Baltimore). 2021;100(50):e28194.
20. Chen F, Chen Z, Cheng Y, Li J, Liao R, Zhao Z, Wu K, Liu J. Meta analysis for insomnia Guizhi Gancao Longgu Muli decoction for insomnia: a meta-analysis. Complement Ther Clin Pract. 2022;47:101550.
21. Cheah KL, Norhayati MN, Husniati Yaacob L, Abdul Rahman R. Effect of Ashwagandha (Withania somnifera) extract on sleep: a systematic review and meta-analysis. PLoS One. 2021;16(9):e0257843.
22. Cheong MJ, Kim S, Kim JS, Lee H, Lyu YS, Lee YR, Jeon B, Kang HW. A systematic literature review and meta-analysis of the clinical effects of aroma inhalation therapy on sleep problems. Medicine (Baltimore). 2021;100(9):e24652.

23. Adib-Hajbaghery M, Mousavi SN. The effects of chamomile extract on sleep quality among elderly people: a clinical trial. Complement Ther Med. 2017;35:109–14.
24. Ngan A, Conduit R. A double-blind, placebo-controlled investigation of the effects of Passiflora incarnata (passionflower) herbal tea on subjective sleep quality. Phytother Res. 2011;25(8):1153–9.
25. Mun S, Lee S, Park K, Lee SJ, Koh BH, Baek Y. Effect of traditional East Asian medicinal herbal tea (HT002) on insomnia: a randomized controlled pilot study. Integr Med Res. 2019;8(1):15–20.
26. Rao TP, Ozeki M, Juneja LR. In search of a safe natural sleep aid. J Am Coll Nutr. 2015;34(5):436–47.
27. Nematolahi P, Mehrabani M, Karami-Mohajeri S, Dabaghzadeh F. Effects of Rosmarinus officinalis L. on memory performance, anxiety, depression, and sleep quality in university students: a randomized clinical trial. Complement Ther Clin Pract. 2018;30:24–8.
28. Lopresti AL, Smith SJ, Metse AP, Drummond PD. Effects of saffron on sleep quality in healthy adults with self-reported poor sleep: a randomized, double-blind, placebo-controlled trial. J Clin Sleep Med. 2020;16(6):937–47.
29. Pachikian BD, Copine S, Suchareau M, Deldicque L. Effects of saffron extract on sleep quality: a randomized double-blind controlled clinical trial. Nutrients. 2021;13(5):1473.
30. Kuratsune H, Umigai N, Takeno R, Kajimoto Y, Nakano T. Effect of crocetin from Gardenia jasminoides Ellis on sleep: a pilot study. Phytomedicine. 2010;17(11):840–3.
31. Umigai N, Takeda R, Mori A. Effect of crocetin on quality of sleep: a randomized, double-blind, placebo-controlled, crossover study. Complement Ther Med. 2018;41:47–51.
32. Pigeon WR, Carr M, Gorman C, Perlis ML. Effects of a tart cherry juice beverage on the sleep of older adults with insomnia: a pilot study. J Med Food. 2010;13(3):579–83.
33. Howatson G, Bell PG, Tallent J, Middleton B, McHugh MP, Ellis J. Effect of tart cherry juice (Prunus cerasus) on melatonin levels and enhanced sleep quality. Eur J Nutr. 2012;51(8):909–16.
34. Yamamura S, Morishima H, Kumano-go T, Suganuma N, Matsumoto H, Adachi H, Sigedo Y, Mikami A, Kai T, Masuyama A, Takano T, Sugita Y, Takeda M. The effect of Lactobacillus helveticus fermented milk on sleep and health perception in elderly subjects. Eur J Clin Nutr. 2009;63(1):100–5.
35. Abbasi B, Kimiagar M, Sadeghniiat K, Shirazi MM, Hedayati M, Rashidkhani B. The effect of magnesium supplementation on primary insomnia in elderly: a double-blind placebo-controlled clinical trial. J Res Med Sci. 2012;17(12):1161–9.
36. Sharifan P, Khoshakhlagh M, Khorasanchi Z, Darroudi S, Rezaie M, Safarian M, Vatanparast H, Afshari A, Ferns G, Ghazizadeh H, Ghayour Mobarhan M. Efficacy of low-fat milk and yogurt fortified with encapsulated vitamin D_3 on improvement in symptoms of insomnia and quality of life: evidence from the SUVINA trial. Food Sci Nutr. 2020;8(8):4484–90.

The Bitter Truth About Artificial Sweeteners

14

Introduction

Mankind has had a fondness for sweet tastes, that is, a "sweet tooth," for millennia. The first known added sweetener in human nutrition was honey, which contains two types of sugar molecules: glucose and fructose. These two sugars are called *monosaccharides*; they contain a single sugar molecule. We know that honey was collected and consumed by ancient civilizations. A cave painting depicting honey collection in the Araña Caves near Valencia, Spain, dates from around 8000 years ago [1].

The most common natural sweetener consumed today is sucrose, which is usually called "sugar." Sucrose is a disaccharide, meaning it has two sugar molecules chemically bonded together, in this case glucose bound to fructose. Like honey, sucrose has also been consumed since antiquity. Sugar cane was cultivated in ancient India and is grown in tropical climates all over the world. In more temperate climates and more recent times, the main agricultural source of sugar is the roots of sugar beets.

Some non-sugar sweeteners are "natural," in the sense that they come from plants, but are not metabolized by humans and are therefore calorie-free [2]. They include monk fruit, which contains a potent sweet chemical called mogroside and grows in China and Thailand, where it has been used to sweeten herbal Chinese medicines for centuries. Another plant-based non-sugar sweetener is stevia, which is native to Brazil and Paraguay, where it has been used for 1500 years by some indigenous peoples to sweeten teas. Stevia is available commercially as a food additive in most countries and is widely used in Europe and Japan.

History of Artificial Sweeteners

Saccharine was the first truly artificial (man-made) sweetener (Fig. 14.1). It was discovered accidentally in 1879 by Constantine Fahlberg and Ira Remsen at John

M. S. Kramer, *Believe It or Not*, https://doi.org/10.1007/978-3-031-46022-7_14

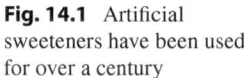
Fig. 14.1 Artificial sweeteners have been used for over a century

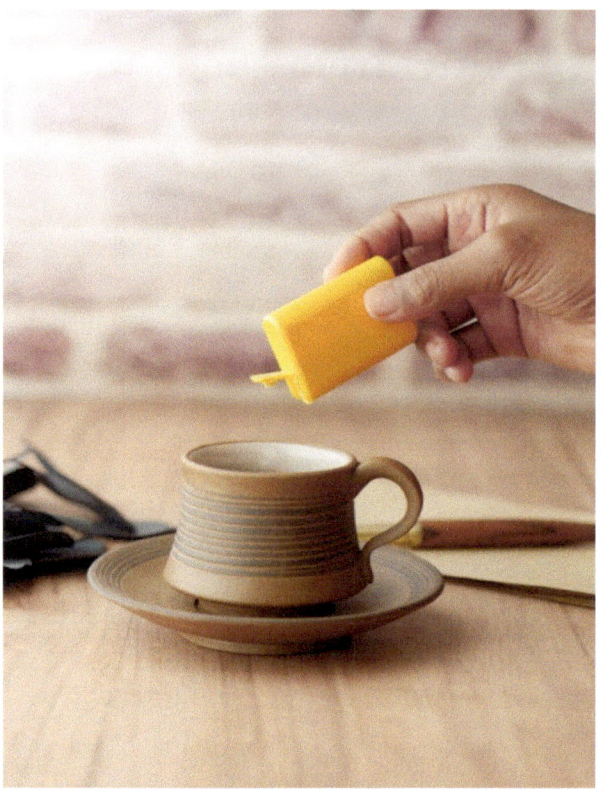

Hopkins University while a searching for a food preservative derived from coal tar derivatives [3]. Saccharine was banned in 1912 in the U.S., because of fear of adding an artificial chemical to food, but was legalized again during World War I owing to a sugar shortage. It remained in common use during the second World War for the same reason. In 1977, however, a Canadian study in rats reported a higher risk of bladder cancer after consuming high doses of saccharine, leading to a ban on its addition to foods and beverages in Canada; the ban remains to this day. Although the U.S. Food and Drug Administration (FDA) proposed a similar ban, the U.S. Congress blocked the ban in response to complaints from the Citizens for Saccharine Committee, who claimed, believe it or not, that "Canadian rats are not the same as American rats" [4]. The FDA did, however, require a label warning on saccharine-containing foods about its carcinogenic (cancer-causing) risk until 2000. Saccharine remains available as an artificial sweetener in the United States.

Some people found that saccharine had a bitter after-taste, and the search for less bitter artificial sweeteners was on. Cyclamate was discovered in 1937 by Michael Sveda, a graduate student at the University of Illinois, while trying to develop a drug to reduce fever—another accidental discovery. It was approved by the FDA as a food additive in 1951. In the U.S. and elsewhere, it was sold as a powder in pink packets under the brand name Sweet 'n Low. The FDA banned its sale in the U.S. in

1969, however, after studies found an increased risk of bladder cancer in rats after ingestion of high doses—a ban that remains in effect, probably because the rats in question this time were "American rats"! In the U.S., a saccharine-based Sweet 'n Low quickly replaced the cyclamate product. Nonetheless, cyclamate continues to be sold and used in many other countries under a variety of brand names, including Sweet 'n Low, Sugar Twin, and Sucaryl.

The third major artificial sweetener to be developed was aspartame in 1965. It too was discovered serendipitously—by James Schlatter, a chemist attempting to develop an anti-ulcer drug at GD Searle and Company. Aspartame is a dipeptide: two amino acids linked together through a chemical bond. It took until 1981, however, for aspartame to be approved by the FDA for use as a food additive. It was marketed and sold by Searle as NutraSweet and remains in use and sold around the world as NutraSweet and Equal, often combined with another artificial sweetener such as acesulfame potassium (Ace-K) or cyclamate to reduce its slightly bitter taste. Ace-K was discovered in 1967 but was not approved by the FDA for use in beverages until 1988 and in other foods in 2003. It is sold and marketed as a stand-alone artificial sweetener under the brand names of Sunett and Sweet One.

Another major artificial sweetener currently in use is sucralose. Sucralose is a chlorinated form of sucrose that was also discovered accidentally—in 1976, through collaborative research carried out by Tate & Lyle, a British sugar company, and University College London. It was approved by the FDA as a food additive in 1999. Sucralose is marketed and sold under the brand name of Splenda. Unlike aspartame, sucralose is heat stable and therefore useful in baking and frying. More recent aspartame derivatives are also heat stable; they include neotame, aclitame, and advantame.

Finally, another class of artificial sweeteners are the sugar alcohols, which include xylitol, sorbitol, and mannitol. They are metabolized by humans and therefore contain utilizable energy, although they are less sweet and supply fewer calories than sucrose. They are used to sweeten chewing gum, candies, and cookies [2].

Current Practices and Beliefs

The only systematic review I was able to find of published population surveys limited its analysis to percentages of acceptable daily intake (ADI), as established by an international Joint Expert Committee on Food Additives [5]. The ADI is based on the highest dose of the food additive that does not produce adverse effects, as observed in experiments on laboratory animals, with an additional 100-fold reduction to provide a safety margin.

In this section, however, I will summarize recent individual-country surveys of representative populations from the U.S., U.K., Australia, China, Brazil, Spain, Portugal, and Lebanon. These surveys describe the proportion of participants who consume artificial sweeteners, the foods and beverages in which they are contained, and the specific types consumed. In addition, most of them assess associations between consumption of artificial sweeteners and characteristics such as age, sex, body weight, ethnic background, and educational level.

For the U.S., the data are based on two 24-h dietary recalls from nearly 17,000 participants in the National Health and Nutrition Examination Survey in 2009–2012 [6]. Among children 2–17 years of age, 25% had consumed at least one source of artificial sweetener: 19% from beverages, 8% from foods, and <1% from added table sweetener powders or liquids; some children consumed more than one source. For adults 18 years of age or older, 41% reported consuming at least one source and 31%, 10%, and 14% reported consuming the same respective source categories cited above for children. In both children and adults, the proportions were higher in females, in non-Hispanic Whites than in Hispanics or Blacks, and in overweight and obese participants and rose with advancing age and higher socioeconomic status. Among adult diabetics, two-thirds reported consuming artificial sweeteners. Specific types of artificial sweeteners were not assessed.

Among 12,000 participants in the 2011–2012 Australian National Nutrition and Physical Activity Survey, artificial sweetener consumption was based on a single 24-h recall [7]. The reported consumption proportions are therefore lower than those reported in the above-noted U.S. survey; 8.5% of children and 18% of adults reported at least one source of artificial sweetener. In both children and adults, beverages were the major source. Yogurt was the second-most common source in children and third-most common in adults; the second-most common source in adults was table sweeteners. Similar associations were seen with sex, age, socioeconomic status, body weight, and diabetes as those reported in the U.S. survey.

A survey of 5800 Nanjing city residents age 6 years or more who participated in the China National Nutrition and Health Study in 2009–2013 used a very different methodology [8]. Instead of asking about consumption of artificial sweeteners, the authors used data from 3 days of 24-h dietary recalls of consumption of processed foods. They then analyzed 1885 locally consumed processed foods for their content of the three most commonly contained artificial sweeteners: saccharine, Ace-K, and cyclamate. Unlike the American and Australian surveys, the major foods responsible for consumption of artificial sweeteners were preserved fruit, processed nuts, and pickled vegetables, followed by soft drinks and other beverages. The authors did not report factors associated with intake of artificial sweeteners.

A representative population survey of nearly 33,000 Brazilian adolescents and adults enquired about food and beverage sweeteners, rather than processed foods to which sweeteners are added [9]. Participants were asked to record all foods, including added sugar and artificial sweeteners, consumed on two non-consecutive days, but not to identify specific types of artificial sweeteners. Overall, 86% of the participants used sugar only, 8% used artificial sweeteners only, 5% used both, and 1.6% used neither. As in the studies summarized above, artificial sweetener consumption was more common in females and in overweight and obese individuals and rose with increasing income. It was also higher in urban areas and southern (more highly developed) regions of the country.

Two small but representative market surveys by the same group of authors examined artificial sweetener use by 507 Spanish and 256 Portuguese adults [10, 11]. Participants were asked to record the average consumption of 65 food and beverage items; sweetener content was obtained from food packaging. The leading source of artificial sweeteners in both countries was non-alcoholic beverages; the second-ranked source was sweets in Spain and milk and dairy products in Portugal. The three main types consumed in both countries were Ace-K, sucralose, and aspartame.

A cross-sectional survey of towns and villages in two areas of Lebanon (Beirut and Mount Lebanon) recruited 376 adults for a dietician-administered food frequency questionnaire [12]. Over 94% had consumed foods or beverages containing artificial sweeteners at least once in the prior 6 months, compared to only 20% consuming the sweeteners in the form of powders or pills. The main sweeteners consumed were aspartame, Ace-K, and sucralose, and the main reason for using them was weight control.

Temporal trends in consumption of artificial sweeteners have been infrequently reported. One recent study analyzed repeated (every 4 years) health behavior surveys of nationally representative samples of European adolescents from four participating countries between 2006 and 2018 [13]. The authors were surprised to observe large relative *reductions* (25–62% in the four countries) in the proportion of adolescents reporting daily consumption of diet soft drinks, despite even larger reductions in daily consumption of sugar-sweetened soft drinks. A recent study from a waste water treatment plant in the state of Queensland, Australia, analyzed changes in concentration of four artificial sweeteners from 2012 to 2018 [14]. Saccharine and sucralose concentrations significantly increased over the period, Ace-K concentrations remained stable, while cyclamate concentrations declined by half.

Health beliefs about artificial sweeteners have been less often studied. A recent web-based survey of over 9000 nationally representative secondary school students in Australia observed that only 20% of the participants believed that diet soft drinks are healthier than sugar-sweetened soft drinks, while 15% believed they are less healthy [15]. Moreover, approximately one-half of them believed that tooth decay, obesity, and diabetes are associated with consumption of diet soft drinks! And a recent survey of 100 physician and dietician students in Mexico City found that half of them disagreed that artificial sweeteners are safe, and half believed that they cause side effects [16].

In summary, the survey results summarized above indicate that consumption of beverages and foods containing artificial sweeteners is frequent, especially among women and overweight and obese persons, and increases with advancing age and education. The latter finding, which appears robust across countries with different dietary preferences, suggests that higher education may provide knowledge about the health benefits and safety of artificial sweeteners relative to sugar. In the following section, I will review the published evidence about the potential benefits and risks of these commonly used food additives.

Key Evidence Points

- Artificial sweeteners have been used for over a century and are a popular weight loss strategy among overweight and obese adults and adolescents in many countries.
- The major dietary sources of artificial sweeteners are diet soft drinks, yogurt, and powder or liquid table sweeteners.
- Strong evidence from randomized trials indicates that artificial sweeteners can lead to weight loss and lower blood sugar and blood pressure in obese adults and youth.
- No beneficial or adverse effects of artificial sweeteners have been demonstrated on "good" (high-density) or "bad" (low-density) cholesterol.
- Xylitol-sweetened gum and candies have been convincingly shown in randomized trials to lower the risk of dental plaque, a known precursor of caries (cavities).
- Despite concerns raised many decades ago about bladder cancer in laboratory studies of rats fed very high doses, no increased risk has been detected in large human studies for bladder, stomach, intestinal, pancreatic, breast, or brain cancer.

Detailed Review of Scientific Evidence[1]

General Principles

A plethora of systematic reviews and meta-analyses have been published, and it was quite a chore to sort through them. Too much information can be as bad as not enough. To help you see the forest instead of a lot of trees, I will first try to establish a few scientific principles, based on the material I summarized in Chaps. 1 and 2 of this book. The first of these principles distinguishes between beneficial, intended effects of artificial sweeteners and adverse effects. The studied beneficial effects include changes in body weight, fat, blood pressure, and blood sugar and lipids (fats such as cholesterol) and reduction in risks of cardiovascular disease, diabetes, and dental caries (cavities). Given the potential for bias due to confounding and reverse causality, I will restrict my review of the common intended benefits of artificial sweeteners to randomized controlled trials (RCTs). Since it is clear from the previous section of this chapter that overweight or obese persons and those of higher socioeconomic status are more likely to consume artificial sweeteners, RCTs are essential to ensure that such consumption *preceded* any change in body weight or fat and that any association is not biased by confounding

---

[1] Readers who prefer to skip the Detailed Review should proceed to the Summary at the end of the chapter.

differences in dietary and other lifestyle factors linked to education or socioeconomic status.

For potential adverse effects of artificial sweeteners, RCTs still provide the strongest evidence for common outcomes (like anxiety, trouble concentrating or sleeping, and diarrhea) but usually are far too small to detect increases in risk of cancer, birth defects, or death. For these health outcomes, I will rely on systematic reviews of observational studies. To reduce the risk of reverse causality, I will emphasize temporal precedence of exposure to artificial sweeteners by excluding cross-sectional studies. For chronic disease outcomes like heart disease, stroke, and type 2 diabetes, the potential confounding by the indication for use of artificial sweeteners, and especially by obesity and other cardiovascular risk factors, is so strong that I will not review evidence from observational studies of these outcomes. The same is true for deaths due to heart disease, stroke, and diabetes, for which studies carry the same potential for confounding by indication. For both beneficial and adverse outcomes, I will rely heavily on the comprehensive systematic review and meta-analysis by Toews and colleagues [17], which analyzed 56 total studies, including 21 randomized trials and 35 observational studies on a wide array of health outcomes.

Finally, I point out another potential source of bias: selective reporting of study results and slanting of conclusions in published reviews of studies in this area, due to industry funding and resulting conflict of interest. Mandrioli and coworkers' systematic review found very strong associations between the results and conclusions of reviews (not necessarily systematic) of studies of artificial sweetener effects on body weight that were sponsored by artificial sweetener manufacturers, as well as those sponsored by the sugar industry [18].

Changes in Body Weight, Fat, and Other Cardio-Metabolic Risk Factors

The main rationale for using artificial sweeteners is to lose weight, or at least to reduce the amount of weight gained. Among overweight or obese adults participating in randomized trials included in the Toews systematic review and meta-analysis [17], those randomized to receive artificial sweeteners lost 2 kg more during the 4-week to 6-month period of follow-up than those randomized to sugar or placebo. No significant difference in weight change was observed, however, in participants of normal weight. In trials comparing artificial sweeteners to sucrose, the change in body mass index was more than half a standard deviation lower among adults randomized to artificial sweeteners. These beneficial effects appear to have been a consequence of significantly lower energy (calorie) intake in participants randomized to artificial sweeteners. In other words, the artificial sweetener did not appear to lead to a hunger-induced compensation for the calories "missing" in the artificial sweeteners.

Results for body weight were similar in randomized trials among children: a non-significantly lower weight gain (by 0.6 kg) in those randomized to artificial sweeteners among normal children, a larger (0.75 kg) reduction among overweight or obese children, and a slightly but significantly smaller increase in body mass index (0.15 standard deviations) in those randomized to artificial versus sucrose sweeteners. Percent body fat and skinfold thicknesses were non-significantly lower in children randomized to the artificial sweetener group in the sole randomized trial reporting those outcomes. A more recent systematic review and meta-analysis of RCTs limited to obese children and adolescents confirmed the beneficial effect of artificial sweeteners on weight gain, with a statistically significantly lower BMI gain by 0.42 kg/m^2 [19].

In the Toews review [17], slightly but significantly lower fasting blood glucose levels were observed in trials comparing artificial sweeteners to sugar in overweight or obese adults. More substantial reductions (5 mmHg) were observed in systolic blood pressure. No significant differences were found in concentrations of high-density ("good") cholesterol or low-density ("bad") cholesterol. In children, no blood pressure differences were observed, and changes in blood sugar were mixed, with some increases and some decreases among those randomized to artificial sweeteners. In a recent systematic review and meta-analysis of 14 RCTs in adults limited to effects on lipids (blood fats) [20], no beneficial or adverse effect of artificial or stevia-based sweeteners was observed on good or bad cholesterol or triglycerides.

Dental Health

High sugar intake is known to increase the risk of dental caries (cavities), but the Toews systematic review [17] mentions only a single non-randomized controlled trial reporting a dental outcome. That trial compared chlorhexidine mouth rinses with stevia, which, as discussed in the first part of this chapter, is a natural (rather than artificial), plant-based sweetener [21]. The chlorhexidine rinses were more effective than stevia in reducing the volume of dental plaque, but caries was not reported. In an RCT not mentioned in the Toews review [22], however, 2600 primary school children in three Puerto Rican communities were randomized by classroom into two groups: no treatment versus chewing of sorbitol/aspartame-sweetened gum for 20 min, three times per day after meals, for 3 years. After 3 years of follow-up, those in the gum-chewing group had a significant reduction in dental caries by examination and X-rays. In the absence of a placebo, blinding of children was of course impossible, but the dentist who performed the follow-up evaluation was apparently unaware of treatment assignment. Of note, the artificially-sweetened gum was *not* compared with sugar-containing gum. Thus, the observed beneficial effect may reflect an increase in flow of saliva or removal of food, rather than an anti-caries effect of the artificial sweetener.

Finally, Söderling and Pienihäkkinen's recent narrative systematic review (without meta-analysis) included 14 randomized trials of xylitol gum or candies in children or adults [23]. In most of these trials, the xylitol gum or candy was compared to sorbitol or maltitol gum or candy, which should provide an adequate placebo control and thus ensure blinding to the treatment allocated. Of the 14 trials, 13 observed a significant reduction in dental plaque, a key precursor of caries. These impressive results suggest a specific benefit of xylitol above and beyond the absence of sugar, salivary flow, or food removal.

Cancer

The main adverse health effect of artificial sweeteners feared by many consumers is cancer. Fortunately, as reviewed in the Toews systematic review [17], the evidence from eight observational studies indicates no increased risk of bladder cancer, the main "red flag" raised by animal studies mentioned earlier in this chapter. Two prospective observational studies with at least 10 years of follow-up found no increased risks of lymphoma or leukemia. One case-control observational study observed a 40% *reduction* in risk of ovarian cancer, and another found an 80% reduction in risk of pancreatic cancer. In children, one observational study found no increased risk of brain cancer.

A recent systematic review and meta-analysis of 38 observational studies by Jatho and coworkers was limited to cancers of the gastrointestinal (GI) tract [24]. No increase in risk of GI cancer overall was observed in participants exposed to artificial sweeteners, nor in cancers of the esophagus, stomach, pancreas, or colon or rectum. A modest (28%) increase was seen for liver cancer, although that analysis was based on only three studies.

A recent article based on a pooled analysis of two U.S. prospective observational studies comprising nearly 600,000 participants was published after, and therefore not included in, the Jatho systematic review [25]. Liver cancer risk was studied in relation to sugar-sweetened and artificially-sweetened sodas and other beverages. Most of the analyses revealed no significant associations, but a very slight increase in risk was observed with sugar-sweetened soda only among participants without diabetes, while a similar slight increase in risk with artificially-sweetened soda was limited to those with diabetes. In both cases, the increased risks barely achieved statistical significance and were limited to participants with shorter follow-up periods. It is difficult to infer a causal relationship from these borderline and contradictory results.

A recent systematic review and meta-analysis of five observational studies found no increased risk of breast cancer associated with consumption of artificial sweeteners, even at the highest doses [26]. Finally, a recent U.S. prospective observational study by Fulgoni and Drewnowski linked dietary data from the National Health and Nutrition Examination Surveys (NHANES) between 1988 and 2018 to 2019 public-use mortality files [27]. No association was observed between consumption of aspartame, saccharine, or all artificial sweeteners and death from cancer.

Nonetheless, highly publicized recent reviews of the scientific evidence by WHO's International Agency for Research on Cancer and the Food and Agricultural Organization led to opposite recommendations about the strength of the evidence linking aspartame to cancer risk [28]. For both organizations, however, the evidence reviewed was based on consumption versus non-consumption of aspartame—not a comparison of sugar-sweetened versus aspartame-sweetened beverages and foods. Obesity itself is a risk factor for liver, colorectal, and breast cancers, and a switch from aspartame to sugar consumption might well do more harm than good. Discontinuation of *all* sweeteners seems an unjustifiable and unattainable public health message.

Adverse Effects on Offspring Due to Exposure During Pregnancy

The Toews review [17] did not include studies of adverse effects of exposure to artificial sweeteners during pregnancy. Cai and colleagues' recent systematic review and meta-analysis included ten observational studies and one RCT of such effects, of which only six observational studies provided quantitative data that could be used in a meta-analysis [29]. Four of the studies provided data on the risk of preterm birth associated with any use of artificial sweeteners during pregnancy; a modest (18%) but statistically significant increase in risk was reported, but no dose-response relationship was observed. That is, the magnitude of the increase did not rise with increasing number of servings per day of artificial sweeteners. Moreover, overweight or obese mothers, who have a higher risk of delivering preterm, were probably more likely to use artificial sweeteners, and thus the increased risk of preterm birth is probably confounded by the reason (indication) for exposure. Finally, the increased risk of preterm birth is not consistent with a small (24 g, just under 1 ounce) *increase* in average birth weight. The Cai review also included a single prospective observational study that observed a higher risk of asthma in the 7-year-old offspring of Danish mothers who consumed artificially-sweetened carbonated soft drinks at 25 weeks of pregnancy, but the diagnosis of asthma was based solely on the mother's report at an interview.

Other Adverse Health Outcomes

Based on the Toews review [17], the evidence is scanty concerning mood, sleep, behavior, and cognitive performance but does not suggest major beneficial or adverse effects on these outcomes in either adults or children. I found one Spanish observational study of risk of male infertility with cyclamate use, in which infertility was based on low sperm counts among 400 men whose partners had been unable to conceive [30]. A similar number of controls were fertile men seeking vasectomies. Neither history of cyclamate use nor cyclamate metabolite urine excretion differed in cases and controls.

Summary

Artificial sweeteners are consumed by many adults and children living in geographically and ethnically diverse regions of the world. They were first discovered in 1879 and have been used regularly since the early twentieth century. Their use is more frequent among women than men and among older and more highly-educated individuals. Consumption also varies consistently with body weight, being much higher among overweight and obese adolescents and adults than among those of normal weight.

Reports of increased risk of bladder cancer when very high doses were administered to laboratory rats led to banning of saccharine and/or cyclamate from a few countries, but large epidemiologic studies have not observed increased risks of bladder cancer in humans consuming food and beverages containing artificial sweeteners. Nor has evidence emerged of increased risks of other cancers, with the possible exception liver cancer.

Conversely, artificial sweeteners have been shown in randomized trials to have modest short-term benefits on body weight, blood sugar levels, and blood pressure, especially in overweight and obese individuals. Xylitol-sweetened gum and candies have also been convincingly shown to reduce the risk of dental plaque, a well-established precursor of caries (cavities). In other words, a population-wide shift from artificial sweeteners to sugar might well do more harm than good.

References

1. Nayik G, Shah T, Muzaffar K, Wani S, Gull A, Majid I, Bhat F. Honey: its history and religious significance: a review. Universal J Pharm. 2014;3:5–8.
2. Sugar substitute. Wikipedia. 6 Apr 2022.
3. Hicks J. The pursuit of sweet. Science History Institute. 2 May 2010.
4. The bittersweet history of sugar substitutes. The New York Times. 29 Mar 1987.
5. Martyn D, Darch M, Roberts A, Lee HY, Yaqiong Tian T, Kaburagi N, Belmar P. Low-/no-calorie sweeteners: a review of global intakes. Nutrients. 2018;10(3):357.
6. Sylvetsky AC, Jin Y, Clark EJ, Welsh JA, Rother KI, Talegawkar SA. Consumption of low-calorie sweeteners among children and adults in the United States. J Acad Nutr Diet. 2017;117(3):441–448.e2.
7. Grech A, Kam CO, Gemming L, Rangan A. Diet-quality and socio-demographic factors associated with non-nutritive sweetener use in the Australian population. Nutrients. 2018;10(7):833.
8. Wang Y, Li C, Li D, Yang H, Li X, Jin D, Xie W, Guo B. Estimated assessment of dietary exposure to artificial sweeteners from processed food in Nanjing, China. Food Addit Contam Part A Chem Anal Control Expo Risk Assess. 2021;38(7):1105–17.
9. Silva Monteiro L, Kulik Hassan B, Melo Rodrigues PR, Massae Yokoo E, Sichieri R, Alves Pereira R. Use of table sugar and artificial sweeteners in Brazil: National Dietary Survey 2008-2009. Nutrients. 2018;10(3):295.
10. Redruello-Requejo M, González-Rodríguez M, Samaniego-Vaesken MDL, Montero-Bravo A, Partearroyo T, Varela-Moreiras G. Low- and no-calorie sweetener (LNCS) consumption patterns amongst the Spanish adult population. Nutrients. 2021;13(6):1845.
11. González-Rodríguez M, Redruello-Requejo M, Samaniego-Vaesken ML, Montero-Bravo A, Puga AM, Partearroyo T, Varela-Moreiras G. Low- and no-calorie sweetener (LNCS) presence and consumption among the Portuguese adult population. Nutrients. 2021;13(11):4186.
12. Daher M, Fahd C, Nour AA, Sacre Y. Trends and amounts of consumption of low-calorie sweeteners: a cross-sectional study. Clin Nutr ESPEN. 2022;48:427–33.
13. Chatelan A, Lebacq T, Rouche M, Kelly C, Fismen AS, Kalman M, Dzielska A, Castetbon K. Long-term trends in the consumption of sugary and diet soft drinks among adolescents: a cross-national survey in 21 European countries. Eur J Nutr. 2022;61(5):2799–813.
14. Li D, O'Brien JW, Tscharke BJ, Choi PM, Ahmed F, Thompson J, Mueller JF, Sun H, Thomas KV. Trends in artificial sweetener consumption: a 7-year wastewater-based epidemiology study in Queensland, Australia. Sci Total Environ. 2021;754:142438.
15. Miller C, Dono J, Scully M, Morley B, Ettridge K. Adolescents' knowledge and beliefs regarding health risks of soda and diet soda consumption. Public Health Nutr. 2022;25(11):3044–53.
16. Romo-Romo A, Brito-Córdova GX, Aguilar-Salinas CA, Cano-García de León C, Farías-Name DE, Reyes-Lara L, Jiménez-Rossainz JM, Del Moral Vidal LP, Gómez-Pérez FJ, Almeda-Valdés P. Beliefs concerning non-nutritive sweeteners consumption in consumers,

non-consumers, and health professionals: a comparative cross-sectional study. Nutr Hosp. 2022;39(5):1086–92.

17. Toews I, Lohner S, Küllenberg de Gaudry D, Sommer H, Meerpohl JJ. Association between intake of non-sugar sweeteners and health outcomes: systematic review and meta-analyses of randomised and non-randomised controlled trials and observational studies. BMJ. 2019;364:k4718.

18. Mandrioli D, Kearns CE, Bero LA. Relationship between research outcomes and risk of bias, study sponsorship, and author financial conflicts of interest in reviews of the effects of artificially sweetened beverages on weight outcomes: a systematic review of reviews. PLoS One. 2016;11(9):e0162198.

19. Espinosa A, Mendoza K, Laviada-Molina H, Rangel-Méndez JA, Molina-Segui F, Sun Q, Tobias DK, Willett WC, Mattei J. Effects of non-nutritive sweeteners on the BMI of children and adolescents: a systematic review and meta-analysis of randomised controlled trials and prospective cohort studies. Lancet Glob Health. 2023;11(Suppl 1):S8.

20. Movahedian M, Golzan SA, Ashtary-Larky D, Clark CCT, Asbaghi O, Hekmatdoost A. The effects of artificial- and stevia-based sweeteners on lipid profile in adults: a GRADE-assessed systematic review, meta-analysis, and meta-regression of randomized clinical trials. Crit Rev Food Sci Nutr. 2023;63:5063–79.

21. Zanela NL, Bijella MF, Rosa OP. The influence of mouthrinses with antimicrobial solutions on the inhibition of dental plaque and on the levels of mutans streptococci in children. Pesqui Odontol Bras. 2002;16(2):101–6.

22. Beiswanger BB, Boneta AE, Mau MS, Katz BP, Proskin HM, Stookey GK. The effect of chewing sugar-free gum after meals on clinical caries incidence. J Am Dent Assoc. 1998;129(11):1623–6.

23. Söderling E, Pienihäkkinen K. Effects of xylitol chewing gum and candies on the accumulation of dental plaque: a systematic review. Clin Oral Investig. 2022;26(1):119–29.

24. Jatho A, Cambia JM, Myung SK. Consumption of artificially sweetened soft drinks and risk of gastrointestinal cancer: a meta-analysis of observational studies. Public Health Nutr. 2021;24(18):6122–36.

25. Jones GS, Graubard BI, Ramirez Y, Liao LM, Huang WY, Alvarez CS, Yang W, Zhang X, Petrick JL, McGlynn KA. Sweetened beverage consumption and risk of liver cancer by diabetes status: a pooled analysis. Cancer Epidemiol. 2022;79:102201.

26. Ye X, Zhang Y, He Y, Sheng M, Huang J, Lou W. Association between consumption of artificial sweeteners and breast cancer risk: a systematic review and meta-analysis of observational studies. Nutr Cancer. 2023;75(3):795–804.

27. Fulgoni VL 3rd, Drewnowski A. No association between low-calorie sweetener (LCS) use and overall cancer risk in the nationally representative database in the US: analyses of NHANES 1988–2018 data and 2019 public-use linked mortality files. Nutrients. 2022;14(23):4957.

28. Riboli E, Beland FA, Lachenmeier DW, Marques MM, Phillips DH, Schernhammer E, Afghan A, Assunção R, Caderni G, Corton JC, de Aragão Umbuzeiro G, de Jong D, Deschasaux-Tanguy M, Hodge A, Ishihara J, Levy DD, Mandrioli D, McCullough ML, McNaughton SA, Morita T, Nugent AP, Ogawa K, Pandiri AR, Sergi CM, Touvier M, Zhang L, Benbrahim-Tallaa L, Chittiboyina S, Cuomo D, DeBono NL, Debras C, de Conti A, El Ghissassi F, Fontvieille E, Harewood R, Kaldor J, Mattock H, Pasqual E, Rigutto G, Simba H, Suonio E, Viegas S, Wedekind R, Schubauer-Berigan MK, Madia F. Carcinogenicity of aspartame, methyleugenol, and isoeugenol. Lancet Oncol. 2023;24(8):848–50.

29. Cai C, Sivak A, Davenport MH. Effects of prenatal artificial sweeteners consumption on birth outcomes: a systematic review and meta-analysis. Public Health Nutr. 2021;24(15):5024–33.

30. Serra-Majem L, Bassas L, García-Glosas R, Ribas L, Inglés C, Casals I, Saavedra P, Renwick AG. Cyclamate intake and cyclohexylamine excretion are not related to male fertility in humans. Food Addit Contam. 2003;20(12):1097–104.

The "Hype" About Sugar and Children's Behavior

15

Introduction

The idea that allergic reactions to food could lead to hyperactivity and other "nervous" behaviors in children can be traced back to 1922, when a series of eight cases was reported by W Ray Shannon, a pediatrician from St. Paul, Minnesota [1]. Shannon used the term "anaphylactic" to refer to non-life-threatening red, scaly (eczematous) or itchy raised (hive) skin reactions that accompanied troublesome behaviors in the eight children, whom he treated with food elimination diets, especially elimination of wheat and egg. These diets were not placebo-controlled or blinded, but Dr. Shannon attributed the apparent success of the diets in improving the child's behavior to food allergy. He inferred that the allergic reactions were caused by some protein in the child's diet.

A quarter century later, TG Randolph, a Chicago-based pediatrician, published another case series of four boys with more systemic allergic symptoms (runny nose, nasal congestion, and cough) accompanied by nervous, jittery behavior, and fatigue [2]. After apparently successful elimination diets, he attributed the respiratory symptoms and abnormal behaviors to allergy to wheat and corn. He insisted that in two of the four cases, the reactions were at least partly caused by corn sugar, that is, glucose, even though glucose is an essential sugar contained in virtually all life forms!

The belief that sugar could lead to hyperactivity and other concerning behaviors received a boost in the 1970s, when Feingold, a pediatrician in Los Angeles, described a child who went "completely wild" when consuming candy, cake, and soft drinks at birthday parties and family gatherings [3]. Feingold, however, believed that food colorings and other additives were responsible for these reactions—not sugar. Feingold attributed the hyperactivity to allergy and devised and marketed the now-famous Feingold elimination diet in search of a cure for hyperactivity and attention disorder. Although the Feingold diet featuring food additive elimination was proven ineffective a few years later, the belief in the sugar "high" or sugar "rush" persisted and even grew over the ensuing decades [3]. I am not sure why;

M. S. Kramer, *Believe It or Not*, https://doi.org/10.1007/978-3-031-46022-7_15

Fig. 15.1 The belief in the sugar "high" has persisted for at least half a century and remains prevalent today

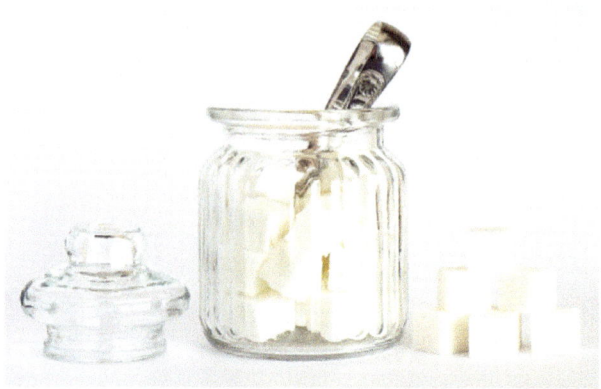

perhaps it was the well-known tendency of groups of school-aged children, and of boys in particular, to go "completely wild" at parties outside of the school setting. The sweets they consumed on such occasions were perhaps an easier target than insufficient parental supervision at the parties! (Fig. 15.1).

How Common Is "Hyper" Behavior?

Young kids get "hyper" from time to time in the right social setting, which doesn't have to be a birthday party. But most school-age children can modulate their behavior when in the classroom or while playing games with friends or watching television at home. A few have great difficulty in doing so, however; they have what is called attention deficit hyperactivity disorder (ADHD).

ADHD is a widely recognized neurologic and behavioral disorder beginning in childhood. Criteria for its diagnosis have been developed by the American Psychiatric Association in its Diagnostic and Statistical Manual (DSM) and by the World Health Organization's International Classification of Diseases (ICD). These criteria have evolved over time in line with the publication of scientific research, but the main characteristics of the disorder are poor attention, distractibility, and excess movement. Although ADHD is sometimes suspected as early as age 2 or 3 years, it is normal for toddlers to be very active and to have limited attention spans. Many cases of ADHD come to light only when the child begins school, as the inattention and disruptive behavior are noted by teachers. The symptoms of ADHD often improve with age, but they persist to some degree into adulthood in a substantial fraction of cases.

ADHD is more likely in children whose parents or siblings have the condition, at least partly due to a genetic contribution, although identified genes explain only a small fraction of cases [4]. Environment certainly plays a role; the family and social (including socioeconomic) environments are probably more important than aspects of the physical environment such as chemical toxins in the air, water, or foods and beverages.

In a 2007 systematic review of 102 studies based on representative study samples from the general population (households, birth registries, or schools), Polanczyk and colleagues estimated a world-wide prevalence of ADHD of 5.3% [5]. The prevalence varied by sex (two-fold higher in boys) and age (two-fold higher in children 6–11 years of age than in adolescents). It also varied geographically, with the lowest rates in the Middle East and Asia, mid-range in Europe and North America, and highest in Africa and South America. The authors argued that cultural differences and use of different diagnostic criteria are likely to explain the geographic differences. In terms of ethnic and racial differences within countries, the 2020 systematic review and meta-analysis of 24 samples in 21 studies by Cénat and coworkers estimated a prevalence of 14.5% in U.S. Blacks, considerably higher than overall U.S. estimates, with even higher rates among those from socioeconomically disadvantaged backgrounds [6].

Why am I bringing up ADHD? For two reasons: first, the condition is common; many parents are aware of it and may worry that children with attention problems or "hyper" behavior are affected by it. Second, parents of children diagnosed with ADHD may believe that sugar aggravates their symptoms.

Sugar Intake and Behavior: Knowledge and Beliefs

Belief that sugar can impair attention and/or lead to "hyper" behavior is widespread, although few studies of this belief have been published. I was unable to locate a systematic review, but in a fascinating study by Macdonald and colleagues, a citizen science website was used to carry out an online survey among adult volunteers in the U.S. with at least some university education [7]. Participants were asked to respond to 32 brief statements about the brain by indicating whether each statement was true or false. The large, but obviously non-representative, sample included 234 participants who had taken at least one university-level course on the brain or neuroscience, 598 educators, and 3045 members of the general public. Of the 32 statements, 15 were so-called "neuromyths," that is, common but false beliefs about the brain and how it functions. One of these neuromyths, the statement "Children are less attentive after consuming sugary drinks and/or snacks," ranked 5th of 15 in the rate of incorrect responses: 59% among the general public, 50% among educators, and 39% among participants with some neuroscience education.

In a qualitative study based on 42 face-to-face interviews with Portuguese parents of primary school children, many parents believed that sugar is addictive [8]. The most common of sugar's adverse effects that they identified related to behavior: hyperactivity, restlessness, and poor attention.

Surprising to me, belief about sugar's adverse effects on children's behavior even extends to the full-blown syndrome of ADHD. From a representative school-based sample of children attending primary school in northern Florida, Bussing and coworkers selected 209 at high risk of ADHD and 165 at low risk and interviewed them and their parents nearly 8 years later, when the children were about 15 years old [9]. Belief that ADHD "is caused by too much sugar in the diet" was similarly frequent among both the teenagers and their parents but was higher in adolescents and parents in whom the child had been deemed at high risk in primary school (around 30%) than those deemed at low risk (around 20%). This belief was far more common in Blacks than in Whites and in low-income participants, independently of their ADHD risk status.

These beliefs apparently extend to teachers, as well as parents. Giannopoulou and colleagues studied two groups of Greek teachers attending an educational seminar on ADHD: 68 nursery- and primary school teachers and 75 private tutors [10]. Prior to the seminar, both groups completed a knowledge questionnaire on ADHD. The teachers were quite knowledgeable about the symptoms, signs, and treatment of ADHD, but much less so about its causes. Nearly 40% of the school teachers and over half of the tutors agreed with the statement that sugar and/or food additives are responsible for the disorder.

Key Evidence Points
- Hyperactivity and inattention are common in toddlers and pre-school children but are more likely to be recognized as problem behaviors at school age.
- The belief that consumption of sugar makes children "hyper" and interferes with their attention and sleep began over 50 years ago and remains highly prevalent among parents, children, adolescents, and teachers.
- Randomized, placebo-controlled trials are necessary to assess the causal effect of sugar on attention, hyperactivity, sleep, and cognitive function.
- Such trials have clearly demonstrated that sugar does *not* affect these outcomes in normal, healthy children, nor in those diagnosed with attention deficit hyperactivity disorder (ADHD).

Detailed Review of the Scientific Evidence[1]

In this section, I will summarize the scientific evidence that sugar intake causes problems with "hyper" behavior, cognitive function, and sleep in children. I will include studies of normal children, children believed by their parents to be particularly sensitive to adverse behavioral effects of sugar, and children with ADHD.

Trying to make solid inferences about adverse effects of sugar on children's behavior and cognitive ability should rely on methodologically rigorous randomized, placebo-controlled trials. As I have mentioned many times in this book, observational studies of cause and effect are prone to two main sources of bias: confounding and reverse causality. In the context of sugar consumption and behavior, observational associations are highly susceptible to confounding by

---

[1] Readers who prefer to skip the Detailed Review should proceed to the Summary at the end of the chapter.

characteristics of the children or their families that influence both diet and behavior. These include genetic factors, such as parents or siblings with ADHD or milder forms of attention deficit or hyperactivity. But they also include non-genetic life-style factors like eating behaviors, television viewing time, reading, and physical activity. Reverse causality is probably an even more important source of bias than confounding, because hyperactive, inattentive children may well have preferences for sweets, or their parents may use sugary drinks, candies, or other sweet foods to mollify the children's behavior. Although cross-sectional studies are particularly prone to this source of bias, even prospective studies can be affected by it, because subtle behaviors can lead parents to offer sweets at an early age, well before those behaviors lead to problems at older ages in school or other settings requiring sustained attention.

Wolraich and colleagues' 1995 systematic review and meta-analysis analyzed 16 published reports of 23 placebo-controlled, blinded crossover trials of sugar versus artificial sweeteners [11]. The trials included three groups of participants: normal children without behavioral or cognitive problems, children judged by their parents as highly sensitive to react to sugar with "hyper" behavior, and children diagnosed with ADHD. None of the behaviors or cognitive function measures differed in any of the three groups of children between the sugar and artificial sweetener treatments.

I was unable to find any additional randomized trials published since the Wolraich review, perhaps attesting to the unusually "settled" evidence base from that review. In 2021, Ward and coworkers' published a systematic review of studies of sleep and diet, most of which were observational studies [12]. The review included a single small Australian randomized crossover trial published in 2011 comparing sleep in children after high-glucose or low-glucose milk consumed 1 h before bedtime [13]. No differences were observed in sleep latency (time to fall asleep), total sleep time, or total wake time between the two treatment conditions.

One might well ask why high-quality scientific studies show no evidence of a sugar "high," while many parents are absolutely convinced of it in their own children. An ingenious, albeit ethically questionable, randomized trial by Hoover and Milich sheds an important light on this contradiction [14]. The investigators randomized 31 boys 5–7 years of age whose behavior their mothers insisted was sugar-sensitive, that is, boys who became hyperactive and more difficult to control after consuming sugar. All of the children consumed an artificially sweetened (with aspartame) Kool-Aid drink half an hour before assessment by their mothers, but half of the mothers were randomized to being (falsely) informed that the drink was sweetened with sugar. That group rated their children as significantly more hyperactive than the group correctly informed that their children's drink had contained the artificial sweetener. In other words, the mothers' expectation of an adverse behavioral reaction became a self-fulfilling prophecy. These results show the importance of confirmation bias: the expectation of an adverse effect of sugar was confirmed in the group told their child had consumed sugar!

Summary

Most kids get "hyper" from time to time, especially in the pre-school years and especially when stimulated by their peers or when playing with adults. But by the time they start primary school, many children can modulate their behavior by focussing their attention on quiet tasks and activities and staying in one place while doing them. The idea that "allergies" or other types of physiological reactions to certain foods could cause behavioral problems began in the early decades of the twentieth century and by the 1970s centered on food additives and sugar. The food additive theory was effectively disproven by randomized, double-blind trials of elimination diets, but the firm belief in the sugar "high" or "rush" has persisted in the face of uniformly negative evidence from many randomized trials of similar design. Sugar does not impair attention, promote hyperactive behavior, or interfere with cognitive function in children who are normal and healthy, those who are judged to be sugar-sensitive by their parents, or even those diagnosed with attention deficit hyperactivity disorder (ADHD). Nor does sugar taken just before bedtime appear to interfere with sleep. Instead, the parents' firm belief in the sugar high appears to create expectations of "hyper" behavior that bias interpretation of their children's behavior after consuming sugar.

References

1. Shannon WR. Neuropathic manifestations in infants and children as a result of anaphylactic reaction to foods contained in their dietary. Am J Dis Child. 1922;24(1):89–94.
2. Randolph TG. Allergy as a causative factor of fatigue, irritability, and behavior problems of children. J Pediatr. 1947;31(5):560–72.
3. Klasco R. Is there such a thing as a "sugar high"? The New York Times. 21 Feb 2020.
4. Ronald A, de Bode N, Polderman TJC. Systematic review: how the attention-deficit/hyperactivity disorder polygenic risk score adds to our understanding of ADHD and associated traits. J Am Acad Child Adolesc Psychiatry. 2021;60(10):1234–77.
5. Polanczyk G, de Lima MS, Horta BL, Biederman J, Rohde LA. The worldwide prevalence of ADHD: a systematic review and metaregression analysis. Am J Psychiatry. 2007;164(6):942–8.
6. Cénat JM, Blais-Rochette C, Morse C, Vandette MP, Noorishad PG, Kogan C, Ndengeyingoma A, Labelle PR. Prevalence and risk factors associated with attention-deficit/hyperactivity disorder among US Black individuals: a systematic review and meta-analysis. JAMA Psychiatry. 2021;78(1):21–8.
7. Macdonald K, Germine L, Anderson A, Christodoulou J, McGrath LM. Dispelling the myth: training in education or neuroscience decreases but does not eliminate beliefs in neuromyths. Front Psychol. 2017;8:1314.
8. Prada M, Saraiva M, Godinho CA, Tourais B, Cavalheiro BP, Garrido MV. Parental perceptions and practices regarding sugar intake by school-aged children: a qualitative study with Portuguese parents. Appetite. 2021;166:105471.
9. Bussing R, Zima BT, Mason DM, Meyer JM, White K, Garvan CW. ADHD knowledge, perceptions, and information sources: perspectives from a community sample of adolescents and their parents. J Adolesc Health. 2012;51(6):593–600.
10. Giannopoulou I, Korkoliakou P, Pasalari E, Douzenis A. Greek teachers' knowledge about attention deficit hyperactivity disorder. Psychiatriki. 2017;28(3):226–33.

11. Wolraich ML, Wilson DB, White JW. The effect of sugar on behavior or cognition in children: a meta-analysis. JAMA. 1995;274(20):1617–21.
12. Ward AL, Jospe M, Morrison S, Reynolds AN, Kuroko S, Fangupo LJ, Smith C, Galland BC, Taylor RW. Bidirectional associations between sleep quality or quantity, and dietary intakes or eating behaviors in children 6-12 years old: a systematic review with evidence mapping. Nutr Rev. 2021;79(10):1079–99.
13. Jalilolghadr S, Afaghi A, O'Connor H, Chow CM. Effect of low and high glycaemic index drink on sleep pattern in children. J Pak Med Assoc. 2011;61(6):533–6.
14. Hoover DW, Milich R. Effects of sugar ingestion expectancies on mother-child interactions. J Abnorm Child Psychol. 1994;22(4):501–15.

Organic Foods: A Healthier Alternative?

16

Introduction

From a strictly chemical perspective, all foods are "organic," because they contain compounds with the element carbon, an essential element in all living organisms, including animals, plants, bacteria, and even viruses. But when most people think or talk about organic foods, they are referring to organic farming methods for producing the foods we eat. Different countries have different regulations governing which foods can be called "organic." Nonetheless, shared criteria across countries include the following:

- No synthetic pesticides, fertilizers, hormones, antibiotics, or preservatives
- No genetically modified organisms (GMOs)
- Proper crop rotations to maintain soil quality and fertility
- Maintenance of adequate and uncontaminated water resources
- Ethical (humane) treatment of animals

These criteria seem highly desirable, don't they? They resonate with many people, especially in high-income Western countries, and organic food sales have approximately doubled globally over the last decade [1]. This increase has occurred despite the 30–40% higher price of organic foods, which is due to lower crop yields, higher labor costs, and high demand. The growing popularity of organic foods appears based on the widespread perception that they have higher nutritional value and health benefits, the evidence for which will be reviewed later in the chapter. Nonetheless, organic foods still account for only about 4% of total food sales, even in the U.S. [2]. Fresh fruit and vegetables comprise about half of those sales, followed by dairy products, processed foods, beverages, and breads and grains. Over 90% organic foods are purchased in conventional food or natural food stores, with the remaining and increasing fraction obtained in farmers' markets (Fig. 16.1).

Fig. 16.1 Organic foods comprise a small but increasing fraction of all food sales in many high-income countries

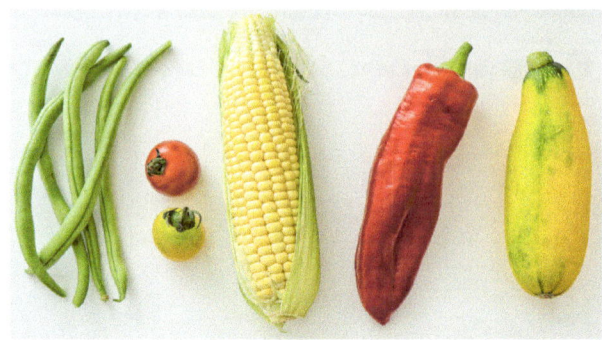

The History of Organic Farming

GMOs are one of the most hotly debated aspects of conventional agriculture, especially in Europe. In fact, however, any deliberate human intervention that interferes with Darwinian natural selection can be considered as genetic modification [3]. Wild wolves were domesticated by our ancestors 30,000 years ago to become the dogs that we know today by artificially selecting, that is, by selectively breeding, those which were more docile and had other desirable traits. The same breeding principles were applied to wheat, other grains, and corn around 10,000 years ago. Selective breeding cannot occur without genetic modification, even though the science of genetics did not exist before Mendel's experiments with peas in the nineteenth century!

True genetic engineering began in 1973 when Boyer and Cohen took a gene that conferred antibiotic resistance in one bacterium and transferred the gene into an antibiotic-susceptible strain, thereby conferring resistance in the recipient [4]. By the 1980s and 1990s, a similar technology was used to improve the texture and shelf life of tomatoes, bacterial pesticide-producing corn, and herbicide-resistant soybeans. This technology was later extended to animals (year-round salmon). Despite the agricultural advantages of GMOs, they have raised fears of mutations "spreading" to humans and given rise to philosophical and religious objections to "playing God" and "messing with Mother Nature." GMO technology is regulated in many countries, including licensing standards for laboratories. Labeling requirements for GMO foods vary considerably. They are voluntary in the U.S. and Canada, for example, whereas Europe requires labeling of all foods containing >0.9% GMOs.

Aspects of organic farming other than exclusion of GMOs began in the wake of the Dust Bowl in the southern plains of the United States, which was caused by poor soil management and prolonged drought [5]. The term "organic farming" was coined by Walter James in his 1940 book, *Look to the Land*, which advocated the concept of dynamic interaction between the soil, plants, and animals. The concept was based on work earlier in the twentieth century in India by the British botanist Sir Albert Howard and in Germany by Rudolph Steiner, emphasizing the use of animal manure and compost to nourish the soil and crops. Over the next half century, the Japanese soil scientist and plant pathologist Masonobu Fukuoka advocated natural, "do-nothing" farming for growing grain and other farm crops. In the U.S., JI Rodale popularized organic gardening for the general public.

Environmental concerns were added to those of soil depletion with the use of herbicides and pesticides developed after World War II. In 1962, Rachel Carson's best-selling book, *Silent Spring*, sounded the alarm about the environmental persistence of DDT, an organochlorine insecticide, which led to thinning of eggs and decline in bird populations in some farming areas. The book led to banning the sale and use of DDT in the U.S. in 1972 and to the creation of both the Environmental Protection Agency and the International Federation of Organic Agricultural Movements. DDT is still used as a farm pesticide in some low-income agricultural countries and to coat mosquito nets for controlling malaria in endemic areas.

In 1990, the U.S. Congress tasked the Department of Agriculture (USDA) to develop national standards for organic food production, and in 2002, the European Union Organic Certification was enacted to enforce similar standards in Europe. In Cuba, the collapse of the Soviet Union and continued U.S. trade embargo made it almost impossible to import chemical fertilizers and heavy agricultural machinery. The result was a state-supported organic farming program called organicopónicos.

Current Beliefs and Practices Concerning Organic Food Consumption

I searched for systematic reviews of studies of the "who" and "why" of organic food consumption: that is, the factors that predict or influence that consumption. Several systematic reviews attempted to identify clusters of underlying attributes among organic food consumers—that is, to shed light on the "why," rather than the "who."

Sebastian-Ponce and colleagues' narrative review focused on labeling of GMOs in 40 studies, most of which were cross-sectional surveys [6]. In most of the studies, consumers expressed a preference for non-GMO foods and for obligatory or voluntary labeling of foods. Most consumers indicated they would be willing to pay a small premium for non-GMO foods.

In a second narrative systematic review, Steinhauser and Hamm did not restrict their review to organic foods but included 66 studies of foods with claims of nutrition, health, or risk reduction ("NHR") advantages [7]. Nutrition knowledge, health motivation, and familiarity with the food were consistently positively associated with study participants' preference and purchase of foods with NHR claims. Female sex and older age were also positively associated with these preferences, but it is unclear whether these associations were independent of their knowledge and attitudes. Educational attainment was inconsistently associated with preferences.

A third narrative systematic review included 89 studies focusing on motives and barriers to organic food consumption [8]. The authors categorized the results of these studies according to underlying constructs; the most commonly investigated of these constructs were health, the environment, and taste. No attempt was made to analyze associations between the underlying constructs and participants' character-istics, however. Finally, a fourth narrative systematic review of "why" was based on 55 studies of organic food product-related factors associated with consumer credi-bility and trust in the product [1]. Labeling, certification, and country of origin were consistently related to consumer trust in organic foods.

Despite the absence of systematic reviews of the "who," several high-quality, population-based surveys paint a fairly clear portrait of which individual character-istics predict or influence the consumption of organic foods. The largest of these is Nutrinet-Santé, a web-based repeated questionnaire survey of over 100,000 French adults, only half of whom provided sufficient data for analysis [9]. The authors compared non-consumers, occasional consumers, and regular consumers of organic foods. Regular consumers were more highly educated and more physically active; ate more plant foods but less sweets, alcoholic beverages, and processed meats; had vitamin and mineral intakes that were closer to recommended nutritional guide-lines; and were less likely to be overweight or obese than non-consumers of organic foods. Only the associations with overweight and obesity were adjusted for con-founding due to other participant characteristics. Occasional consumers of organic foods had characteristics that were generally intermediate between those of regular consumers and non-consumers.

In a statewide, computer-assisted telephone survey in Tennessee, 1838 adults (out of 9339 households contacted) responded to questions about their characteris-tics and their consumption of organic foods [10]. About half of the respondents were organic food consumers, of whom only 22% consumed them on a daily basis. Organic food consumers were older, more likely to be White, and had higher educa-tion and income than non-consumers. No differences were observed in sex between the two groups. Consumers were significantly more likely to believe that organic foods taste better and contain fewer hormones and antibiotics than conventional (non-organic) foods. None of these associations were mutually adjusted; that is, they are not necessarily statistically independent of one another.

A representative population-based, interviewer-administered survey included 1710 adults living in Campinas, a Brazilian city near Sao Paulo [11]. Slightly more than one-quarter of the participants reported at least some consumption of organic foods. Increased schooling and income were significantly associated with organic food consumption, which was also more frequent in women than in men. No signifi-cant differences were found between seniors and non-senior adults.

In a randomly selected population sample from nine cities in central Ecuador, Moreno-Miranda and coworkers conducted face-to-face, questionnaire-based inter-views with 382 heads of households to identify factors contributing to their inten-tion to purchase organic foods [12]. Purchasing intent was similar in men and women but was significantly higher in younger respondents and in those with higher education and income.

Finally, in a much larger population-based face-to-face food consumption survey of 3300 adults in South Korea, Han and Lee investigated socioeconomic factors influencing participants' reported frequency of their consumption of organic foods [13]. Women reported significantly higher frequency of consumption than men;

other factors significantly associated with more frequent consumption were younger age, higher education and income, and living in Seoul.

Key Evidence Points
- Organic food consumption has increased markedly in recent years.
- Consumers of organic foods tend be younger, better educated, and wealthier than non-consumers.
- Preference for organic over conventional foods is based on beliefs about its better taste, improved nutritional value, lower exposure to environmental chemical contaminants, and greater respect for animal welfare.
- Rigorous, blinded taste tests have shown no taste preference for organic foods.
- Organic foods contain lower amounts of pesticides and a higher content of antioxidant nutrients and of omega-3 fatty acids than conventional foods.
- Organic meat is less likely to be contaminated by pathogenic (disease-producing) bacteria that are resistant to antibiotics, which contribute to selection for antibiotic resistance in the community.
- No beneficial health effects of the above-noted differences in content have been documented in consumers of organic foods.
- Observational studies of potential health benefits are confounded (biased) by differences in lifestyle factors between consumers of organic versus conventional foods, and large randomized trials are required to demonstrate such benefits.

Detailed Review of the Evidence on Health Benefits of Organic Foods[1]

In the sections below, I will review the published evidence on the following purported benefits of organic food consumption:

- Better taste
- Lower exposure to chemical contaminants
- Difference in exposure to pathogenic (disease-causing) bacteria
- Improved nutrient content
- Improved health

---

[1] Readers who prefer to skip the Detailed Review should proceed to the Summary at the end of the chapter.

Do Organic Foods Taste Better?

Blinded experiments are essential to rigorously compare the taste of organic versus conventional (non-organic) foods, because of the obvious confirmation bias favoring organic food among people who consume those foods. I was unable to find a systematic review on this issue, but Bourn and Prescott's 2002 narrative, non-systematic review provides a balanced summary of research before that date [14]. The authors describe three categories of studies: discrimination, i.e., the ability to distinguish the two food types (organic vs. conventional); comparative ratings of qualitative descriptors, such as bitterness, sweetness, or juiciness; and overall taste preference of one food type over the other. The studies reviewed evaluated several fruit and vegetables, including tomatoes, carrots, spinach, grapes, corn, grapefruit, beetroot, kale, apples, lettuce, green beans, and potatoes. Most of the studies observed an inability to discriminate, similar descriptor ratings, and no clear preference between organic and conventional foods. The few results favoring the organic product were counterbalanced by others favoring the conventional product. For example, one study observed a preference for the organic tomato of one variety but for the conventional tomato of another variety [15]. Similarly, a second study from the same research group compared descriptive ratings of organic and conventional carrots from two different growing seasons [16]. The observed result was less sweetness and overall flavor for organic carrots in the first year, but no difference in sweetness and more aftertaste in the second year! [16]. The authors also point out the lack of control for possible differences in harvest time and modes of distribution of organic versus conventional foods.

In the two decades since the Bourn and Prescott review [14], studies have done little to alter the review's findings and conclusions. Lester and colleagues compared organic and conventional pink grapefruit juice in blinded taste tests [17]. The organic juice was rated as significantly more tart by the tasting panel, while the conventional juice was judged to be significantly sweeter and significantly higher on overall acceptance. Brown and coworkers compared the taste of chicken breasts in randomized and blinded taste tests among four different conditions: standard breeding, maize-fed, free-range, and organic [18]. Chickens with standard rearing were the most preferred, while organic chickens were the least preferred.

Kresova and coworkers carried out taste tests of a convenience sample of 138 walk-by volunteers in Kiel, Germany, to compare their preference for organic versus conventional fresh milk under both blinded and unblinded conditions [19]. Under blinded conditions, a clear preference for organic milk was expressed by 48% of the sample, while 41% clearly preferred the fresh milk, and the remaining 11% were indifferent between the two. The order of tasting the two milk types was fixed, however, rather than randomized. Moreover, the difference was significantly augmented in the unblinded taste tests, suggesting that confirmation bias due to unblinding had a larger effect than any true difference in taste preference. In contrast, however, a similar study of 174 volunteers from Raleigh, North Carolina, observed that a preference for organic over conventional milk in blinded (and randomized) taste tests was slightly blunted in unblinded tests [20].

Sorqvist and coworkers studied Swedish volunteers' preference for "eco-friendly" versus conventional coffee in randomized, blinded taste tests of two identical cups of coffee [21]. The participants were deliberately misled by the investigators by being told which of the cups contained eco-friendly coffee. Of the 44 participants, 27 preferred the coffee labeled as eco-friendly over the identical but conventionally-labeled alternative. This preference was more marked among participants who scored above the median on a brief questionnaire related to their purchase of eco-friendly products. In a recent blinded and randomized taste test in 108 volunteers from Nova Scotia, Canada, no significant differences were observed in preference for organic versus conventional arugula [22].

Unsurprisingly, confirmation bias due to non-blinding seems especially strong in children. In Soldavini and colleagues' study of 47 fourth- and fifth-grade students in Northern California, 72% of the children preferred the taste of cookies labeled as reduced-fat, 67% preferred crackers labeled as whole-grain, and 54% preferred fruit punch labeled as 100% juice over the *identical* product without the health claim of "reduced-fat," "whole-grain," or "100% juice" [23].

Do Organic Foods Provide Lower Exposure to Chemical Contaminants?

A systematic review and meta-analysis by Smith-Spangler and coworkers observed a 30% reduction in the detection of *any* pesticide among organic versus conventional crop foods (fruits, vegetables, and grains) [24]. Three of the included studies reported very low proportions of crop foods with pesticide levels exceeding maximal allowable European Union limits. No studies reported on pesticide contamination of meat, poultry, eggs, or milk. Two of the studies observed significantly lower levels of organophosphate pesticide metabolites in children on organic food diets than in those consuming conventional diets, but health effects of those differences were not examined. Baranski and colleagues' 2014 systematic review and meta-analysis evaluated 62 studies comparing cadmium concentrations in organic versus conventional crop foods and observed significantly lower concentrations of cadmium in the organic crops [25]. No significant differences were found in 34 studies comparing lead concentrations, nor in 3 studies comparing arsenic concentrations.

A recent narrative systematic review by Bergman and Pandhi focused on organic versus conventional rice [26]. The authors emphasize the lack of control for differences in soil conditions and length of time that fields were exposed to organic farming methods, as well as insufficient specification of rice variety. They found no consistent differences in arsenic, mercury, cadmium, chromium, or lead levels in studies comparing organic and conventional rice, although organic rice was far less likely to contain organochlorine, carbamate, or pyrethrin pesticide residues.

Do Organic and Conventional Foods Differ in Bacterial Contamination?

The Smith-Spangler systematic review and meta-analysis cited in the previous section also compared organic and conventional foods with respect to contamination by enteric (gastrointestinal) bacteria [24]. The main disease-causing enteric bacteria of concern are *E. coli*, *Campylobacter*, *Salmonella*, and *Listeria*. The authors found no difference in *E. coli* contamination of organic versus conventional crop foods. No published study in the review detected other enteric pathogens in produce, but detection rates of all four bacteria were much higher in meat, poultry, and eggs, with no statistically significant differences between organic and conventional foods. I was surprised by these results, given that conventional animal farming frequently uses feed containing antibiotics. Less surprising were the results comparing antibiotic-resistant bacterial contamination between organic and conventional pork and chicken. Five studies reported a one-third reduction in contaminants resistant to ampicillin (a commonly used antibiotic) in the organic meats, as well as a one-third reduction in contaminants resistant to three or more antibiotics.

Do Organic Foods Have a Better Nutrient Content?

Dangour and coworkers' 2009 systematic review and meta-analysis of 55 high-quality studies documented higher phosphorus and lower nitrogen concentrations in organically-grown food crops than in those grown conventionally [27]. These differences are almost certainly attributable to the high nitrogen content of commercial fertilizers used in conventional farming and the high phosphorus content of manure and plant-based fertilizers used in organic farming. The more limited studies of animal livestock products observed no significant nutrient differences.

The above-cited systematic review and meta-analysis by Smith-Spangler and colleagues [24] confirmed the higher phosphorus content and also found significantly higher levels of phenolic compounds in 153 studies comparing organic and conventional crops. Phenolic compounds are known antioxidants with potential, but unproven, benefits in human disease prevention. The previously cited, and slightly more recent, systematic review and meta-analysis by Baranski and coworkers confirmed the higher concentration of phenolic compounds, including individual differences in flavonoids, flavonols, anthocyanins, and carotenoids [25]. The above-mentioned narrative systematic review by Bergman and Pandhi found inconsistent differences between organic and conventional rice in content of calcium, iron, zinc, or flavonoid or other phenolic compounds [26].

The Smith-Spangler review reported no significant differences in vitamin content in the few studies comparing organic and conventional meats but did observe higher omega-3 long-chain polyunsaturated fatty acid (PUFA) levels in organic milk and organic chicken relative to their conventional counterparts [24]. The more recent systematic review and meta-analysis by Srednicka-Tober and coworkers was restricted to meat [28]. The authors observed a 20% higher omega-3 PUFA content and a slightly smaller difference in omega-6 PUFA in organic versus conventional meats. The differences were larger for poultry than for beef, pork, and lamb.

Does Organic Food Consumption Improve Health?

Vigar and colleagues' 2020 narrative systematic review (without meta-analysis) of the human health effects of organic food consumption included 35 publications: 15 publications based on 13 experimental trials and 20 publications based on 13 observational studies [29]. Some of the trials are labeled as "RCTs" (randomized controlled trials), but it is unclear whether or not the unlabeled trials randomized their treatment allocation. The observational studies (which the authors erroneously label as "observational cohorts") include many cross-sectional studies and at least one case-control study.

Of the trials, several were single-dose substitution of an organic versus a conventional food or beverage. No differences in blood or urine nutrient levels were observed in those trials. In whole-diet substitution trials lasting 4–5 days in children and up to 22 days in adults, however, marked reductions were found in urine pesticide metabolite concentrations in both children and adults consuming organic versus conventional food diets, as well as increases in blood antioxidant levels. In one non-randomized, unblinded Italian crossover trial, 100 healthy men were prescribed a conventional Mediterranean diet for 2 weeks, followed by an organic Mediterranean diet for 2 weeks. Fat mass was reported as over 6 kg lower, and percent body fat 10.5% lower, along with even larger increases in lean body mass, after only 2 weeks on the organic diet! Since no differences were observed in body weight, these enormous changes in body composition in 2 weeks are simply not credible. Inflammatory blood makers were also reported as markedly reduced after the organic diet.

Observational studies relating organic diets to health outcomes are plagued by bias due to confounding by the enormous lifestyle differences between consumers of organic versus conventional foods. These include quantitative and qualitative differences in intake of energy (calories), fruits and vegetables, whole-grain cereals and breads, as well as physical activity, smoking, alcohol consumption, and mental health. In addition, the potential for publication bias is substantial, since investigators are unlikely to submit observational studies showing no association between diet and disease outcome, and those submitted are unlikely to be accepted for publication. In Vigar and coworkers' narrative systematic review [29], disease outcomes studied include obesity, diabetes, cancer, and abnormal sperm counts in healthy adults; pre-eclampsia (high blood pressure and protein in the urine) in pregnant women; and hypospadias (a congenital anomaly of the penis), eczema, wheezing, and ear infections in children. No consistent benefits were demonstrated in the included studies of these disease outcomes. A more recent systematic review of four observational studies by Bhagavathula and colleagues, however, focused on obesity and also included a meta-analysis [30]. The authors observed a modest (11%) but statistically significant reduction in risk of obesity associated with organic diets, although the potential for confounding by lifestyle factors associated with organic food consumption creates a large potential for biasing this association.

Finally, a recent narrative systematic review by Liu and coworkers was limited to four observational studies of consumption of organic foods during pregnancy [31]. Only one of those studies was published after the above-mentioned Vigar review [29]. That study observed no significant difference in risk of gestational diabetes among mothers consuming an organic food diet during pregnancy [32].

Summary

Organic food consumption has increased markedly over the last several decades. Consumers of organic foods are younger, better educated, and wealthier than non-consumers. Their reasons for preferring organic over conventional foods are varied and numerous, including better taste, improved nutritional value, lower exposure to environmental chemical contaminants (pesticides, herbicides, and fertilizers), and greater respect for animal welfare. Most organic food consumers are willing to pay a somewhat higher price for their organic food products.

My review of the scientific evidence revealed no taste preference for organic foods in rigorous, blinded taste tests. Organic foods contain markedly lower amounts of pesticides and a higher content of antioxidant nutrients and of omega-3 fatty acids. But healthy diets with adequate intakes of fruits, vegetables, and fish provide ample quantities of these nutrients. Moreover, no health benefits have been demonstrated for these differences in pesticide and nutrient contents. Conventional meats are more likely to be contaminated by pathogenic (disease-producing) bacteria that are resistant to antibiotics. These bacteria are important from a public health perspective—not because eating the meat is a cause of human infection, but because strains that are resistant to currently available antibiotics will be more difficult to treat if they infect humans through other routes of infection.

Randomized trials comparing health outcomes in consumers of organic versus conventional diets have been variable in their methodologic quality. The trials report lower blood and urine levels of pesticide metabolites and higher levels of antioxidants but no convincing differences in health outcomes. Given the enormous differences in diet, physical activity, and other lifestyle factors between consumers of organic versus conventional diets, observational studies contribute little or nothing to the scientific evidence base. Large, rigorous randomized trials are required. Based on the available evidence, organic foods do not appear to confer health benefits but may be preferred by some consumers for environmental reasons.

References

1. Nagy LB, Lakner Z, Temesi Á. Is it really organic? Credibility factors of organic food—a systematic review and bibliometric analysis. PLoS One. 2022;17(4):e0266855.
2. U.S. Department of Agriculture Economic Research Service. Organic market summary and trends. 6 May 2022.

3. Rangel G. From corgis to corn: a brief look at the long history of GMO technology. Science in the News. 9 Aug 2015.
4. Genetically modified organism. https://en.wikipedia.org/w/index.php?title=Genetically_modified_organism&oldid=1088923067.
5. History of organic farming. https://en.wikipedia.org/w/index.php?title=History_of_organic_farming&oldid=1055774076.
6. Sebastian-Ponce MI, Sanz-Valero J, Wanden-Berghe C. Consumer reaction to information on the labels of genetically modified food. Rev Saude Publica. 2014;48(1):154–69.
7. Steinhauser J, Hamm U. Consumer and product-specific characteristics influencing the effect of nutrition, health and risk reduction claims on preferences and purchase behavior: a systematic review. Appetite. 2018;127:303–23.
8. Kushwah S, Dhir A, Sagar M, Gupta B. Determinants of organic food consumption: a systematic literature review on motives and barriers. Appetite. 2019;143:104402.
9. Kesse-Guyot E, Péneau S, Méjean C, Szabo de Edelenyi F, Galan P, Hercberg S, Lairon D. Profiles of organic food consumers in a large sample of French adults: results from the Nutrinet-Santé cohort study. PLoS One. 2013;8(10):e76998.
10. Gwira Baumblatt JA, Carpenter LR, Wiedeman C, Dunn JR, Schaffner W, Jones TF. Population survey of attitudes and beliefs regarding organic, genetically modified, and irradiated foods. Nutr Health. 2017;23(1):7–11.
11. Medina LPB, Barros MBA, Fisberg RM, de Assumpção D, Barros Filho AA. Sociodemographic inequalities in eating practices and concerns. Public Health Nutr. 2021;24(14):4514–21.
12. Moreno-Miranda C, Franco-Crespo C, Pachucho I, Uño K, Gordillo A, Ortiz J. Socioeconomic characteristics, purchasing preferences and willingness to consume organic food: a cross-location comparison of nine cities in Central Ecuador. Foods. 2022;11(24):3979.
13. Han S, Lee Y. Analysis of the impacts of social class and lifestyle on consumption of organic foods in South Korea. Heliyon. 2022;8(10):e10998.
14. Bourn D, Prescott J. A comparison of the nutritional value, sensory qualities, and food safety of organically and conventionally produced foods. Crit Rev Food Sci Nutr. 2002;42(1):1–34.
15. Johansson L, Haglund A, Berglund L, Lea P, Risvik E. Preference for tomatoes, affected by sensory attributes and information about growth conditions. Food Qual Pref. 1999;10:289–98.
16. Haglund A, Johansson L, Berglund L, Dahlstedt L. Sensory evaluation of carrots from ecological and conventional growing systems. Food Qual Pref. 1999;10:23–9.
17. Lester GE, Manthey JA, Buslig BS. Organic vs. conventionally grown Rio Red whole grapefruit and juice: comparison of production inputs, market quality, consumer acceptance, and human health-bioactive compounds. J Agric Food Chem. 2007;55(11):4474–80.
18. Brown SN, Nute GR, Baker A, Hughes SI, Warriss PD. Aspects of meat and eating quality of broiler chickens reared under standard, maize-fed, free-range or organic systems. Br Poult Sci. 2008;49(2):118–24.
19. Kresova S, Gutjahr D, Hess S. German consumer evaluations of milk in blind and nonblind tests. J Dairy Sci. 2022;105(4):2988–3003.
20. Harwood WS, Drake MA. The influence of automatic associations on preference for milk type. J Dairy Sci. 2020;103(12):11218–27.
21. Sörqvist P, Hedblom D, Holmgren M, Haga A, Langeborg L, Nöstl A, Kågström J. Who needs cream and sugar when there is eco-labeling? Taste and willingness to pay for "eco-friendly" coffee. PLoS One. 2013;8(12):e80719.
22. Barker S, Moss R, McSweeney MB. Identification of sensory properties driving consumers' liking of commercially available kale and arugula. J Sci Food Agric. 2022;102(1):198–205.
23. Soldavini J, Crawford P, Ritchie LD. Nutrition claims influence health perceptions and taste preferences in fourth- and fifth-grade children. J Nutr Educ Behav. 2012;44(6):624–7.
24. Smith-Spangler C, Brandeau ML, Hunter GE, Bavinger JC, Pearson M, Eschbach PJ, Sundaram V, Liu H, Schirmer P, Stave C, Olkin I, Bravata DM. Are organic foods safer or healthier than conventional alternatives? A systematic review. Ann Intern Med. 2012;157(5):348–66.
25. Barański M, Srednicka-Tober D, Volakakis N, Seal C, Sanderson R, Stewart GB, Benbrook C, Biavati B, Markellou E, Giotis C, Gromadzka-Ostrowska J, Rembiałkowska E, Skwarło-Sońta K, Tahvonen R, Janovská D, Niggli U, Nicot P, Leifert C. Higher antioxidant and lower

cadmium concentrations and lower incidence of pesticide residues in organically grown crops: a systematic literature review and meta-analyses. Br J Nutr. 2014;112(5):794–811.

26. Bergman C, Pandhi M. Organic rice production practices: effects on grain end-use quality, healthfulness, and safety. Foods. 2023;12(1):73.
27. Dangour AD, Dodhia SK, Hayter A, Allen E, Lock K, Uauy R. Nutritional quality of organic foods: a systematic review. Am J Clin Nutr. 2009;90(3):680–5.
28. Średnicka-Tober D, Barański M, Seal C, Sanderson R, Benbrook C, Steinshamn H, Gromadzka-Ostrowska J, Rembiałkowska E, Skwarło-Sońta K, Eyre M, Cozzi G, Krogh Larsen M, Jordon T, Niggli U, Sakowski T, Calder PC, Burdge GC, Sotiraki S, Stefanakis A, Yolcu H, Stergiadis S, Chatzidimitriou E, Butler G, Stewart G, Leifert C. Composition differences between organic and conventional meat: a systematic literature review and meta-analysis. Br J Nutr. 2016;115(6):994–1011.
29. Vigar V, Myers S, Oliver C, Arellano J, Robinson S, Leifert C. A systematic review of organic versus conventional food consumption: is there a measurable benefit on human health? Nutrients. 2019;12(1):7.
30. Bhagavathula AS, Vidyasagar K, Khubchandani J. Organic food consumption and risk of obesity: a systematic review and meta-analysis. Healthcare (Basel). 2022;10(2):231.
31. Liu B, Curl CL, Brantsæter AL, Torjusen H, Sun Y, Du Y, Lehmler HJ, Balentine A, Snetselaar LG, Bao W. Perspective: organic food consumption during pregnancy and the potential effects on maternal and offspring health. Adv Nutr. 2023;14(1):12–21.
32. Simões-Wüst AP, Moltó-Puigmartí C, van Dongen MCJM, Thijs C. Organic food use, meat intake, and prevalence of gestational diabetes: KOALA birth cohort study. Eur J Nutr. 2021;60(8):4463–72.

Protein Supplements: Bulk or Bilk?

17

Introduction

For many years, I have worked out in gyms in a not-very-successful battle to avoid or reduce loss of muscle mass as I age. Before and after my work-outs, I have witnessed many teenage boys and young men in their early twenties consuming large quantities of thick, opaque liquids. (I hope they taste better than they look, but I fear the reverse may be true!) They usually drink these liquids from large plastic containers that they keep in their gym lockers and vigorously shake before consuming their contents.

But more interesting to me than the visual spectacle of the shaking and drinking are the discussions I have heard about which brands are best, what portion size is optimal, and when (before or after weightlifting and other resistance exercise) the protein shakes are most effective. If you have read this far in the book, you will not be surprised to learn that my fascination on hearing these conversations was tinged with extreme skepticism. The boys and men I saw and overheard were certainly not protein-deficient; their diets likely contained ample amounts of meat, fish, milk, and soy and other plant protein. How could drinking a slurry of protein, protein hydrolysates (partially digested protein), or amino acids help them bulk up, that is, help build up their muscle mass above and beyond the effects of their exercise? Nothing I had learned about biochemistry, nutrition, or protein metabolism in medical school or my pediatrics residency suggested that such practice would be beneficial in their quest to bulk up. Skepticism is a good way to start, but it is no substitute for rigorous scientific evidence (Fig. 17.1).

Proteins are one of the three major macronutrients ("macro" from the Greek word meaning large), along with carbohydrates and fats, contained in the foods we eat. They are macronutrients because their quantities in the diet are measured in grams (or ounces) and kilograms (pounds), as opposed to the micronutrients like vitamins, minerals, and essential fatty acids, which are measured in milligrams or micrograms, that is, thousandths or even millionths of an ounce. The building blocks of proteins are called amino acids, which contain atoms of carbon, nitrogen,

Fig. 17.1 Protein
supplement "shakes" are
very popular among body
builders

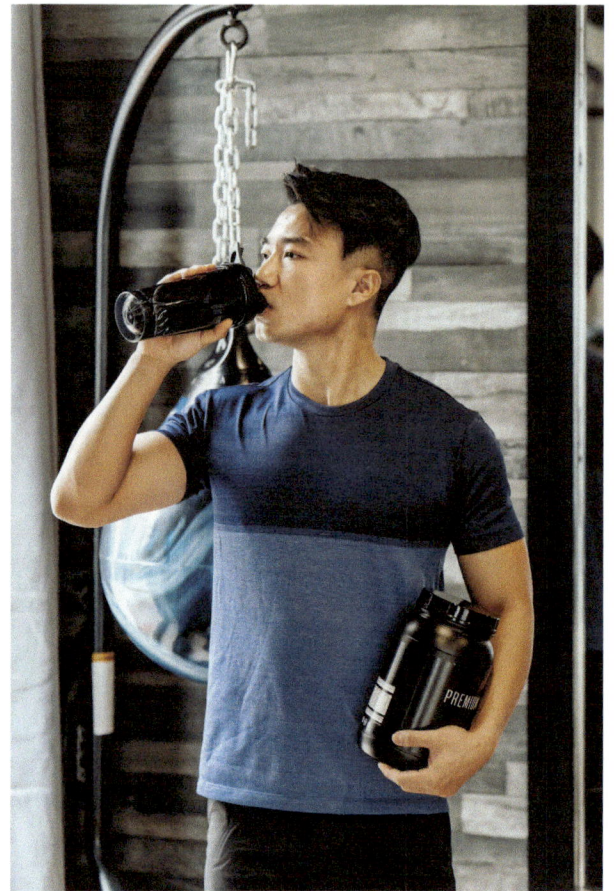

oxygen, and hydrogen. Carbohydrates are foods containing carbon, oxygen, and hydrogen in the form of sugars and starches, but no nitrogen. Fats also contain carbon, oxygen, and hydrogen without nitrogen, in the form of fatty acids and molecules called triglycerides, which contain three fatty acids bound to an alcohol called glycerol. Excess dietary carbohydrate can be stored in small quantities in the liver and muscle as a starch called glycogen but can also be converted to triglycerides and stored in large fat depots under the skin and in the abdominal cavity. Protein can be used for energy, but unlike carbohydrates and fats, excessive protein intake cannot be stored and must be metabolized to urea in the liver, which is then excreted by the kidneys into the urine.

Protein Supplements to Increase Muscle Mass and Strength: A Brief History

In ancient Greece, Spartan warriors were given extra-large meals to boost their size and strength. Milo of Croton, a sixth-century BC Greek wrestler, supplemented his training by consuming 9 kg of meat, 9 kg of bread, and 18 pints of wine *per day*! [1].

In the 1910s, Eugen Sandow, widely touted as the first modern bodybuilder, advocated consumption of Plasmon, a German whey protein, which is derived from milk after removing the curd (casein) protein [1, 2]. Sandow moved to England, but Plasmon's popularity there fell during World War I because of anti-German sentiment. In the 1950s and 1960s, bodybuilding gained widespread popularity. Irvin Johnson, Robert Hoffman, and Joe Weider combined their reputations as bodybuilders with considerable marketing skills and financial ambition to champion egg and milk protein powders [2]. It goes without saying that rigorous scientific evidence was *not* a component of their pitch. Photographs of muscle-bound men, along with a few apocryphal before-and-after testimonials, were all that was required to sell their products. In more recent years, heavily marketed powders with improved consistency and taste, bearing such names as Met RX, Muscle Milk, and Craze, have led to skyrocketing sales. Current global sales have been estimated at $20 billion per year [3].

In the U.S., where consumption of protein supplements is the highest, the Food and Drug Administration (FDA) never required manufacturers of dietary supplements to show evidence of their effectiveness, as they do with drugs. Since 1994, the FDA no longer even requires evidence of safety. It is unsurprising, therefore, that some protein supplements have been adulterated with illegal ingredients, including anabolic steroids with known muscle- and performance-enhancing properties [4]. In 2015, *Consumer Reports* reported unsafe levels of several toxic heavy metals in the protein powders they tested, including arsenic, cadmium, lead, and mercury. Craze, which is sold by both Walmart and Amazon, was even found to contain a methamphetamine-like stimulant, which led several athletes to fail their drug tests [5].

Current Beliefs and Practices Concerning Protein Supplements

I started this chapter by recounting the conversations I overheard at my local gym by teenage boys and young men who kept protein shakers in their gym lockers and discussed the best brands, the best timing before or after weightlifting, and other niceties of protein supplement shakes. As in other chapters in this book, I do not want readers to be limited by my experiences and anecdotes. In this section, therefore, I will summarize the scientific literature I found on who consumes protein supplements, their principal reasons for consuming them, and which regimens they prefer.

The only systematic review I was able to find on these topics was a narrative review limited to five studies of high school rugby players in South Africa [6]. The five studies reported a range of 30–54% sport supplement use, of which the most frequently consumed were protein supplements. The remainder of studies I located were all individual studies.

Whitehouse and Lawlis administered written questionnaires to 87 male and female athletes aged 13–18 years recruited from sports clubs in Canberra, Australia [7]. These athletes trained in their specific sport from 3 to 12 or more hours per week. Overall, 60% reported taking protein supplements. A slightly higher percentage of boys reported using the supplements, and boys and girls over age 16 were significantly more likely to consume them than younger teens. Coaches were the major provider of information on supplements. The most common types of supplements used were whey protein powders, protein bars, and pre-mixed protein drinks. The major reasons cited for supplement use were muscle "recovery," improved performance, and injury prevention. Timing was most often after training or competition. Most of the participants consumed the supplement daily or a few days per week. More than half of the respondents believed that supplement use carried some risks; some were worried about contaminating ingredients, others about weight gain, but many had only vague concerns about adverse effects on health.

Manore and colleagues surveyed 535 high school soccer players from 13 schools and 24 soccer teams in Oregon about their nutrition knowledge and behaviors [8]. Written questionnaires were completed in the schools. Some nutritional supplement use was reported by nearly half of the participants; 30% reported consuming a protein shake or beverage. The latter were one-third more likely to be used by boys than girls, and Latino participants were 80% more likely than Whites to use protein supplements.

Among adults, Austin and coworkers reported two cross-sectional surveys, each recruiting around 1000 personnel from 10 U.S. army bases in 2006–07 and 11 bases in 2010–11 [9]. In both surveys, protein or amino acid supplements were the second most common (after multivitamins) type of nutritional supplement consumed, and prevalence of their use was higher in men than in women. Reported use of protein supplements rose from 24% to 30% among men in the 4 years between the two surveys but fell from 13% to 6% among women.

Since my initial exposure to protein supplements was in gyms, I was particularly interested in the survey by Sánchez Oliver and colleagues, who recruited 415 adult participants (260 men, 155 women) from four gyms in Seville [10]. Every third client was asked to complete a questionnaire at the gym on weekdays, evenings, and weekends. Of the men, 43% reported using protein powder supplements, compared to only 3% of the women participants. Most of the supplements were derived from whey protein, and about 20% each consumed them before, after, or both before and after training, with the remainder consuming them in the morning and/or evening irrespective of training.

Tsitsimpikou and coworkers distributed questionnaires to 329 clients (180 men, 149 men) at the reception desk of 11 gyms in Athens, Greece [11]. Over 40% reported using nutritional supplements, among whom protein or amino acid supplements were the most common type (62.5%), especially among the men. Finally, a recent study by Brisebois and colleagues recruited over 2500 CrossFit gym users by distributing flyers at the gyms, mostly in the U.S. [12]. Participants agreed to complete an online questionnaire; over 80% of them reported using one or more nutritional supplements, and over half of those consumed a protein supplement. The most common reasons cited (by 40–50% of participants) for consuming supplements overall were to speed recovery, improve overall health, increase muscle mass or strength, and improve CrossFit performance.

Protein supplement use is common even among physically impaired athletes. Graham-Paulson and coworkers recruited 255 elite and 144 non-elite impaired athletes attending competitions or training camps in the U.K., Canada, USA, Switzerland, and Germany [13]. Protein supplements in the form of powders, liquids, or bars were the most common type of supplement consumed (26%), exceeding use of hydrating sports drinks (20%) and multivitamins (14%). Common reasons given for consuming performance-enhancing supplements (not restricted to protein) were to support "exercise recovery," boost energy, and increase strength.

Key Evidence Points
- Nutritional supplements have been used by elite athletes since Greek antiquity.
- Protein supplements have been "promoted" and financially profitable for body building for over a century.
- Protein supplements are largely unregulated, despite several well-documented instances of adulterated products.
- Randomized trials have clearly shown that protein supplements are effective in improving muscle mass, strength, and other aspects of physical performance, when combined with resistance training.
- These benefits have been demonstrated in healthy young adults, postmenopausal women, and the elderly.
- The type or source of protein has not been proven to be important, but higher doses (in terms of grams of protein per kg of body weight) appear to have larger effects.
- In younger adults, protein supplements have also been shown to speed recovery of muscle after resistance training and, when combined with aerobic (endurance) exercise training, to increase aerobic fitness.

Detailed Review of Scientific Evidence[1]

Individuals who consume protein supplements to improve their muscle mass and strength and athletic performance are likely to differ from non-consumers of supplements in their participation in physical activities such as weightlifting, other resistance training, and aerobic exercise. They may also differ in their diets, as well as in

---

[1] Readers who prefer to skip the Detailed Review should proceed to the Summary at the end of the chapter.

smoking, alcohol consumption, and drug use. These differences will confound any positive associations between consumption of protein supplements and muscle mass, strength, or fitness. It is difficult to imagine how all of these potential confounding factors could be accurately measured and controlled for in observational studies. Even in randomized trials, the use of a non-supplemented control group, or one based on water or a flavored beverage, prevents blinding and creates a strong potential for bias due to a placebo effect. Placebo-controlled trials with look- and taste-alike control supplements are therefore highly desirable for studying the causal effects of protein supplements. Unfortunately, however, in almost all of the trials included in the systematic reviews summarized below, the control group received no supplement or received a control supplement that could be easily distinguished from the protein supplement.

I will nonetheless summarize the evidence from systematic reviews of randomized supplementation trials in the remainder of this chapter. I will divide my evidence summary according to the goal and target population for protein supplementation by separating reviews of trials in healthy adults wishing to improve their muscle mass, strength, and performance from trials in the elderly. In the latter population, the goal is to correct or reduce aging-induced loss of muscle mass and strength and thereby prevent, delay, or slow the onset of frailty.

Protein Supplements in Healthy Adults

Two recent and comprehensive systematic reviews with meta-analyses by Tagawa and colleagues reported separately on lean body mass (which includes muscle but also internal organs, bone, and water) [14] and muscle strength [15]. The lean body mass review examines 105 randomized trials in over 5000 participants; half the trials combined weightlifting or other resistance training (in both the protein supplement and control groups), whereas the other half studied the effect of supplements in the absence of such training. The muscle strength review includes 82 randomized trials in nearly 4000 participants, with 70% of the trials combining resistance training and protein supplementation and the other 30% studying supplements alone. The supplements were given for at least a 2-week period, and the doses of supplemental protein varied over a fairly wide range. Overall, the supplemented group had an increase in muscle mass (usually measured as lean body mass or fat-free mass) of half a kilogram (1.1 pounds) relative to the control group and was similar in those trials with or without inclusion of resistance training [14]. The increase in muscle mass was even higher (0.8 kg, or 1.8 lb) in those studies using a higher dose of protein in their supplement.

In the muscle strength review [15], the combined supplement plus training group had a modest (2%) but statistically significant increase in strength, while those receiving supplements alone had no increase. As with muscle mass, a dose–response effect on muscle strength was noted with increasing amounts of protein: 0.7% increase per 0.1 g of protein per kg of body weight up to 1.5 g per kg, after which no further increase was observed. Morton and coworkers' earlier systematic review and meta-analysis of trials that combined resistance training and protein supplementation for at least 6 weeks observed a significant increase in muscle strength of 2.5 kg (5.5 lb), i.e., the supplemented participants were able to lift weights that were heavier by that amount [16]. To put that difference in context, however, the increase in muscle strength observed due to the resistance training alone was 27 kg, that is, over ten times higher.

A fourth systematic review and meta-analysis by Lin and colleagues focused on randomized trials of the effects of protein supplementation on aerobic fitness, as determined by peak oxygen consumption [17]. The 19 trials in the Lin review included 1162 participants and combined protein supplementation with endurance (aerobic) training like running, cycling, or brisk walking, rather than weightlifting or other resistance training. A statistically significant increase in aerobic fitness was observed in the participants randomized to the protein supplement. The magnitude of the difference was about 25% of the increase observed with the aerobic training alone.

Other systematic reviews of protein supplement trials have focused on the type of protein supplemented. These include trials of beef protein versus whey protein [18], hydrolyzed (chemically digested) protein versus other supplements [19], and trials restricted to supplementation with whey protein [20]. The results of these systematic reviews were consistent with those detailed above and did not reveal any novel effects of protein supplementation.

A recent systematic review and meta-analysis of 29 randomized trials by Pearson and coworkers focused on a different outcome: recovery of muscle after a bout of resistance training [21]. Protein supplementation before or right after training resulted in substantial (around half a standard deviation) and statistically significant increases in muscle contraction measures and reduction in muscle damage, as reflected by blood concentration of the muscle enzyme creatine kinase, from 24 to 72 h after resistance exercise.

On the other hand, Kloby Nielsen and colleagues' systematic review and meta-analysis of trials comparing combined protein and carbohydrate supplements to carbohydrate-only supplements supports my concern about the potential for bias due to non-blinding in virtually all protein supplementation trials [22]. Improvements in athletic performance were significantly larger in analyses of all trials comparing participants randomized to supplements combining protein and carbohydrates to those randomized to carbohydrate-only supplements. (Carbohydrate-only supplements were given to the control group in many of the supplementation trials included in the reviews I have summarized in this section.) No difference was observed, however, in those trials in which the combined protein and carbohydrate supplements and carbohydrate-only supplements had the same energy (calorie) content. This result could suggest that the protein content has no beneficial effect on performance beyond providing additional calories!

Despite these concerns, it is difficult to understand how bias due to non-blinding could affect objective outcomes like muscle mass measured by dual-energy X-ray absorption (DEXA). Knowledge of treatment received might affect effort in outcomes like lifting weights or fitness tests, but not DEXA results, especially in the absence of concomitant resistance training. Even if the mechanism by which protein supplementation improves outcomes is incompletely understood, the evidence strongly suggests beneficial effects. The magnitude of those effects is probably smaller, however, than those of training.

Protein Supplements in the Elderly

Several systematic reviews and meta-analyses have been published on the effects of protein supplementation, alone or combined with a training program, on muscle mass, strength, and physical performance in the elderly. A few of the randomized trials included in those reviews have focused on preventing the decline in these outcomes that usually occurs with aging, but the majority have attempted to rectify, at least partially, losses that have already occurred. Those losses increase the risks of falls and their consequences, including disability and death. Given the aging of the population in most industrialized countries, these adverse consequences constitute an important global public health burden.

Kuo and colleagues' recent systematic review focused on randomized trials of whey protein supplementation, either alone or in combination with resistance training, in postmenopausal women 55 years of age or more [23]. As summarized above for trials in young, healthy adults, protein supplementation in combination with resistance training resulted in a substantial (0.7 standard deviations) increase in biceps muscle strength and a large (1.1 standard deviations) increase in lower-limb lean mass, which includes muscle, bone, and water. No effect on either outcome was observed for protein supplementation alone in the absence of resistance training.

A recent narrative, non-quantitative "umbrella review" (a review of reviews) by Gielen and coworkers included 15 systematic reviews of randomized trials of protein and other nutritional supplements in men and women 65 years of age or older [24]. Four of the systematic reviews were restricted to trials of protein supplementation alone, with positive effects on muscle mass but equivocal results for muscle strength and physical performance. Four systematic reviews of trials of protein supplementation combined with resistance training observed positive effects on muscle strength as well as muscle mass, but not on physical performance. Four other systematic reviews of protein supplementation combined with variable combinations of balance training, walking, aerobic exercise, and resistance training found positive intervention effects on muscle mass, but not on muscle strength or physical performance.

Hou and coworkers' 2019 systematic review and meta-analysis of randomized trials of protein supplementation [25], with resistance training in both the supplemented and control groups, was not included in the Gielen review. The Hou review provides quantitative meta-analytic estimates of the effects of protein supplementation when added to resistance training. Supplementation led to small but highly statistically significant increases in fat-free (lean) body mass (which includes internal organs, bone, muscle, and water) by 0.23 kg, or half a pound; limb (arm and leg) muscle mass by 0.39 kg, or nearly a pound; both handgrip and leg strength by about

0.3 kg; but no effect on measures of physical function, including gait speed or time to stand up from a chair. A more recent systematic review and meta-analysis by Kirwan and colleagues included trials of protein supplementation with and without resistance training and found slightly higher, and statistically more significant, benefits of supplementation among those trials that incorporated resistance training than in trials of supplementation alone [26]. Negm and coworkers' recent so-called network meta-analysis is based on mathematical modeling of comparisons of three or more interventions studied in separate randomized trials of pairs of interventions. It attempts to compare the effects of supplementation, resistance training, aerobic exercise, and other forms of physical activity in adults with sarcopenia (reduced muscle mass and strength) but is not restricted to the elderly [27]. Their analysis confirms the value of these interventions on muscle mass, strength, and physical performance.

I will not separately summarize the systematic reviews included in the above-mentioned umbrella and network reviews. Instead, I will limit my comments to recent reviews and trials not included above. Tu and colleagues' 2021 systematic review included randomized trials of protein and other types of supplements in the elderly [28]. The authors do not explicitly mention a physical activity component, but several of the trials did include such a component in both the supplemented and control groups. One of the trials published in 2020 included an exercise program 5 days per week in both the supplemented and control groups and observed strong positive effects of the protein supplement on muscle mass, handgrip strength, and the Short Physical Performance Battery, which incorporates components testing balance, gait speed, and standing up from a chair [29].

Evidence from laboratory studies suggests that branched-chain amino acids like leucine, isoleucine, and valine may offer advantages over straight-chain amino acids in stimulating protein synthesis in human muscle. A recent systematic review of 35 randomized trials of supplementation of older adults with branched-chain amino acids, or of proteins such as whey protein that are rich in branched-chain amino acids, compared these supplements to placebo or carbohydrate-containing supplements—but not to other protein supplements without enrichment of branched-chain amino acids [30]. Most of the trials also included an exercise program in both the supplementation and control groups. Given the results summarized so far, it is not surprising that the meta-analysis demonstrated moderate effects on muscle mass, strength, and physical performance. But the absence of a head-to-head comparison with other protein supplements makes it impossible to infer any "special" or extra effect of branched-chain amino acid-enriched proteins on these outcomes. Another recent systematic review and meta-analysis of leucine-rich protein supplements was restricted to six small randomized trials in elderly adults with sarcopenia (low muscle mass) [31]. Again, these supplements were not compared to other types of protein supplements, and half of the trials also included a training or exercise component. The authors observed a significant increase in muscle strength in the supplemented group, but no "special" effect of leucine-rich protein supplements can be inferred.

Finally, a 2020 systematic review and meta-analysis by Oktaviana and colleagues of eight randomized trials was restricted to frail elderly participants (at least 65 years of age), based on recognized criteria for frailty, or elderly adults living in residential care [32]. In other words, healthy seniors were excluded from the trials reviewed. No significant differences between the supplemented and control groups were observed in lean body mass, muscle strength, or physical performance. Nonetheless, most of the differences favored the supplemented group, and the magnitude of those differences was similar to those reported in the meta-analyses summarized above. Moreover, the trials were small (the largest recruited 100 participants), and the only three trials that also included an exercise program in both the supplemented and control groups observed significant differences favoring the protein-supplemented group. It would be unjustified, therefore, to infer that protein supplement is ineffective in frail, elderly persons.

Summary

Protein supplements have been popular among body builders and other athletes for over a century and remain largely unregulated, despite several well-documented instances of adulteration. The popularity of protein shakes has increased in recent years, especially among men. When combined with resistance training, randomized trials of protein supplementation have observed modest increases in muscle mass, strength, and physical performance in healthy young adults, postmenopausal women, and the elderly. The effects on muscle mass and strength show a dose-response relationship, that is, the increase is larger when the daily dose of protein supplement is higher, but no clear evidence from randomized trials indicates differences in effect according to the type or source of protein. In younger adults, protein supplements have also been shown to speed recovery of muscle after resistance training, and positive effects on aerobic fitness have been observed when the supplements are combined with aerobic (endurance) training.

The control groups in these trials are prone to bias due to non-blinding, since the control groups usually receive either no supplementation or a supplement that is easily distinguishable by appearance or taste from the protein supplement. Nonetheless, it is difficult to argue that non-blinding can lead to bias in ascertaining an objective outcome like muscle mass, which is usually measured by an X-ray technique like dual-energy X-ray absorptiometry (DEXA) or by bioelectrical impedance. Thus even though the physiological and biochemical mechanisms of the beneficial effect remain unclear, protein supplementation may be useful for increasing muscle mass and strength and physical performance among athletes and other healthy persons and for delaying the decline in these outcomes that accompanies normal aging.

References

1. Mackenzie C. This history of protein supplements. Healthy for Men. 3 July 2018.
2. Schinetsky R. The complete history of protein powder. Tiger Fitness. 2 Oct 2018.

3. Miller J. The complete (and unusual) history of protein powder. Body Nutrition. 23 Aug 2021.
4. Savino G, Valenti L, D'Alisera R, Pinelli M, Persi Y, Trenti T, WDPP, Working Group Doping Prevention Project. Dietary supplements, drugs and doping in the sport society. Ann Ig. 2019;31(6):548–55.
5. Bodybuilding supplement. https://en.wikipedia.org/w/index.php?title=Bodybuilding_supplem ent&oldid=1092360271.
6. Harmse B, Noorbhai H. Sport supplement use among high school rugby players in South Africa: a scoping review. S Afr J Sports Med. 2022;34(1):v34i1a13348.
7. Whitehouse G, Lawlis T. Protein supplements and adolescent athletes: a pilot study investigating the risk knowledge, motivations and prevalence of use. Nutr Diet. 2017;74(5):509–15.
8. Manore MM, Patton-Lopez MM, Meng Y, Wong SS. Sport nutrition knowledge, behaviors and beliefs of high school soccer players. Nutrients. 2017;9(4):350.
9. Austin KG, Price LL, McGraw SM, McLellan TM, Lieberman HR. Longitudinal trends in use of dietary supplements by U.S. Army personnel differ from those of civilians. Appl Physiol Nutr Metab. 2016;41(12):1217–24.
10. Sánchez Oliver A, Miranda León MT, Guerra-Hernández E. Prevalence of protein supplement use at gyms. Nutr Hosp. 2011;26(5):1168–74.
11. Tsitsimpikou C, Chrisostomou N, Papalexis P, Tsarouhas K, Tsatsakis A, Jamurtas A. The use of nutritional supplements among recreational athletes in Athens, Greece. Int J Sport Nutr Exerc Metab. 2011;21(5):377–84.
12. Brisebois M, Kramer S, Lindsay KG, Wu CT, Kamla J. Dietary practices and supplement use among CrossFit® participants. J Int Soc Sports Nutr. 2022;19(1):316–35.
13. Graham-Paulson TS, Perret C, Smith B, Crosland J, Goosey-Tolfrey VL. Nutritional supplement habits of athletes with an impairment and their sources of information. Int J Sport Nutr Exerc Metab. 2015;25(4):387–95.
14. Tagawa R, Watanabe D, Ito K, Ueda K, Nakayama K, Sanbongi C, Miyachi M. Dose-response relationship between protein intake and muscle mass increase: a systematic review and meta-analysis of randomized controlled trials. Nutr Rev. 2020;79(1):66–75.
15. Tagawa R, Watanabe D, Ito K, Otsuyama T, Nakayama K, Sanbongi C, Miyachi M. Synergistic effect of increased total protein intake and strength training on muscle strength: a dose-response meta-analysis of randomized controlled trials. Sports Med Open. 2022;8(1):110.
16. Morton RW, Murphy KT, McKellar SR, Schoenfeld BJ, Henselmans M, Helms E, Aragon AA, Devries MC, Banfield L, Krieger JW, Phillips SM. A systematic review, meta-analysis and meta-regression of the effect of protein supplementation on resistance training-induced gains in muscle mass and strength in healthy adults. Br J Sports Med. 2018;52(6):376–84.
17. Lin YN, Tseng TT, Knuiman P, Chan WP, Wu SH, Tsai CL, Hsu CY. Protein supplementation increases adaptations to endurance training: a systematic review and meta-analysis. Clin Nutr. 2021;40(5):3123–32.
18. Valenzuela PL, Mata F, Morales JS, Castillo-García A, Lucia A. Does beef protein supplementation improve body composition and exercise performance? A systematic review and meta-analysis of randomized controlled trials. Nutrients. 2019;11(6):1429.
19. Shen M, Zhang W, Wu G, Zhu L, Qi X, Zhang H. A systematic review and meta-analysis: effects of protein hydrolysate supplementation on fat-free mass and strength in resistance-trained individuals. Crit Rev Food Sci Nutr. 2023;63:964–74.
20. Sepandi M, Samadi M, Shirvani H, Alimohamadi Y, Taghdir M, Goudarzi F, Akbarzadeh I. Effect of whey protein supplementation on weight and body composition indicators: a meta-analysis of randomized clinical trials. Clin Nutr ESPEN. 2022;50:74–83.
21. Pearson AG, Hind K, Macnaughton LS. The impact of dietary protein supplementation on recovery from resistance exercise-induced muscle damage: a systematic review with meta-analysis. Eur J Clin Nutr. 2023;77(8):767–83. https://doi.org/10.1038/s41430-022-01250-y.
22. Kloby Nielsen LL, Tandrup Lambert MN, Jeppesen PB. The effect of ingesting carbohydrate and proteins on athletic performance: a systematic review and meta-analysis of randomized controlled trials. Nutrients. 2020;12(5):1483.

23. Kuo YY, Chang HY, Huang YC, Liu CW. Effect of whey protein supplementation in post-menopausal women: a systematic review and meta-analysis. Nutrients. 2022;14(19):4210.
24. Gielen E, Beckwée D, Delaere A, De Breucker S, Vandewoude M, Bautmans I, Sarcopenia Guidelines Development Group of the Belgian Society of Gerontology and Geriatrics (BSGG). Nutritional interventions to improve muscle mass, muscle strength, and physical performance in older people: an umbrella review of systematic reviews and meta-analyses. Nutr Rev. 2021;79(2):121–47.
25. Hou L, Lei Y, Li X, Huo C, Jia X, Yang J, Xu R, Wang X. Effect of protein supplementation combined with resistance training on muscle mass, strength and function in the elderly: a systematic review and meta-analysis. J Nutr Health Aging. 2019;23(5):451–8.
26. Kirwan RP, Mazidi M, Rodríguez García C, Lane KE, Jafari A, Butler T, Perez de Heredia F, Davies IG. Protein interventions augment the effect of resistance exercise on appendicular lean mass and handgrip strength in older adults: a systematic review and meta-analysis of randomized controlled trials. Am J Clin Nutr. 2022;115(3):897–913.
27. Negm AM, Lee J, Hamidian R, Jones CA, Khadaroo RG. Management of sarcopenia: a network meta-analysis of randomized controlled trials. J Am Med Dir Assoc. 2022;23(5):707–14.
28. Tu DY, Kao FM, Tsai ST, Tung TH. Sarcopenia among the elderly population: a systematic review and meta-analysis of randomized controlled trials. Healthcare (Basel). 2021;9(6):650.
29. Rondanelli M, Cereda E, Klersy C, Faliva MA, Peroni G, Nichetti M, Gasparri C, Iannello G, Spadaccini D, Infantino V, Caccialanza R, Perna S. Improving rehabilitation in sarcopenia: a randomized-controlled trial utilizing a muscle-targeted food for special medical purposes. J Cachexia Sarcopenia Muscle. 2020;11(6):1535–47.
30. Bai GH, Tsai MC, Tsai HW, Chang CC, Hou WH. Effects of branched-chain amino acid-rich supplementation on EWGSOP2 criteria for sarcopenia in older adults: a systematic review and meta-analysis. Eur J Nutr. 2022;61(2):637–51.
31. Lee SY, Lee HJ, Lim JY. Effects of leucine-rich protein supplements in older adults with sarcopenia: a systematic review and meta-analysis of randomized controlled trials. Arch Gerontol Geriatr. 2022;102:104758.
32. Oktaviana J, Zanker J, Vogrin S, Duque G. The effect of protein supplements on functional frailty in older persons: a systematic review and meta-analysis. Arch Gerontol Geriatr. 2020;86:103938.

Prevention and Treatment of Jet Lag: What Works?

18

Introduction

The first mention of the term "jet lag" is attributed to Horace Sutton, a journalist writing in the *Los Angeles Times* in 1966. "If you're going to be a member of the Jet Set and fly off to Katmandu for coffee with King Mahendra," he wrote, "you can count on contracting Jet Lag, a debility not unakin to a hangover. Jet Lag derives from the simple fact that jets travel so fast they leave your body rhythms behind" [1]. Prior to air travel, it was not possible for humans to cross many time zones in a short period. And it is the crossing of at least five time zones that leads to a severe disruption in the body's physiologic functions, many of which are closely linked to the dark-light cycle. That cycle is of course finely tuned to the time of day. Crossing several time zones "confuses" the body's biological clock and diurnal, or circadian, rhythm of sleep, wakefulness, hunger, and body temperature, along with other brain functions and secretion of key hormones like cortisol [2].

In 1980, at the request of the U.S. Congress, the Federal Aviation Association (FAA) and the National Aeronautics and Space Administration collaborated in studying jet lag in over 500 airline pilots. The researchers found that the biological clock is tuned to a 25-h day, rather than the expected 24 h [1]. [The term "circadian" is derived from Latin: *circa* (near, approximate) + *diem* (day).] More recent studies have indicated a slightly shorter period of about 24.5 h [3]. Caucasian-Americans have been shown to have a slightly but statistically significantly longer circadian period than African-Americans [4].

Eastward travel is more likely to cause symptoms of jet lag than westward travel, probably because it is harder to advance our biological clock than to delay it [5]. Going westward, it usually takes about half the number of days as time zones to recover from jet lag. Going eastward, the general rule is about two-thirds as many days as the number of time zones crossed. But the earth is round, of course, so a trip half-way around the world results in the same severity and duration of jet lag symptoms, regardless of east- or westward flight path. I have traveled many times to

M. S. Kramer, *Believe It or Not*, https://doi.org/10.1007/978-3-031-46022-7_18

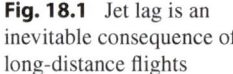
Fig. 18.1 Jet lag is an inevitable consequence of long-distance flights

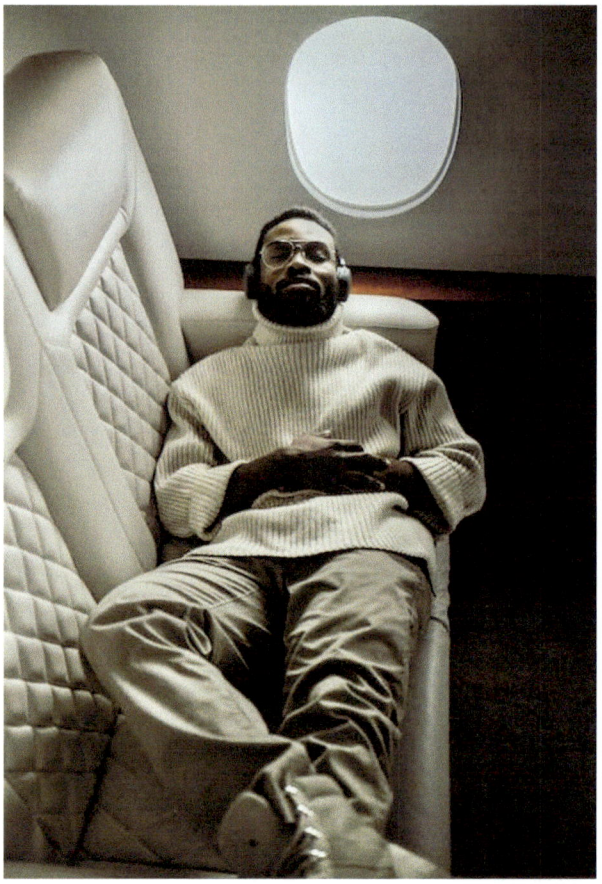

Singapore, sometimes flying east from Montreal across the Atlantic, other times west across the Pacific, with total travel times similar at about 24 h. Singapore is 12 h later than Montreal (13 h in winter, after daylight savings time ends), and it takes me about 5–6 days to adjust to the new time zone, regardless of which direction I fly.

Our biological clock is closely linked to the light-dark cycle created by the orbit of the earth around the sun [2, 5]. The control center for this clock is located in a part of the brain called the hypothalamus, in a collection of nerve cells called the supra-chiasmatic nucleus, just above (supra-) the crossing (chiasm) of the optic nerves from both eyes, which transmit light signals from the eyes to the brain. The nerve cells in this nucleus communicate with the pineal gland, which secretes the hormone melatonin in the absence of light (that is, at night). Melatonin secretion makes us sleepy. Persons with rigid sleep schedules and those over 60 years of age tend to have more difficulties with jet lag [3], but no significant differences have been noted between adolescents and adults (Fig. 18.1) [6].

Current Beliefs and Practices: Who Gets Jet Lag and What Do They Do About It?

Beh and colleagues' recent narrative systematic review comprises 22 studies of nearly 4000 adult air travelers, including passengers and flight crews, with a variety of study objectives and research designs [7]. Most of the studies focused on participants' travel priorities, knowledge about jet lag and travel fatigue, and self-reported strategies for managing those problems. Given the "mixed" bag of objectives, methods, and reported outcomes, it is difficult to extract much in the way of useful information from this review about the risks and risk factors for jet lag and about current beliefs and practices. I will therefore summarize some pertinent findings from several individual studies.

In a questionnaire-based survey of 140 international business travelers who worked in the oil and gas industry in western Canada, three-quarters reported jet lag and two-thirds reported difficulty sleeping during overseas trips [8]. In an online questionnaire-based survey of 107 Australian business travelers recruited through social media, two-thirds reported having experienced jet lag symptoms always or "fairly often" on their trips [9]. On the other hand, two-thirds of all respondents claimed that they were very good or good at managing jet lag on their trips. The most popular pre-flight measures they reported were sleeping well and exercising prior to leaving. During the flight, the most common measures were consuming extra water, napping, and using noise-canceling headphones. After arrival, the most cited measures were staying awake until bedtime, exposure to bright light, exercise, and use of melatonin or prescription sleep medication.

Bin and colleagues recruited a convenience sample of 460 adults taking flights of eight or more hours on Qantas Airways into or out of Australia, who were recruited online in the week prior to departure and contacted again 2–3 days after their arrival [10]. Acceptance (participation) rates were not reported. Participants were asked what strategies (from a list developed by the investigators) they used before, during, and after the flight to reduce jet lag. The most common strategies used were naps (especially during the flight, by 60%); deliberately altered sleep times (usually after the flight, 50%); consumption (47%) or avoidance (29%) of caffeinated drinks before, during, and/or after the flight; and consumption (47%) or avoidance (34%) of alcohol before, during, and/or after the flight. Nearly half altered the size of their meals, while 20% consumed vitamins or other dietary supplements. Fifteen percent took a prescription or over-the-counter sleep medication, but only 8% took oral melatonin.

In a recent questionnaire-based study carried out in 200 French military pilots and flight crew members, over 60% reported being affected by jet lag, a frequency that was lower in pilots and higher among flight crew members [11]. These reported rates did not differ significantly by age, but women reported being affected more frequently than men: 77% versus 57%. The most commonly used measures to combat jet lag were adjustment of sleep, additional exercise, increased exposure to sunlight, use of stimulants like caffeine, and consumption of melatonin or sleep medications.

Key Evidence Points
- Jet lag is a recent phenomenon (due to jet airplane travel) that occurs with the rapid crossing of five or more time zones and causes disruption of sleep and other bodily functions that are tuned to our "biological clock" and the light-dark cycle.
- Jet lag symptoms occur in the majority of travelers and are more severe and of longer duration after flights in the eastward than in the westward direction.
- Most international travelers manage their own jet lag symptoms, and many measures are used before, during, or after the flight to prevent those symptoms or treat them after they occur.
- Placebo-controlled randomized trials have shown beneficial effects on sleep of melatonin and of prescription Z-drugs taken for several nights after arrival.
- Non-drug measures such as bright light exposure, physical activity, and altered timing of meals require rigorous randomized trials of prevention and treatment.

Detailed Review of Scientific Evidence on Prevention or Treatment of Jet Lag[1]

What can be done to prevent jet lag in persons who are planning a long-haul flight, either before or during the flight? What can be done after arrival at the destination to treat jet lag symptoms once they occur? Considering the high probability of jet lag symptoms when crossing multiple time zones during long-haul flights, I assumed that preventive and treatment interventions would have been extensively studied. Nothing could be further from the truth! The dearth of studies is rivaled only by their poor quality. If you have read previous chapters in this book, and especially Chap. 1, you will understand why placebo-controlled randomized trials, preferably with blinding of both participants and investigators, are essential to avoid biases, especially confounding and reverse causality.

My search for systematic reviews of randomized trials to prevent or treat jet lag underlined the dearth of research on this topic. I was surprised to observe that most of the treatments tested in randomized trials focused on interventions initiated after arrival to relieve sleep difficulties and other jet lag symptoms, rather than initiated prior to travel and intended to prevent those symptoms. I was unable to find any systematic reviews or individual randomized trials of increased physical activity or changing the timing (advancing or delaying) of meals.

---

[1] <Footnote ID="Fn1"><Para ID="Par16">Readers who prefer to skip the Detailed Review should proceed to the Summary at the end of the chapter.</Para></Footnote>

The best and most complete systematic review of drug treatments, albeit somewhat dated, is the narrative review by Herxheimer in 2014 [12]. This review includes Herxheimer's older Cochrane review (with meta-analysis) of melatonin treatment [13], as well as published randomized trials (without meta-analyses) of the so-called Z-drugs, sleep medications whose names begin with or contain the letter "z" and function as stimulators of receptors for a related group of drugs called benzodiazepines. The most commonly used Z-drugs are zolpidem and zopiclone, and they share many of the side effects and some of the addictive potential as the benzodiazepines but are very short-acting, which means they work rapidly and wear off rapidly. That is especially true for sublingual zolpidem, which is placed under the tongue and is absorbed directly into the bloodstream.

For melatonin and the Z-drugs, the effects of the interventions were generally favorable. Six randomized trials of melatonin versus placebo administered before, during, and/or after long-haul flights compared subjective jet lag scores (on a scale of 0 to 100) among 142 travelers flying eastward (four trials) and 90 flying westward (two trials). In meta-analyses, moderate differences of 17–20 points on this scale favored both groups of participants randomized to melatonin over those randomized to placebo. One trial observed a statistically significant improvement in sleep quality in participants randomized to melatonin, but no quantitative results were reported. It is unclear whether higher doses of melatonin result in a larger reduction in jet lag symptoms, although that appears to be the case when melatonin is used to treat chronic sleep disorders [14]. Yet, only about 15% of orally administered melatonin is absorbed [15].

In the Herxheimer review [12], three randomized trials compared Z-drugs to placebo; the drugs or placebo were administered for the first three to four nights after the flight. In the larger of the two trials that reported on overall jet lag symptoms, a statistically significant reduction was observed in participants randomized to the Z-drugs. The results on sleep duration and quality significantly favored travelers randomized to Z-drugs in the two trials reporting those outcomes. One of the three trials also included a group who received both a Z-drug and melatonin but observed no difference in overall jet lag symptoms versus those receiving the Z-drug alone.

Non-medication treatments have been less well studied than melatonin and Z-drugs but benefit from several systematic reviews. The above-cited Herxheimer systematic review [12] also includes one small randomized trial of bright light, which reported a 1-h delay in melatonin secretion in the bright light group but no significant effect on self-reported sleep quality. A more recent narrative systematic review by Bin and coworkers [16] included seven controlled studies of bright light interventions, including three small RCTs, two very small non-randomized trials, and one small observational study, most of which found no significant difference favoring the intervention. An additional, larger RCT by Jurvelin and colleagues was also included in the review [17]. That trial studied trans-cranial (through the skull) bright light versus inactive light placebo 4 times per day in the first week after arrival in 55 men taking trans-Atlantic flights from or back to Finland. The authors observed a significant reduction in subjective jet lag symptoms and sleepiness but no change in sleep as recorded in diaries. The Bin review also includes one small non-randomized trial and two small observational controlled studies of increased physical activity, but the small sample sizes and poor design prevent any rigorous inferences [16]. Also included in the Bin review is a larger but uninterpretable observational study of the Argonne diet (alternate days of feasting and fasting). The Bin review also includes one small randomized trial that compared chiropractic versus sham manipulation and a small crossover trial of a multi-component intervention that had no placebo control; neither trial observed any significant intervention effect.

Finally, a recent systematic review and meta-analysis by Chan and colleagues examined controlled studies of the so-called functional foods (foods containing physiologically active ingredients beyond their nutrient content), beverages, and nutrient supplements claiming to reduce the adverse effects of long-haul air travel [18]. The review was not restricted to placebo-controlled randomized trials, and the effects examined were not limited to jet lag but also included leg edema (swelling) and flight performance by pilots. The review confirmed the substantial beneficial effects of melatonin on jet lag symptoms observed in the above-cited Herxheimer reviews [12, 13], but the various herb and plant extracts, caffeine, and extra fluid studied focused on leg swelling and pilot performance, rather than jet lag symptoms.

Summary

Melatonin and Z-drug sleep medications are clearly helpful in reducing the sleep disruption that occurs following long-haul flights, especially those in an eastbound direction. Most of the evidence is based on treatment during the first 3–4 days after arrival at the flight destination; the evidence base is very thin regarding the use of these medications preventively before or during the flight. Most studies of bright light exposure after arrival have been too small to show significant benefits, although the encouraging results of the Jurvelin trial [17] and the known effects of bright light on inhibiting endogenous melatonin secretion suggest that walking or other outdoor physical activity during the "droopy" afternoons in the first few days after landing may be beneficial; they are almost certainly harmless. Extra fluid, alteration of mealtimes, and consumption of specific foods have been inadequately studied, either as prevention before or during the light, or as treatment after arrival. The field would greatly benefit from large, placebo-controlled trials of these interventions.

References

1. Maksel R. When did the term "jet lag" come into use? And has anybody found a cure? Smithsonian Magazine. 17 June 2008.
2. Winget CM, DeRoshia CW, Markley CL, Holley DC. A review of human physiological and performance changes associated with desynchronosis of biological rhythms. Aviat Space Environ Med. 1984;55(12):1085–96.

3. Waterhouse J, Reilly T, Atkinson G, Edwards B. Jet lag: trends and coping strategies. Lancet. 2007;369(9567):1117–29.
4. Eastman CI, Tomaka VA, Crowley SJ. Circadian rhythms of European and African-Americans after a large delay of sleep as in jet lag and night work. Sci Rep. 2016;6:36716.
5. Jet lag. https://en.wikipedia.org/w/index.php?title=Jet_lag&oldid=1098747405.
6. Pupaibool J, Walaliyadda H, Tasevac B, Brintz BJ, Park IK, Graves M, Benson LS, Hale P, Powell J, Leung DT. Travel-related behaviors and health outcomes of adolescents compared with adults on short-term international service missions. Am J Trop Med Hyg. 2022;106(1):345–50.
7. Beh SF, Lee SKM, Bin YS, Cheung JMY. Travelers' perceptions of jetlag and travel fatigue: a scoping review. Chronobiol Int. 2022;39(8):1037–57.
8. Rogers HL, Reilly SM. A survey of the health experiences of international business travelers: part one—physiological aspects. AAOHN J. 2002;50(10):449–59.
9. Rigney G, Walters A, Bin YS, Crome E, Vincent GE. Jet-lag countermeasures used by international business travelers. Aerosp Med Hum Perform. 2021;92(10):825–30.
10. Bin YS, Ledger S, Nour M, Postnova S, Stamatakis E, Cistulli PA, de Chazal P, Allman-Farinelli M, Caillaud C, Bauman A, Simpson SJ. How do travelers manage jetlag and travel fatigue? A survey of passengers on long-haul flights. Chronobiol Int. 2020;37(11):1621–8.
11. Guiu G, Monin J, Perrier E, Manen O. Travel health study in commercial aircrew members. Travel Med Infect Dis. 2022;45:102209.
12. Herxheimer A. Jet lag. BMJ Clin Evid. 2014;4:2303.
13. Herxheimer A, Petrie KJ. Melatonin for the prevention and treatment of jet lag. Cochrane Database Syst Rev. 2002;2:CD001520.
14. Ferracioli-Oda E, Qawasmi A, Bloch MH. Meta-analysis: melatonin for the treatment of primary sleep disorders. PLoS One. 2013;8(5):e63773.
15. DeMuro RL, Nafziger AN, Blask DE, Menhinick AM, Bertino JS Jr. The absolute bioavailability of oral melatonin. J Clin Pharmacol. 2000;40(7):781–4.
16. Bin YS, Postnova S, Cistulli PA. What works for jetlag? A systematic review of non-pharmacological interventions. Sleep Med Rev. 2019;43:47–59.
17. Jurvelin H, Jokelainen J, Takala T. Transcranial bright light and symptoms of jet lag: a randomized, placebo-controlled trial. Aerosp Med Hum Perform. 2015;86(4):344–50.
18. Chan V, Wang L, Allman-Farinelli M. Efficacy of functional foods, beverages, and supplements claiming to alleviate air travel symptoms: systematic review and meta-analysis. Nutrients. 2021;13(3):961.

High Sugar Consumption and Diabetes Risk: A Sweet Lie

19

Introduction

Many people believe that they should avoid eating "too much" sugar, because it will increase their risk of developing diabetes. A 2016 quote from Pope Francis is illustrative: "It's sweet, we like it, and it goes down easily. But then we get sick! We come to a nasty end! When we have too much sugar, we end up with diabetes, and our country ends up being diabetic!" [1]. It is common knowledge that diabetes is characterized by high blood levels of glucose. Glucose is one of the two components (along with fructose) of sucrose, that is, table sugar, the main sweetening ingredient in sodas and juices. It seems only logical that consuming less sugar will lower your blood sugar, right? Logical, perhaps, but almost certainly wrong! (Fig. 19.1)

The full name of the disease is "diabetes mellitus," from the Greek "*diabetes*" (meaning passing through, which refers to the large urine output common in patients with diabetes) and the Latin "*mellitus*" (denoting sweet or honeyed). The excess urine is caused by the kidney's attempt to lower the body's glucose load, which requires excretion of water. Healthy persons without diabetes do not need to regulate their blood glucose through their kidneys; instead, they rely on the pancreas to secrete the hormone insulin whenever the blood sugar rises. The insulin helps transport glucose from the bloodstream into cells in the liver, muscle, and fat and keeps the blood glucose level within a narrow range that optimizes the body's need for glucose to move, think, and carry out other essential functions, while avoiding the high levels that would lead to excess urine excretion and to damage of the arteries, nervous system, and kidneys.

Two types of diabetes can be distinguished. Type 1 diabetes is due to immune auto-destruction of insulin-producing cells of the pancreas. It is the less common of the two types and usually starts in childhood or adolescence and requires daily administration of insulin injections to replace the loss of insulin from the pancreas. Type 2 diabetes is not caused by an insufficient supply of insulin from the pancreas, but rather by the resistance of liver, muscle, and fat cells to the action of insulin. Fat cells in particular are resistant to insulin, and the majority of patients with type 2

Fig. 19.1 Does high sugar consumption increase the risk of diabetes? Many people believe it does

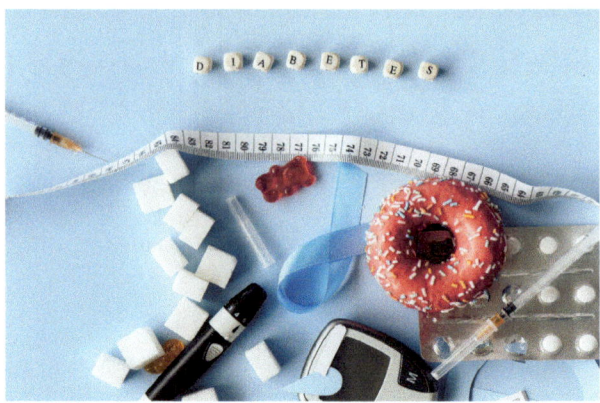

diabetes are overweight and carry excess fat. Type 2 diabetes typically occurs in middle-age or elderly adults but has become more common in adolescents and even school-age children with the recent obesity epidemic. Physical inactivity also contributes to insulin resistance. Type 2 diabetes can be treated with weight loss, exercise, and oral medications that increase the pancreas's secretion of insulin, but it may require insulin injections if those treatments prove insufficient. Nearly 9% of the world's population is affected by diabetes, 90% of whom have type 2, and the disease is responsible for about 4 million deaths per year [2].

Historical Background

A condition resembling diabetes was described in ancient Egypt around 1500 BC [2, 3]. The first apparent use of the term "diabetes" can be traced to Apollonius in Memphis, around 230 BC. The condition was also recognized by ancient Indian physicians, who observed that ants were attracted to the sweet urine excreted by affected persons. The two types of diabetes were first distinguished by Chinese and Indian physicians in the fifth century AD, with one (now known as type 1) observed among young, thin individuals and the other (type 2) among older, wealthy, overweight adults. In 1889, von Mering and Minkowski discovered that dogs whose pancreas had been removed developed diabetes. The pancreatic hormone insulin was discovered by Banting and Best at the University of Toronto in 1921, when they observed that an extract from healthy dog pancreas reversed the condition in diabetic dogs whose pancreas had been removed [4]. Within a year of that discovery, insulin had been purified and used to successfully treat a teenager with type 1 diabetes.

Current Beliefs and Behaviors Concerning Sugar Consumption and Diabetes

I was unable to locate any systematic reviews of population-based studies of beliefs about sugar consumption as a cause of diabetes. Even individual studies are uncommon, although several surveys have been reported from populations at high risk of type 2 diabetes, including indigenous North Americans, South Asians, and Pacific Islanders. One qualitative study (no quantitative data are reported) was based on themes that emerged from interviews with key informants from a northwestern Ontario community of Ojibway and Cree, including traditional healers, local leaders, native health workers, and diabetics from the community [5]. These key informants commonly believed that diabetes was caused by consumption of sugar, a non-native food substance. In fact, the Ojibway-Cree word for diabetes, *sho-goh-wah-pee-nay*, means "sugar disease." In one quantitative study based on interviews of 161 male and female household heads from urban and remote areas of the Marshall Islands in the South Pacific, 78% of the respondents believed that eating sweets caused diabetes [6].

In a randomized trial of a culturally-adapted intervention to reduce diabetes risk among 198 Pakistani immigrant women in Oslo, Norway, a baseline (prior to intervention) questionnaire showed that sugar was the leading food (reported by two-thirds) that the women believed should be consumed in limited amounts [7]. In a study of 121 South Asian immigrants in the Vancouver area who had immigrated to Canada after the age of 18 years, over one-third of the participants reported having increased their consumption of both sugar-sweetened soft drinks and candies or sweet desserts since they had immigrated [8]. These changes since immigration suggest an adverse effect of acculturation on prevailing dietary customs.

I found few published studies of sugar consumption in general population samples. In a nationally representative sample of over 1500 adolescents and young adults who participated in a Belgian food consumption survey in 2014, participants living in households in which the highest education level did not go beyond secondary schooling reported the highest consumption of sugar-sweetened beverages (SSBs) [9]. A recent study was based on repeated nationally representative health behavior surveys of adolescent consumption of SSBs in 14 Eastern European countries from 2002 to 2018 [10]. Most of the participating countries showed a favorable reduction in SSB consumption over the 16-year span. But the rate of decrease was significantly steeper in adolescents from wealthier families, leading to reversal of the disparity in consumption between adolescents from the wealthiest families and those from the poorest families in 5 of the 14 countries.

Finally, a recent nationally representative sample of over 9000 Australian secondary school students participated in a web-based survey during class time about their consumption of sugar-containing soft drinks (sodas) and their beliefs about the health effects of that consumption [11]. Nearly 80% of the participants reported at least some consumption of soda, more than half of whom limited their consumption to less than one cup (250 mL) per week. More than 87% of the participants believed that regular (sugar-containing) soda was likely to cause future health problems, and over 70% believed it would cause diabetes. The latter percentage was significantly higher in girls than in boys and rose significantly with age and with socioeconomic advantage of the neighborhood in which they lived.

Key Evidence Points
- Type 2 diabetes is caused by reduced cellular sensitivity to insulin, usually due to increased body weight and fat.
- Diabetes is increasing in prevalence world-wide as a result of the obesity epidemic and is a major cause of heart disease and mortality.
- Many adults and adolescents believe that high sugar intake causes diabetes.
- Observational studies linking sugar consumption to later diabetes are hopelessly confounded by cultural, ethnic, and socioeconomic factors.
- Sugar intake (especially via sugar-sweetened beverages, SSBs) is a known cause of overweight and obesity, but randomized trials in which sugar was replaced by calorically equivalent nutrients found no differences in weight change.
- Randomized trials of diets with high versus low sugar content have shown no difference in blood sugar in the groups following the two diets.
- Reducing sugar consumption does not help prevent diabetes unless the reduced sugar calories are not compensated for by increasing the intake of other nutrients.

Detailed Review of Evidence on Sugar Consumption and Risk of Diabetes[1]

In a 2016 article in *The Guardian*, Leslie opined that scientists who claimed that increasing fat intake was largely responsible for the rise in diabetes and cardiovascular diseases constituted a "conspiracy" against those who argued that increasing sugar consumption was the major culprit [12]. The article quotes scientists on both "sides" of the argument but provides no cogent scientific arguments favoring either the fat or sugar theories.

In this section, I will examine the published evidence on the effect of sugar consumption on the risk of developing diabetes. My focus here will be on type 2 diabetes, since the insulin deficiency due to immune-mediated destruction or damage to insulin-producing cells in the pancreas that characterizes type 1 diabetes is itself a clear cause of high blood glucose (sugar) levels. As discussed early in this chapter, type 2 diabetes is closely linked to body weight, and especially body fat, which impairs insulin's ability to promote the influx of glucose into the muscle, liver, and fat cells and hence its metabolism. Moderate and vigorous physical activity is also

---

[1] Readers who prefer to skip the Detailed Review should proceed to the Summary at the end of the chapter.

important in promoting insulin sensitivity, above and beyond its effect on body weight or fat.

Most of the evidence on sugar ignores its effect of overweight and obesity. Sugar and other kinds of carbohydrates are important sources of calories (energy), and excess caloric intake is the major cause of excess body weight and fat. But the question is whether sugar has any *unique* effect on causing diabetes above and beyond its caloric content. Fat has an even greater caloric content, gram for gram, than sugar or other carbohydrates. Yet, it does not carry the same stigma for causing diabetes, perhaps because the link between dietary fat intake and blood sugar does not seem as obvious as the link with sugar intake.

Demonstrating a causal link between high sugar consumption and diabetes requires a comparison with equal caloric intake from non-sugar sources. In other words, increased sugar consumption must be compared to increased consumption of non-sugar foods with respect to subsequent diabetes risk. The same is true for reducing sugar intake; the effects on diabetes risk must be compared with reducing intake of other foods with equivalent caloric content.

Moreover, high versus low sugar consumption cannot be validly compared in observational studies; such studies are hopelessly confounded by factors that affect diet and also affect diabetes risk independently of diet. As we saw in the previous section of this chapter, people who consume high sugar diets differ in many respects from those who consume low sugar diets with respect to cultural, ethnic, and socio-economic factors. Although less well documented, they are also likely to differ in physical activity. In other words, randomized trials are essential for making causal inferences about high versus low sugar diets and subsequent risk of diabetes.

Given these methodologic issues, it is not surprising that several recent systematic reviews and meta-analyses based on prospective observational studies have observed a modest but statistically significant association between sugar-sweetened beverages (SSBs) and type 2 diabetes in adults [13, 14]. But a causal effect of SSB consumption on risk of diabetes, independent of its effect on body weight and fat, simply cannot be inferred from observational studies. This problem is clearly illustrated by the recent systematic review of prospective observational studies by Li and colleagues [14]. The authors compared the risk of developing type 2 diabetes among participants who consumed SSBs at the highest 10% of the combined studies versus those consuming at the lowest 10%. The authors observed a 27% increased risk for high SSB consumption, but also a 32% *increased* risk for high consumption of artificially-sweetened beverages!

These principles of appropriate research methods are also demonstrated in Te Morenga and colleagues' 2012 systematic review of 30 randomized trials assessing the effects of changes in dietary sugar intake on body weight [15]. Five trials in adults comparing low sugar versus usual or high sugar diets showed a reduction of 0.8 kg (nearly 2 lb) in participants randomized to the low sugar diet. In ten trials of adults randomized to high sugar versus usual diets, a similar-size increase in body weight was observed in those receiving the high sugar diets. But in 11 trials in which the group randomized to a low sugar diet received non-sugar carbohydrates or other nutrients of equal caloric content as the removed sugar, absolutely no difference in body weight was observed between the two randomized groups. In other words, any effect on body weight of reduced or added sugar in the diet is entirely explained by the reduced or added calories due to the sugar—*not* to a specific effect of sugar.

Five randomized trials in children were also included in the Te Morenga systematic review [15]. These trials did not compare two different diets, but rather advice (vs. no advice) to reduce the intake of sugar-sweetened beverages (SSBs) and other sources of added dietary sugar. Such advice is notoriously associated with poor compliance on the part of the children and their parents, so it is no surprise that no difference in body weight was observed between the two randomized groups.

A Dutch randomized trial [16] published in 2012 was not included in the Te Morenga review. That trial was a double-blind comparison of sugar-sweetened versus artificially-sweetened beverages distributed daily over an 18-month period as single 250 mL (one cup) cans to 641 children 4–11 years of age who attended eight Amsterdam schools. Children in the SSB group increased their obesity measures to a significantly greater extent than those in the artificially-sweetened beverage group. The differences were substantial: 0.13 standard deviation units for BMI, just over 1 kg for weight, 6.6 mm for waist circumference (a measure of central-body fat), and 1% for percent body fat. To my knowledge, no randomized trials in children have provided a calorically equivalent dietary intervention to the control group.

A recent Cochrane Review of randomized trials in adults by Bergwall and coworkers provides strong evidence against any effect of sugar consumption on blood glucose (sugar) levels [17]. The review does not compare weight outcomes in the randomized groups, but randomization to diets with high versus low sugar consumption in 16 trials resulted in no difference in blood sugar between the two groups, whether the control diet was ad libitum (no change to usual diet) or a diet with replacement of sugar by a calorically equivalent substitute.

Finally, mechanistic studies have suggested that fructose (which is the main sugar in fruit and in corn syrup) may increase insulin resistance to a greater degree than glucose or sucrose (sucrose, or table sugar, is a disaccharide in which glucose is bound to fructose) [18]. Nonetheless, Tsilas and colleagues' 2017 systematic review of prospective observational studies found no evidence of increased risk of new cases of type 2 diabetes associated with fructose, sucrose, or total sugars [19]. I found no randomized trials (or systematic reviews of trials) of interventions to reduce or increase fructose intake.

Summary

Diabetes is characterized by high blood glucose levels, and many people therefore believe that excess sugar consumption can cause diabetes. This belief is particularly widespread among indigenous and immigrant groups at increased genetic risk of type 2 diabetes. Obesity and high body fat have been convincingly shown to increase the risk of type 2 diabetes, as has physical inactivity. The best scientific evidence from randomized intervention trials makes it clear that sugar-sweetened beverages and other dietary sources of sugar are an important cause of obesity, but trials of diets substituting sugar with non-sugar dietary components of equal caloric content demonstrate no difference in body weight or in blood sugar levels.

Maintaining a healthy body weight and engaging in regular physical activity are the best ways to prevent diabetes. Avoiding or reducing sugar consumption may help to control body weight (and improve dental health) but has no impact on preventing diabetes unless the reduced sugar calories are not compensated for by increasing the intake of other nutrients.

References

1. Lean ME, Te Morenga L. Sugar and type 2 diabetes. Br Med Bull. 2016;120(1):43–53.
2. Diabetes. https://en.wikipedia.org/w/index.php?title=Diabetes&oldid=1110085175.
3. Higuera V. Diabetes: past treatments, new discoveries. Med News Today. 17 June 2020.
4. Polonsky KS. The past 200 years in diabetes. N Engl J Med. 2012;367(14):1332–40.
5. Gittelsohn J, Harris SB, Burris KL, Kakegamic L, Landman LT, Sharma A, Wolever TM, Logan A, Barnie A, Zinman B. Use of ethnographic methods for applied research on diabetes among the Ojibway-Cree in northern Ontario. Health Educ Q. 1996;23(3):365–82.
6. Cortes LM, Gittelsohn J, Alfred J, Palafox NA. Formative research to inform intervention development for diabetes prevention in the Republic of the Marshall Islands. Health Educ Behav. 2001;28(6):696–715.
7. Råberg Kjøllesdal MK, Hjellset VT, Bjørge B, Holmboe-Ottesen G, Wandel M. Food perceptions in terms of health among Norwegian-Pakistani women participating in a culturally adapted intervention. Int J Public Health. 2011;56(5):475–83.
8. Lesser IA, Gasevic D, Lear SA. The association between acculturation and dietary patterns of South Asian immigrants. PLoS One. 2014;9(2):e88495.
9. Desbouys L, De Ridder K, Rouche M, Castetbon K. Food consumption in adolescents and young adults: age-specific socio-economic and cultural disparities (Belgian Food Consumption Survey 2014). Nutrients. 2019;11(7):1520.
10. Chatelan A, Rouche M, Dzielska A, Lebacq T, Fismen AS, Kelly C, Zaborskis A, Kopcakova J, Tsareva A, Kalman M, Castetbon K. Time trends in consumption of sugar-sweetened beverages and related socioeconomic differences among adolescents in Eastern Europe: signs of a nutrition transition? Am J Clin Nutr. 2021;114(4):1476–85.
11. Miller C, Dono J, Scully M, Morley B, Ettridge K. Adolescents' knowledge and beliefs regarding health risks of soda and diet soda consumption. Public Health Nutr. 2022;25(11):3044–53.
12. Leslie I. The sugar conspiracy. The Guardian. 7 Apr 2016.
13. Santos LP, Gigante DP, Delpino FM, Maciel AP, Bielemann RM. Sugar sweetened beverages intake and risk of obesity and cardiometabolic diseases in longitudinal studies: a systematic review and meta-analysis with 1.5 million individuals. Clin Nutr ESPEN. 2022;51:128–42.
14. Li B, Yan N, Jiang H, Cui M, Wu M, Wang L, Mi B, Li Z, Shi J, Fan Y, Azalati MM, Li C, Chen F, Ma M, Wang D, Ma L. Consumption of sugar sweetened beverages, artificially sweetened beverages and fruit juices and risk of type 2 diabetes, hypertension, cardiovascular disease, and mortality: a meta-analysis. Front Nutr. 2023;10:1019534.
15. Te Morenga L, Mallard S, Mann J. Dietary sugars and body weight: systematic review and meta-analyses of randomised controlled trials and cohort studies. BMJ. 2012;346:e7492.
16. de Ruyter JC, Olthof MR, Seidell JC, Katan MB. A trial of sugar-free or sugar-sweetened beverages and body weight in children. N Engl J Med. 2012;367(15):1397–406.
17. Bergwall S, Johansson A, Sonestedt E, Acosta S. High versus low-added sugar consumption for the primary prevention of cardiovascular disease. Cochrane Database Syst Rev. 2022;1(1):CD013320.

18. Stanhope KL. Sugar consumption, metabolic disease and obesity: the state of the controversy. Crit Rev Clin Lab Sci. 2016;53(1):52–67.
19. Tsilas CS, de Souza RJ, Mejia SB, Mirrahimi A, Cozma AI, Jayalath VH, Ha V, Tawfik R, Di Buono M, Jenkins AL, Leiter LA, Wolever TMS, Beyene J, Khan T, Kendall CWC, Jenkins DJA, Sievenpiper JL. Relation of total sugars, fructose and sucrose with incident type 2 diabetes: a systematic review and meta-analysis of prospective cohort studies. CMAJ. 2017;189(20):E711–20.

Part V

Pregnancy and Childhood

Born Too Soon: What's in a Number?   **20**

Introduction

It was my mother-in-law who first informed me about her firm belief that preterm ("premature") babies born in the seventh month were more likely to be healthy and survive than those born in the eighth month of pregnancy. She told me that she had learned this while growing up in Morocco and that the belief was widely shared by both the Jewish and Arab (Muslim) communities there.

I don't recall the precise time she first told me about this, but it must have been after my 1981 marriage to her daughter Claire. I had been trained as both a pediatrician and an epidemiologist and had already done some research in perinatal epidemiology on topics relating to pregnancy, birth, and infant health. So, she knew this was an area of my interest and expertise, and I knew that her belief was untrue. But it was not until I started writing this book that I learned how long the belief has persisted and how geographically widespread it is.

Because the belief is so illogical and so easy to disprove, I have decided to reverse the usual order of the chapters in this book, in which I first discuss the origins and prevalence of medical beliefs and then summarize the scientific evidence bearing on them. Instead, I will start with the evidence about the belief and only then summarize the fascinating story of its roots. But first, you will need a primer on the terminology of pregnancy, how the dating of pregnancy is established nowadays, and how the practices and terms used by older civilizations have changed over time.

When Does Pregnancy Begin?

This question seems simple enough to answer, at least from a biological standpoint. Pregnancy begins with fertilization: a male sperm cell enters and fuses with ("invades") the ovum, the egg released from the ovary at the time of ovulation. The fusion of the ovum and sperm in the Fallopian tube creates what is called the *zygote*, which divides several times as it descends the tube and implants into the lining of the uterus several days later. It is then referred to as an *embryo*. Within 2 or 3 months after implantation, the word *fetus* replaces embryo, and if the fetus is born alive, as a newborn *baby* after the birth. Most mothers and prenatal care providers, however, refer to the fetus as a baby once the pregnancy is documented by a positive pregnancy test.

How do we (or the mother) know when fertilization takes place? Ovulation is assumed to occur *around* 2 weeks after the onset of the previous menstrual period, but that assumption depends on the regularity of the mother's periods. And, since delayed ovulation is more common than early ovulation, it is slightly more likely to occur on day 15 or 16 than on day 12 or 13 of the normal 28-day menstrual cycle. And sperm within the Fallopian tube may be viable up to 5 days, which further adds to variability in estimating the day of fertilization. Although Hippocrates and other ancient physicians maintained that women somehow "knew" when they became pregnant, that seems highly improbable. Variations between women and within the same woman in the day of ovulation, the frequency of sexual intercourse in the days before and after ovulation, and the number of days between sperm release and fertilization are the major sources of the uncertainty.

Partly because of these variations, it has become customary to date pregnancies not from the day of fertilization, but from the first day of the previous menstrual period. This day can usually be pinpointed readily by the pregnant woman, especially if she and her partner are trying to conceive. It can also be defended biologically, because the mother's egg undergoes growth and maturation during the 2 weeks between the onset of the previous menstrual period and the day of ovulation.

How Long Does Pregnancy Last?

The duration of gestation (pregnancy) is highly variable. It varies among all mammals, including humans, and even within the same healthy mother from one pregnancy to the next. And of course, illness or poor nutrition in the mother and complications of the pregnancy itself can also affect the duration of pregnancy.

But a more fundamental problem is the *unit* used to denote time. Should pregnancy duration be expressed in days? In weeks? In months? Until fairly recently, the general public and pregnant women tended to report their stage of pregnancy in months. But months can vary in duration from 28 to 31 days, and much can change in the pregnant women and her fetus over a month. In ancient times, "months" generally referred to lunar months (about 28 days). Since the reign of Julius Caesar, however, the Julian (solar) calendar has replaced the lunar calendar. As we shall see later in the chapter, the belief in the non-viability of the eighth-month baby originated well before the time of Caesar.

Moreover, the belief concerns the seventh versus the eighth months. The *"th"* is key here, because the seventh month of pregnancy begins as soon as the pregnancy reaches 6 months. And pregnancy enters its eighth month once seven complete months have elapsed. Weeks have gradually replaced months for dating pregnancy, but this change has created its own problems. Only the month of February has exactly 4 weeks, and even then, only in non-leap years. A seventh-month baby can therefore be up to 4.4 weeks younger than a 7-month baby, and an eighth-month baby can be up to 4.4 weeks younger than an 8-month baby.

The "normal" duration of pregnancy is approximately 40 completed weeks (9 completed months plus another completed week), or 280 days. In the absence of obstetric intervention (induction of labor or pre-labor cesarean delivery), most healthy women give birth between 38 and 42 completed weeks. Pregnancy complications like high blood pressure, pre-eclampsia (high blood pressure combined with protein in the urine), and gestational diabetes can lead to earlier delivery, either spontaneously or because of obstetric intervention. Delivery before 37 completed weeks (259 days) is referred to as preterm birth (commonly called "prematurity"). Delivery at or after 42 completed weeks (294 days) is called post-term birth, and most obstetricians will intervene around that time to reduce the risk of stillbirth, a fetus who dies before birth and has no signs of life at birth; this risk rises sharply in late pregnancy, perhaps owing to aging of the placenta.

Review of Scientific Evidence

It is inherently illogical to believe that preterm babies born in the seventh month are less likely to die or to suffer from serious illnesses, in both the short and long term, than babies born in the eighth month. Immature lungs, brains, and immune systems are well known to threaten the health and survival of preterm babies, and the lower their gestational age at birth, the higher the risk of these adverse health outcomes. As I discussed in Chap. 1, belief is a poor substitute for scientific evidence. But logic can also mislead and run contrary to evidence. Many "logical" arguments were offered in the past for treatments that were subsequently found to be useless or even harmful. And some counter-intuitive remedies, such as walking instead of bed-rest soon after undergoing orthopedic surgery, have proven to have important benefits.

I was unable to find a systematic review of the published literature on the risks of death or other adverse health outcomes as a function of gestational duration. Moreover, the outcomes of preterm babies have improved progressively over the last half century with the advent of neonatal intensive care and specific treatments to prevent and treat the many illnesses to which preterm infants are predisposed. As a perinatal epidemiologist who has published hundreds of peer-reviewed research articles on preterm birth and infant mortality, I have *never* encountered a published study whose data support the belief in the "advantages" of birth in the seventh month versus the eighth month.

To illustrate the evidence, I have chosen to graph data published in tabular form on neonatal deaths (deaths in the first 4 weeks after birth) among all singleton (one baby, thereby excluding twins, triplets, etc.) live births in the USA from 1995 to 1997, taken from a study by Alexander and colleagues published in 2003 [1]. More than 10 million births were included in the study, and the data were separated by the

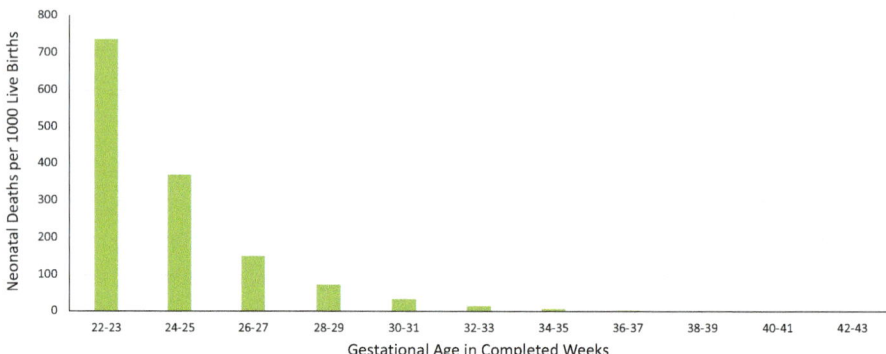

Fig. 20.1 Neonatal mortality (death before 28 completed days of life) according to gestational age (duration of pregnancy) among infants born alive to White non-Hispanic mothers in the USA, 1995–1997 [1]

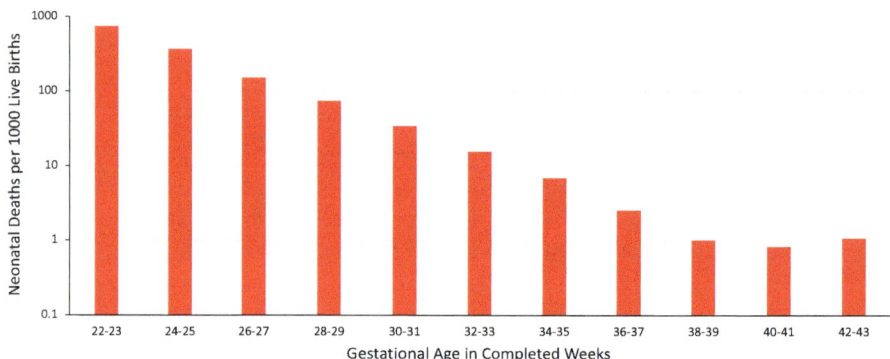

Fig. 20.2 Neonatal mortality (death before 28 completed days of life) according to gestational age (duration of pregnancy) among infants born alive to White non-Hispanic mothers in the USA, 1995–1997 [1]. The data have been transformed using a logarithmic scale to visually reduce the apparent magnitude of differences in neonatal mortality with rising gestational age

mother's ethnicity into White non-Hispanic, Black non-Hispanic, and Hispanic. The data graphed below in Fig. 20.1 are based on the 6.7 million White non-Hispanic births, and the results shown are grouped by 2-week intervals of gestational age, beginning at 22 completed weeks.

The data in Fig. 20.1 show a rapidly declining risk of neonatal death as the duration of gestation increases. The differences are very hard to discern after 30 weeks (the beginning of the eighth month), however, so the same data are graphed using a logarithmic scale in Fig. 20.2.

On this scale, the vertical (y) axis shows equal distances between neonatal mortality rates that differ tenfold. We can now see that the neonatal mortality rate continues to fall beyond 30 weeks, reaching a minimum at 40–41 weeks before rising slightly at 42–43 weeks. No "bump up" in mortality risk is seen in the eighth month

(30–33 completed weeks), which is much lower than the risk during the seventh month (26–29 completed weeks). Although these data are limited to neonatal death, a similar pattern has been repeatedly observed seen for lung disease, infection, and brain damage.

History and Cultural Origins

The earliest known written document on viability of the eighth- versus seventh-month baby is attributed to the ancient Greek physician Hippocrates in his treatise entitled *Peri Octamanou (On the eighth-month fetus)*, written in the fifth century BC. According to Hanson [2], the belief was based on numerology: the mystical importance attached to the number 7. Beyond numerology, Reiss and Ash quote some rather convoluted physiologic arguments by Hippocrates to "explain" the paradoxical viability of the seventh-month fetus [3]. Aristotle was apparently skeptical, however, and wondered whether the reasoning was circular, that is, a self-fulfilling prophecy: the strong belief that all eighth-month babies were doomed led to their not being fed or cared for! [3].

The belief in the enhanced viability of seventh-month babies remained strong in the ensuing centuries, despite Aristotle's skepticism. The ancient Greeks did not keep complete and accurate records of births, estimated gestational ages, and infant deaths, so data were no substitute for Greek wisdom. Even several centuries later, renowned Greek physicians like Galen and Soranos continued to subscribe to the belief in eighth-month non-viability [3]. The belief was also shared by rabbis. Those who contributed to the Talmud, commentaries on Jewish law based on the torah (Old Testament), also accepted its validity [4]. In fact, they allowed desecration of the Sabbath to save the life, or even to perform a circumcision, for a seventh-month baby but not for an eighth-month baby. Moreover, the viability of seventh-month babies was used to "determine" paternity when a woman permitted to remarry 2.5 months after the death of her first husband gave birth gave birth 7 months later.

The belief in the non-viability of the eighth-month baby continued to be promulgated by Muslim, Christian, and Jewish authorities throughout the Middle Ages. It was endorsed by Ambroise Paré, a renowned surgeon in sixteenth-century France [5], and by John Sadler in a well-respected medical text published in seventeenth-century England [6]. I was unable to locate any published survey investigating the prevalence of this belief or of factors affecting it. The persistence of the belief among women into the modern era, however, was encountered by Reiss and Ash among Indian immigrants, Russian and German grandmothers, and Ozark midwives [3]. Reiss and Ash do not cite my mother-in-law, but her conviction of the validity of the belief, even in the face of empirical data like those I presented in the previous section, reminds us that long-held convictions "do not go gently into that good night."

Key Evidence Points

- The belief that preterm babies born in the seventh month of pregnancy were more likely to survive than those born in the eighth month originated at least 2500 years ago.
- That belief was probably based on numerology, the mystic importance attached to the number 7.
- The belief is not supported by population-based studies of risks of mortality or severe illness in relation to the gestational age (duration of pregnancy) at birth, which clearly show lower risks in the eighth versus seventh month and even lower risks in the ninth month.
- Despite the absence of scientific evidence supporting the belief, it has persisted into modern times in some cultures, religions, and geographic regions.

References

1. Alexander GR, Kogan M, Bader D, Carlo W, Allen M, Mor J. US birth weight/gestational age-specific neonatal mortality: 1995-1997 rates for whites, hispanics, and blacks. Pediatrics. 2003;111(1):e61–6.
2. Hanson AE. The eight months' child and the etiquette of birth: obsit omen! Bull Hist Med. 1987;61(4):589–602.
3. Reiss RE, Ash AD. The eighth-month fetus: classical sources for a modern superstition. Obstet Gynecol. 1988;71(2):270–3.
4. Talmudology.   talmudology.com/jeremybrownmdgmailcom/2014/11/16/-an-eight-month-fetus-cannot-survive-rashi-yevamot-42a.
5. Paré A. Oeuvres complètes, vol. 2. Geneva: Slatkine Reprints; 1970.
6. Sadler J. The Sicke Womans private looking-Glasse. London: 1936 Facsimile Edition, National Library of Medicine.

Take Your Shots? Parents' Fear of Adverse Effects of Vaccines

21

Introduction

My previous book was entitled *Beyond Parenting Advice: How Science Should Guide Your Decisions on Pregnancy and Child-Rearing* [1]. It provided a systematic review of published evidence bearing on decisions made by pregnant women and new parents. The book contained two chapters on vaccines: one on vaccines offered to pregnant women, the other on childhood vaccines. In the latter chapter, I review the evidence on whether measles vaccine causes autism and whether receipt of many vaccines during early childhood has long-term adverse effects on the immune system. Some of the material from my first book will be repeated here, along with an update that includes studies published since that book. In addition, however, this chapter will summarize the literature on parents' beliefs about vaccine adverse effects. This update is timely, given the recent acrimonious conflict around vaccinating children against COVID-19, public health mandates, and vaccine misinformation, especially on social media.

Historical Context

The under-5 mortality rate is defined as the proportion of all children born in a given population or community who die before their fifth birthday. It is a valuable health indicator used by the World Health Organization (WHO) and the United Nations Children's Fund (UNICEF) to compare countries at any point in time and to assess progress (reductions) across time. In 1800, nearly half of all the world's children died before their fifth birthday. Even by 1900, the proportion was one-third and remained 25% at the end of World War II. Since then, however, it has declined sharply, reaching 3.7% by 2020. But the huge reduction in the global rate hides very wide disparities among countries: from near 10% in the poorest sub-Saharan countries to under 0.5% in the high-income countries of Europe, North America, Australia, and New Zealand. WHO's Sustainable Development Goal 3.2.1 is to

Fig. 21.1 Child receiving a vaccine

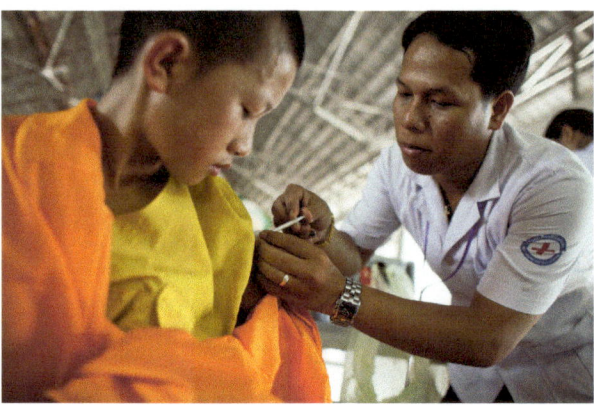

reach a level of 2.5% or less in *every* country of the world by the year 2030—a target that is probably unreachable but worth striving for.

A major contributor to the fall in under-5 mortality since World War II is the reduction in deaths from infectious diseases due to vaccines and antibiotics. Infectious diseases like tetanus, diphtheria, whooping cough, polio, and meningitis have very high mortality rates but are rare today because of vaccination. Most parents in high-income countries today have never seen a child who has died of these diseases (Fig. 21.1).

But childhood deaths can also occur from more common infectious diseases like measles, rotavirus diarrhea, influenza (the flu), and other respiratory viruses. These diseases are far less likely to be fatal than the ones listed above, but their very high incidence (frequency) nonetheless translates into a large total number of childhood deaths. As recently as 1990, for example, measles killed more than half a million young children. And in 2018, a huge increase in measles deaths worldwide occurred after parents stopped vaccinating their children against the disease after fraudulent reports of a link with autism. I will return to that issue later in the chapter.

Although childhood vaccines have saved millions of lives, it would be naïve and irresponsible not to acknowledge their adverse effects, several of which are detailed in my previous book [1]. One of the earliest of these to be recognized was caused by an error in Cutter Laboratories' production of a large batch of its polio vaccine in 1955 by inadequate inactivation of the live poliovirus. Some 200,000 children were injected with the live virus, leading to 40,000 cases of polio, 200 cases of persistent paralysis, and 10 deaths [2].

A second historical example of adverse vaccine effects was inconsolable crying, beginning 2–8 h after receipt of the diphtheria, tetanus, and pertussis (whooping cough) vaccine, which persisted for up to 24 h. This adverse reaction was traced to the pertussis component of the vaccine and disappeared when whole-cell pertussis bacteria were removed from the vaccine in the 1990s and replaced by an acellular pertussis component containing only two pertussis antigens [2].

Finally, a third notable example of adverse reactions to vaccines occurred with RotaShield, the original vaccine developed in the late 1990s to prevent rotavirus [1].

Rotavirus is the world's most common cause of gastroenteritis (diarrheal disease), which is responsible for many infant and child deaths in low-income countries. Although several randomized trials prior to its licensure showed that RotaShield was highly effective in preventing rotavirus infection, two large observational studies published in 2001 (after the vaccine's licensure) reported a large increase in risk of intussusception. Intussusception is a very dangerous intestinal condition in infants and toddlers in which part of the intestine telescopes into another part, causing intestinal blockage and interruption of the intestinal blood supply. Over the last two decades, new rotavirus vaccines have been developed and tested in randomized trials large enough to detect an increased risk of intussusception. No such increase has been found [3], and the newer rotavirus vaccines have saved many lives in low-income countries and have reduced illnesses across the world, along with consequent absences from child daycare and school and parental work.

Parents' Beliefs About the Risks and Benefits of Vaccination

In summarizing what parents believe and fear when deciding about vaccinating their children, I will rely heavily on several recent systematic reviews. Some of the reviews have analyzed qualitative studies, that is, studies that summarize or extract the main themes raised by parents when interviewed using open-ended questions posed in one-on-one interviews or in small focus groups. Most of the reviews, however, included or were restricted to quantitative studies, which use fixed-choice response alternatives that can be quantified, statistically analyzed, and pooled (meta-analyzed). Some of the reviews of quantitative studies are narrative descriptions of the included studies, that is, do not include a meta-analysis.

Qualitative Studies

Wilson and colleagues systematically reviewed qualitative studies that inquired about barriers to vaccination among "newcomers" (that is, migrants, refugees, and students) [4]. The main barriers identified in 21 such studies were cultural norms and influences by family and friends, knowledge gaps, insufficient access to health care, and vaccine hesitancy due to fear of adverse effects and perceived low vaccine effectiveness.

Gidengil and colleagues' 2019 systematic review included 71 published qualitative studies carried out in the USA, most (67) restricted to parents [5]. Nearly one-third of the studies involved minority groups, and over half were limited to the human papilloma virus (HPV) vaccine. The authors identified the following seven themes, in decreasing order of frequency with which they were addressed in the 71 studies: adverse effects, mistrust, lack of necessity, pro-vaccine opinions, skepticism about effectiveness, desire for autonomy, and morality concerns (with respect to HPV vaccine). The four most frequently expressed beliefs all related to adverse effects: vaccines cause illnesses or diseases (36 of 71 studies), too many vaccines overload the immune system (13 studies), vaccines contain harmful ingredients (12 studies), and young children are more susceptible to vaccine risks (9 studies). The specific adverse effects reviewed in the studies included autism and autoimmune diseases.

Another systematic review of qualitative studies by Díaz Crescitelli and coworkers focused on vaccine hesitancy or refusal among parents of children 0–6 years of age [6]. A total of 27 studies were included from around the world; unsurprisingly, fear of adverse effects was among the most prominent themes arising from parental interviews. High among the specific risks mentioned were autism, "toxic ingredients" in the vaccines, and compromise or disruption of the immune system.

Skafle and colleagues' recent systematic review of qualitative studies was restricted to COVID-19 vaccines and focused on misinformation [7]. Among the 45 studies included in the review, 23 were carried out on social media platforms, while the remainder used more conventional methods based on questionnaires and interviews. The main themes identified in both sets of studies were conspiracy claims, medical misinformation (including adverse vaccine effects), and perceived "problems" in vaccine development.

Forster and coworkers systematically reviewed eight qualitative studies investigating beliefs among Black and Asian ethnic minority parents in the UK [8]. The major factors mentioned by participants in these studies, most of which tended to reduce the parents' willingness to vaccinate their children, were religious beliefs, language/communication problems, and belief that their ethnicity made them more biologically susceptible to vaccine side effects.

I briefly mentioned above the recent resurgence of measles following reduction in vaccination against measles in many countries. Wilder-Smith and Qureshi systematically reviewed 20 qualitative European studies of parental beliefs about the measles-mumps-rubella (MMR) vaccine [9]. The major reasons for parents' hesitancy to have their children receive the MMR vaccine were concerns about vaccine safety and effectiveness, belief that measles is not a dangerous disease, and mistrust of experts.

Before summarizing systematic reviews of quantitative studies, I first want to mention one recent individual qualitative study, rather than a systematic review, because the study focuses on autism, one of the major outcomes examined in the next section of the chapter. Anderson-Chavarria and Turner interviewed 35 parents (mostly mothers) of autistic children living in Puerto Rico [10]. The majority of the parents (32 of 35) believed autism to be the result of genetic risks combined with one or more "trigger" factors. Half of the parents did not believe vaccines were responsible for their child's autism, but three attributed the autism entirely to vaccines, while another 14 believed vaccines to be one of the several possible triggers.

Quantitative Studies

Smith and coworkers systematically reviewed 64 quantitative observational studies of parents of children 5 years or younger that reported associations between parental beliefs or other psychological factors and the uptake (receipt) of one or more childhood vaccines [11]. The review does not provide quantitative data on the magnitude of associations reported in the included studies, nor any meta-analyses, but merely tabulates the number of studies investigating specific beliefs and the number reporting a statistically significant association with non-receipt of vaccine. The most frequently reported associations with non-receipt were beliefs that the vaccine is unsafe; that the vaccine causes side effects; that the vaccine is not effective; that the child is at low risk of the disease vaccinated against; the perceived low severity of the disease vaccinated against; confusion about the vaccine schedule; and logistical barriers.

Karafillakis and colleagues' 2017 systematic review was restricted to studies in European countries but included both qualitative and quantitative studies [12]. Participants were not limited to parents but included older adults and health care workers; 145 total studies were included. The authors presented their results by tabulating frequencies of vaccine beliefs, although they did compare beliefs across European countries and by vaccine. By far, the most commonly observed concern was related to vaccine safety. Other beliefs were that the vaccines were unnecessary or ineffective and that the risk or severity of the disease prevented was low. Misunderstanding or lack of information was also a common theme. Participants' concerns did not differ greatly among countries but were more frequent for HPV and influenza vaccines than for other vaccines.

Périères and coworkers' recent narrative systematic review also included both quantitative and qualitative studies but was restricted to 37 studies from urban and rural areas in 11 sub-Saharan African countries [13]. The authors focused on reasons for non-vaccination or under-vaccination of children and adolescents. Respondents in most of the studies were parents. Interestingly, vaccine safety was not the leading reason given for incomplete vaccination (non- or under-vaccination). In declining frequency, the major reported reasons cited were time constraints (cited in 27 of the 37 studies), insufficient information (26 studies), unavailable vaccines or personnel (26 studies), child illness or other missed opportunities for vaccination (25 studies), fear of minor side effects (23 studies), poor access to vaccination services (21 studies), and beliefs about serious adverse effects (17 studies).

Bocquier and colleagues' 2017 narrative systematic review (without meta-analysis) included 43 studies that investigated socioeconomic status (SES) differences in childhood vaccine uptake and/or knowledge and beliefs about childhood vaccines in high-income countries [14]. Unsurprisingly, the vast majority of the included studies reported higher vaccine uptake in groups with high SES based on income, education, and/or occupation category than in those with low SES. High SES was also strongly associated with greater confidence in vaccine safety, although a reverse direction was observed for MMR vaccine in one study from Germany. Tabacchi and coworkers' systematic review and meta-analysis of 26 European studies was limited to MMR vaccine uptake [15]; ethnic minorities had a significantly lower uptake in Southern Europe, but less consistent associations were observed in Northern and Western Europe.

Chen and coworkers systematically reviewed and meta-analyzed 29 quantitative studies of parents' willingness to vaccinate their children against COVID-19 [16]. All 29 studies were published in 2020 or 2021 (most before vaccines were available), and thus the "willingness" was not based on actual vaccination rates. Among the studies reviewed, prevalence rates of willingness varied widely, ranging from 22% to 91%; the pooled overall rate was 61%. The most common reasons for parents' hesitancy were concerns about safety and side effects (61%), the novelty of the vaccine (54%), and effectiveness (24%), whereas the main reason offered for willingness to vaccinate was to protect children and their contacts (55%). Significant predictors of willingness were parents' age of 30 years or more and their history of having provided routine childhood vaccines or seasonal flu vaccine.

Similar findings were reported in Bianchi and colleagues' 2023 systematic review and meta-analysis limited to nine quantitative studies of COVID-19 vaccine hesitancy among Italian parents, all published in 2021 or 2022 (after vaccines were available) [17]. Hesitancy prevalence, that is, the proportion of children who had not received COVID-19 vaccine, was 55% overall and varied from 31% to 83% among the studies. The authors also reported on risk factors associated with hesitancy among those studies reporting on such associations. The odds of hesitancy increased significantly in parents of children 5–11 years of age versus parents of adolescents; in parents with higher education; in those who were less afraid of the disease; and especially among parents who had not themselves been vaccinated against COVID.

Abu El Kheir-Matraria and coworkers' recent systematic review and meta-analysis also analyzed parental self-reported acceptance to vaccinate their children against COVID-19 but restricted their focus to low- and middle-income countries [18]. Acceptance rates were highly variable among the 13 studies included in the review, ranging from 5% to 91%, but the authors did not attempt to explain the factors responsible for the variability. The pooled acceptance was just under 50%. The most common reasons given by parents for non-acceptance were concerns about vaccine efficacy, safety, and side effects, but no quantitative results were presented.

Several other systematic reviews of quantitative studies have been limited to "controversial" vaccines other than measles and COVID, such as HPV and influenza. For HPV vaccine, Newman and coworkers systematically reviewed 79 studies including over 840,000 parents of children and adolescents living in 15 countries [19]. The overall uptake rate was only 41.5%, and the rate was twice as high for girls as for boys. The reason for the sex discrepancy is almost certainly that the disease vaccinated against (cervical cancer) is restricted to women. But HPV is sexually transmitted, and public health recommendations for universal HPV vaccination apply to both sexes. Factors significantly favoring uptake included physician recommendation, receipt of a recent check-up, and belief in the value of vaccines in general; factors negatively associated with uptake were safety concerns and out-of-pocket costs. Finally, Kang and colleagues' narrative systematic review included 11 studies of parents' attitudes and beliefs about school-based influenza vaccine programs in the USA [20]. Significant facilitators of flu vaccination included no or low cost, belief in the efficacy of the vaccine, and perceived severity of influenza. The principal barriers identified were concerns about vaccine safety and side effects and distrust of the school setting.

In summary, the evidence reviewed above demonstrates that many parents believe that vaccines can be dangerous, and some mistrust the medical and pharmaceutical "establishment" sufficiently to delay or even withhold vaccination in their young children. The major reason for these beliefs is fear of adverse vaccine effects. Among the most prominent specific adverse effects feared are autism, autoimmune disease, and weakening or "overwhelming" the immune system to the point of increasing susceptibility to ordinary infections. In the next section, I will review the scientific evidence bearing on these specific adverse effects.

Key Evidence Points
- Parents' fear of adverse childhood vaccine effects is a major contributor to vaccine hesitancy in high-income countries, especially among ethnic minorities.
- Autism, autoimmune disease, and weakening or "overwhelming" the immune system are among the specific adverse effects mentioned by parents.
- Based on large, population-based studies, the risk of autism is not increased in children who receive measles (or MMR) vaccine or other childhood vaccines.
- Despite the large number of childhood vaccines currently recommended, fully vaccinated children are at lower overall risk of death and no increase in risk of infections unrelated to the bacteria or viruses vaccinated against.
- Autoimmune diseases like type 1 diabetes, Crohn's disease, ulcerative colitis, rheumatic diseases, and multiple sclerosis are not caused by childhood vaccination.
- Multisystem inflammatory disease and myocarditis do occur in children who receive COVID-19 vaccine, but at a much lower rate than in the unvaccinated.

Detailed Review of Scientific Evidence Behind Parents' Beliefs[1]

Autism

Autism is a brain disorder characterized by disabilities in language development and social interaction in childhood. Although the signs of autism can be observed during the first year of life in severe cases, they may be delayed to the second year or even later in less severe forms of the disease. The disorder persists into adulthood. Autism affects at least 1% of all children, a much higher prevalence than previously thought. No blood or brain imaging tests can accurately identify autism,

---

[1] Readers who prefer to skip the Detailed Review should proceed to the Summary at the end of the chapter.

and the recent rise in prevalence is likely due to increased awareness of the condition and a broader clinical spectrum that now includes milder cases; hence, the now frequent term *autism spectrum disorder*, or ASD. A true increase in occurrence cannot be excluded, however.

The age period when autism signs and symptoms are often first noted is the same period at which most children receive the large majority of their vaccines. It is therefore likely that one or more vaccines were received in the days or weeks prior to the first observed autistic traits. In other words, a chance *temporal association* with vaccination is likely to lead some parents to infer that a recently received vaccine was the *cause* of the child's autism. In 1998, Andrew Wakefield and his colleagues published an article in the *Lancet*, a prestigious British medical journal, describing what the authors claimed was a new syndrome in 12 children. The new syndrome combined what the authors referred to as "regressive autism" and "non-specific colitis" (inflammation of the large intestine) after the children received the combination measles-mumps-rubella (MMR) vaccine [21].

Some years later, a British investigative journalist named Brian Deer helped uncover the fraud that underlay Wakefield's new syndrome. Deer found out that many of the parents of the children described in the *Lancet* article had been coached prior to their evaluation by Wakefield and his team, that the intestinal biopsies claimed as showing colitis were mostly entirely normal when reviewed by independent experts, that several of the children had clearly shown autistic symptoms *before* their MMR vaccination, and that Dr. Wakefield had received several hundred thousand pounds in consulting fees from a lawyer who was coordinating a lawsuit against the vaccine manufacturer. In light of these revelations, the UK's General Medical Council undertook an extensive review of the evidence. As a result, Dr. Wakefield's license to practice medicine was revoked, and the *Lancet* published a retraction of the 1998 article [21]. Mr. Deer published a summary of these events in a 2011 article in the *British Medical Journal* [22].

Unrelated to the Wakefield episode, but occurring around the same time, theoretical concerns were raised about organic mercury in vaccines. Thimerosal is a mercury-based preservative that had been added to vaccine vials intended to provide multiple doses of the vaccine. The thimerosal helps prevent growth of bacteria that might get into the vial with multiple needle accesses. Health concerns about mercury were based on the known human toxicity of methylmercury, not the ethylmercury in thimerosal. Nonetheless, in 2001, the U.S. Food and Drug Administration took the cautious approach of requiring removal of thimerosal from all childhood vaccines. The publicity around thimerosal, however, along with the increase in reported prevalence of autism, led some parents of autistic children to blame their children's condition on the child's prior receipt of thimerosal-containing vaccine. A 2014 systematic review and meta-analysis of observational studies by Taylor and colleagues, however, found no increased risk of autism or ASD with MMR, mercury- or thimerosal-containing vaccines, or vaccines in general [23]. More recent systematic reviews of MMR vaccine have confirmed those findings for MMR [3, 24].

Several recent systematic reviews have observed higher blood, urine, or hair levels of mercury, lead, arsenic, cadmium, or aluminum among children and adults with autism or ASD than among non-autistic controls [25–28]. These heavy metal levels were all obtained *after* the autism diagnosis was made, however, and sometimes many years after the diagnosis. Moreover, no evidence from the studies included in these reviews documents the source of the heavy metals, nor implicates vaccines. It is possible that autistic children and adults may eat or drink products (other than conventional foods and beverages) containing high levels of these metals, and some of the authors have speculated about differences in metabolism as the reason for their findings.

Adverse Effects on the Immune System

When I was a young child, the only routinely administered vaccines were DTP and smallpox. Smallpox has now been eliminated, so that vaccine is no longer given. Polio vaccines were introduced when I was in primary school. I have distinct memories of being ill with measles, mumps, German measles (rubella), and chickenpox. Vaccines against those diseases are now routine in most high-income countries, as are vaccines to prevent rotavirus, two different types of bacterial meningitis, bacterial pneumonia, hepatitis A and B, influenza, COVID-19, and HPV.

As mentioned in the previous section, many parents fear that the large number of vaccines recommended for babies and toddlers may overwhelm or "shut down" the immune system. Most parents are probably not aware, however, that babies and young children are exposed to far more bacterial and viral antigens than those contained in vaccines. Antigens are the proteins that stimulate the immune system to produce antibodies and enhance immune cells to recognize and fight invading germs. Most food contains bacteria, and both bacteria and viruses commonly colonize (live in) the mouth, nose, ears, skin, and intestinal tract. Of course, those germs are not injected, as the vaccines are.

Glanz and coworkers carried out a prospective observational study of nearly half a million children followed in six health care organizations participating in the U.S. Centers for Disease Control and Prevention's Vaccine Safety Link, a national surveillance network set up to monitor vaccine safety [29]. The authors formed two groups of children: those with (the cases) and those without (the controls) health care visits between 2 and 4 years of age for infections caused by bacteria or viruses not contained in recommended vaccines. The two groups were then compared with respect to the number of vaccine antigens to which they had been exposed in the first 2 years of life. The number of vaccine antigens was virtually identical in the cases and controls: 241 and 243, respectively.

Higgins and colleagues' 2016 systematic review and meta-analysis evaluated randomized trials of BCG (Bacillus Calmette-Guérin) and measles-containing vaccines for their effect on mortality [30]. BCG is a vaccine frequently administered in low- and middle-income countries to prevent tuberculosis. The deaths that occurred in the included studies could be from any cause, including vaccine-related or vaccine-unrelated infections, accidents, or cancer. Randomized trials are helpful for this type of analysis to reduce confounding by the *reasons* for not receiving the vaccines, since children with chronic diseases or other risk factors are more likely not to be vaccinated. Based on five randomized controlled trials (RCTs) of BCG, mortality was reduced by 30%. Meta-analysis of four RCTs of measles-containing vaccines found the mortality risk to be reduced by 24%, but the reduction was not statistically significant.

What about parents' concerns about autoimmune diseases? These diseases are caused by immune system inflammation and damage to the body's normal organs and tissues. They include type 1 diabetes; intestinal diseases like ulcerative colitis, Crohn's disease, and celiac disease; rheumatoid arthritis and lupus; and neurological diseases like multiple sclerosis and Guillain-Barré syndrome. These diseases are fairly rare, and therefore randomized trials are usually too small to provide sufficient statistical power to detect an increased risk. Pineton de Chambrun and colleagues' 2015 systematic review of 11 observational studies found no increased risk of Crohn's disease or ulcerative colitis in children who received DTP, influenza, or measles-containing vaccines [31]. Mailand and Fredriksen's 2017 systematic review observed no increased risk of multiple sclerosis associated with DTP, polio, MMR, or BCG vaccines [32]. Zhang and coworkers' recent systematic review and meta-analysis of 7 studies of nearly 6 million children found no increase in risk of type 1 diabetes or celiac disease in recipients of rotavirus vaccine [33].

Wang and coworkers' 2017 systematic review and meta-analysis reported an increased risk of both rheumatoid arthritis and lupus (a multisystem rheumatic disease) after vaccination, but the 16 studies included in the review focused on vaccines administered to adolescents and adults, such as HPV, influenza, and herpes zoster (shingles) vaccines, rather than those administered to children [34]. In more recent systematic reviews limited to HPV, however, no increase in risk of autoimmune diseases was observed overall or with Guillain-Barré syndrome [35, 36].

Finally, two recently discovered autoimmune diseases have been described in recipients of COVID-19 mRNA vaccines: multisystem inflammatory syndrome in children (MIS-C, an inflammation of the skin, kidneys, heart, and intestines) and myocarditis (inflammation of the heart muscle). Watanabe and coworkers' recent systematic review of these diseases after receipt of COVID vaccines included two randomized trials and 15 observational studies involving nearly 11 million vaccinated children and 2.6 million unvaccinated (control) children [37]. MIS-C was observed after COVID vaccine in children but its risk was *reduced* 20-fold compared to unvaccinated children, because MIS-C, although uncommon, is known to occur in children with COVID infection, which of course is more likely to develop in unvaccinated children. Myocarditis was observed in 1.3 children per million children vaccinated following the first dose of COVID vaccine and 1.8 per million after the second dose. These rates are too low to compare to those in the unvaccinated group, although a large, population-based Israeli study in older adolescents and adults observed a threefold *reduction* in myocarditis among participants vaccinated versus unvaccinated against COVID-19 [38].

Summary

Vaccines have prevented many millions of deaths over the last 75 years. Nonetheless, the large increase in number of recommended vaccines for children and the growth of social media have led to a rise in parental concerns about vaccine safety, particularly the risks of autism and adverse effects on the immune system. Concerns about autism focused on the measles-mumps-rubella (MMR) vaccine, leading to a marked fall in MMR vaccination and consequent rise in measles infections and deaths in many high-income countries. High-quality systematic reviews and meta-analyses have found no increase in risks of autism, infection by bacteria or viruses not included in the vaccines, death from all causes, or autoimmune diseases associated with MMR or other childhood vaccines. HPV and other vaccines administered to adolescents and adults, however, may increase the risk of rheumatic diseases.

References

1. Kramer MS. Beyond parenting advice: how science should guide your decisions on pregnancy and child-rearing. Springer Nature: Cham; 2021.
2. Institute of Medicine. Adverse events associated with childhood vaccines: evidence bearing on causality. Washington, DC: The National Academies Press; 1994. https://doi.org/10.17226/2138.
3. Gidengil C, Goetz MB, Newberry S, Maglione M, Hall O, Larkin J, Motala A, Hempel S. Safety of vaccines used for routine immunization in the United States: an updated systematic review and meta-analysis. Vaccine. 2021;39(28):3696–716.
4. Wilson L, Rubens-Augustson T, Murphy M, Jardine C, Crowcroft N, Hui C, Wilson K. Barriers to immunization among newcomers: a systematic review. Vaccine. 2018;36(8):1055–62.
5. Gidengil C, Chen C, Parker AM, Nowak S, Matthews L. Beliefs around childhood vaccines in the United States: a systematic review. Vaccine. 2019;37(45):6793–802.
6. Díaz Crescitelli ME, Ghirotto L, Sisson H, Sarli L, Artioli G, Bassi MC, Appicciutoli G, Hayter M. A meta-synthesis study of the key elements involved in childhood vaccine hesitancy. Public Health. 2020;180:38–45.
7. Skafle I, Nordahl-Hansen A, Quintana DS, Wynn R, Gabarron E. Misinformation about COVID-19 vaccines on social media: rapid review. J Med Internet Res. 2022;24(8):e37367.
8. Forster AS, Rockliffe L, Chorley AJ, Marlow LAV, Bedford H, Smith SG, Waller J. Ethnicity-specific factors influencing childhood immunisation decisions among Black and Asian Minority Ethnic groups in the UK: a systematic review of qualitative research. J Epidemiol Community Health. 2017;71(6):544–9.
9. Wilder-Smith AB, Qureshi K. Resurgence of measles in Europe: a systematic review on parental attitudes and beliefs of measles vaccine. J Epidemiol Glob Health. 2020;10(1):46–58.
10. Anderson-Chavarria M, Turner J. Searching for the 'Trigger': an ethnographic analysis of parental beliefs regarding autism causation and vaccination in Puerto Rico. Vaccine. 2023;41(2):540–6.
11. Smith LE, Amlôt R, Weinman J, Yiend J, Rubin GJ. A systematic review of factors affecting vaccine uptake in young children. Vaccine. 2017;35(45):6059–69.
12. Karafillakis E, Larson HJ, ADVANCE Consortium. The benefit of the doubt or doubts over benefits? A systematic literature review of perceived risks of vaccines in European populations. Vaccine. 2017;35(37):4840–50.

13. Périères L, Séror V, Boyer S, Sokhna C, Peretti-Watel P. Reasons given for non-vaccination and under-vaccination of children and adolescents in sub-Saharan Africa: a systematic review. Hum Vaccin Immunother. 2022;18(5):2076524.
14. Bocquier A, Ward J, Raude J, Peretti-Watel P, Verger P. Socioeconomic differences in child-hood vaccination in developed countries: a systematic review of quantitative studies. Expert Rev Vaccines. 2017;16(11):1107–18.
15. Tabacchi G, Costantino C, Napoli G, Marchese V, Cracchiolo M, Casuccio A, Vitale F, The Esculapio Working Group. Determinants of European parents' decision on the vaccination of their children against measles, mumps and rubella: a systematic review and meta-analysis. Hum Vaccin Immunother. 2016;12(7):1909–23.
16. Chen F, He Y, Shi Y. Parents' and guardians' willingness to vaccinate their children against COVID-19: a systematic review and meta-analysis. Vaccines (Basel). 2022;10(2):179.
17. Bianchi FP, Stefanizzi P, Cuscianna E, Riformato G, Di Lorenzo A, Giordano P, Germinario CA, Tafuri S. COVID-19 vaccination hesitancy among Italian parents: a systematic review and meta-analysis. Hum Vaccin Immunother. 2023;19(1):2171185.
18. Abu El Kheir-Mataria W, Saleh BM, El-Fawal H, Chun S. COVID-19 vaccine hesitancy among parents in low- and middle-income countries: a meta-analysis. Front Public Health. 2023;11:1078009.
19. Newman PA, Logie CH, Lacombe-Duncan A, Baiden P, Tepjan S, Rubincam C, Doukas N, Asey F. Parents' uptake of human papillomavirus vaccines for their children: a systematic review and meta-analysis of observational studies. BMJ Open. 2018;8(4):e019206.
20. Kang GJ, Culp RK, Abbas KM. Facilitators and barriers of parental attitudes and beliefs toward school-located influenza vaccination in the United States: systematic review. Vaccine. 2017;35(16):1987–95.
21. Wakefield AJ, Murch SH, Anthony A, Linnell J, Casson DM, Malik M, Berelowitz M, Dhillon AP, Thomson MA, Harvey P, Valentine A, Davies SE, Walker-Smith JA. Ileal-lymphoid-nodular hyperplasia, non-specific colitis, and pervasive developmental disorder in children. Lancet. 1998;351(9103):637–41. Retraction in: Lancet. 2010;375(9713):445.
22. Deer B. How the case against the MMR vaccine was fixed. BMJ. 2011;342:c5347.
23. Taylor LE, Swerdfeger AL, Eslick GD. Vaccines are not associated with autism: an evidence-based meta-analysis of case-control and cohort studies. Vaccine. 2014;32(29):3623–9.
24. Di Pietrantonj C, Rivetti A, Marchione P, Debalini MG, Demicheli V. Vaccines for measles, mumps, rubella, and varicella in children. Cochrane Database Syst Rev. 2020;4(4):CD004407.
25. Jafari T, Rostampour N, Fallah AA, Hesami A. The association between mercury levels and autism spectrum disorders: a systematic review and meta-analysis. J Trace Elem Med Biol. 2017;44:289–97.
26. Sulaiman R, Wang M, Ren X. Exposure to aluminum, cadmium, and mercury and autism spectrum disorder in children: a systematic review and meta-analysis. Chem Res Toxicol. 2020;33(11):2699–718.
27. Amadi CN, Orish CN, Frazzoli C, Orisakwe OE. Association of autism with toxic metals: 2 systematic review of case-control studies. Pharmacol Biochem Behav. 2022;212:173313.
28. Shiani A, Sharafi K, Omer AK, Kiani A, Karamimatin B, Massahi T, Ebrahimzadeh G. A sys-tematic literature review on the association between exposures to toxic elements and an autism spectrum disorder. Sci Total Environ. 2023;857(Pt 2):159246.
29. Glanz JM, Newcomer SR, Daley MF, DeStefano F, Groom HC, Jackson ML, Lewin BJ, McCarthy NL, McClure DL, Narwaney KJ, Nordin JD, Zerbo O. Association between estimated cumulative vaccine antigen exposure through the first 23 months of life and non-vaccine-targeted infections from 24 through 47 months of age. JAMA. 2018;319(9):906–13.
30. Higgins JP, Soares-Weiser K, López-López JA, Kakourou A, Chaplin K, Christensen H, Martin NK, Sterne JA, Reingold AL. Association of BCG, DTP, and measles containing vaccines with childhood mortality: systematic review. BMJ. 2016;355:i5170.
31. Pineton de Chambrun G, Dauchet L, Gower-Rousseau C, Cortot A, Colombel JF, Peyrin-Biroulet L. Vaccination and risk for developing inflammatory bowel disease: a meta-analysis of case-control and cohort studies. Clin Gastroenterol Hepatol. 2015;13(8):1405–15.

32. Mailand MT, Frederiksen JL. Vaccines and multiple sclerosis: a systematic review. J Neurol. 2017;264(6):1035–50.
33. Zhang X, Xu XF, Jin J. Rotavirus vaccination and the risk of type 1 diabetes and celiac disease: a systematic review and meta-analysis. Front Pediatr. 2022;10:951127.
34. Wang B, Shao X, Wang D, Xu D, Zhang JA. Vaccinations and risk of systemic lupus erythematosus and rheumatoid arthritis: a systematic review and meta-analysis. Autoimmun Rev. 2017;16(7):756–65.
35. Genovese C, La Fauci V, Squeri A, Trimarchi G, Squeri R. HPV vaccine and autoimmune diseases: systematic review and meta-analysis of the literature. J Prev Med Hyg. 2018;59(3):e194–9.
36. Boender TS, Bartmeyer B, Coole L, Wichmann O, Harder T. Risk of Guillain-Barré syndrome after vaccination against human papillomavirus: a systematic review and meta-analysis, 1 January 2000 to 4 April 2020. Euro Surveill. 2022;27(4):2001619.
37. Watanabe A, Kani R, Iwagami M, Takagi H, Yasuhara J, Kuno T. Assessment of efficacy and safety of mRNA COVID-19 vaccines in children aged 5 to 11 years: a systematic review and meta-analysis. JAMA Pediatr. 2023;177(4):384–94.
38. Barda N, Dagan N, Ben-Shlomo Y, Kepten E, Waxman J, Ohana R, Hernán MA, Lipsitch M, Kohane I, Netzer D, Reis BY, Balicer RD. Safety of the BNT162b2 mRNA Covid-19 vaccine in a nationwide setting. N Engl J Med. 2021;385(12):1078–90.

Does Teething Cause Fever, Rash, and Other Signs of Illness?

22

Introduction

A baby's first teeth emerge around 6–8 months of age, and tooth eruption continues through the rest of infancy and toddlerhood. A full set of 20 primary (baby) teeth is usually achieved between 24 and 30 months. Parents can often observe red or bluish-red firm ridges on the gum before each tooth erupts, often accompanied by redness and swelling of the surrounding gum. Toward the end of toddlerhood (after 2 years), most children are talking and can tell their parents if they are experiencing pain or other symptoms. But during the first year or 18 months, drooling, fussiness, and disturbed sleep are the main indications that the baby is experiencing some discomfort.

Hard rubber or plastic teething rings are often offered to the baby to chew on, sometimes chilled in the refrigerator or freezer, but I was unable to find any placebo-controlled randomized trials demonstrating their effectiveness in relieving the discomfort. Hard raw vegetables like carrots or celery are sometimes used instead, but the danger of breakage and choking raises questions of safety. Acetaminophen (Tylenol) and ibuprofen (Advil, Motrin) syrups are proven pain relievers, although I found no randomized trials of their use for teething. In any case, the discomfort usually lasts only a few days and resolves soon after the tooth breaks through the gum (Fig. 22.1).

Historical Perspective

The recognition that emerging teeth are a source of pain and discomfort for the infant can be traced back at least 5000 years to the Sumerians, and the issue was mentioned in the Atharva Veda (Hindu) prayers and hymns in ancient India from around 1000 BC [1]. Hippocrates, often called the "father" of modern medicine, wrote what is apparently the first treatise on teething, in which he wrote that teething causes serious illnesses, including fever, diarrhea, and convulsions [1].

© The Author(s), under exclusive license to Springer Nature Switzerland AG 2023
M. S. Kramer, *Believe It or Not*, https://doi.org/10.1007/978-3-031-46022-7_22

Fig. 22.1 Hard rubber or plastic toys are often used to relieve teething symptoms

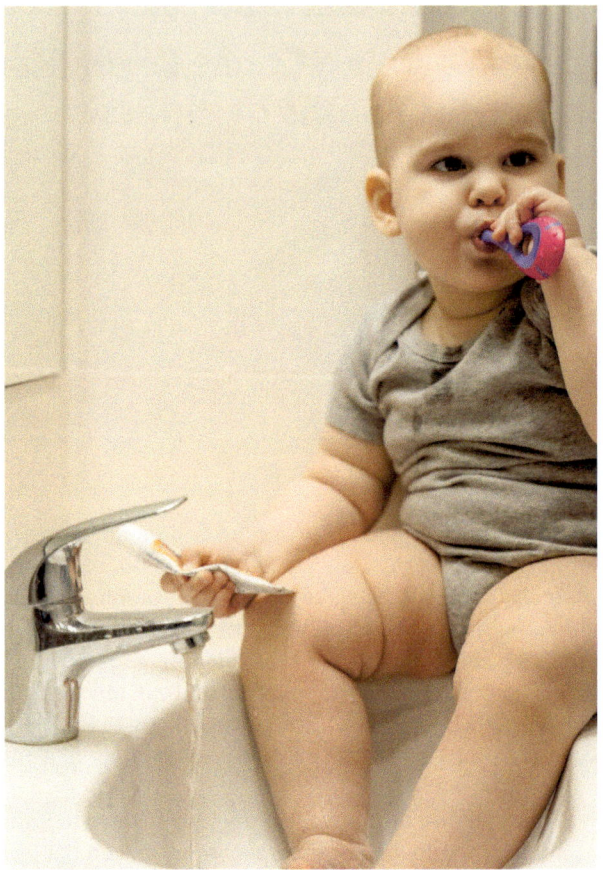

In Roman times, Soranus of Ephesus (Turkey) was the first of many physicians to recommend smearing hare's brain on the gum of the teething infant, a remedy that persisted until the seventeenth century [1]. (This may be the origin of the modern term "hare-brained scheme.") Other topical treatments popular in the Middle Ages included chewing on red coral or animal teeth. In the nineteenth century, other concoctions replaced hare brain for topical (applied to the gum) treatment. Some of them became big business. The manufacturers of Mrs. Winslow's Soothing Syrup advertised the syrup as follows: "Depend on it, Mothers, it will give rest to yourselves and relief and health to your babies" [2]. The syrup may well have provided those benefits, since it contained both morphine and alcohol, although I shudder to think about the deaths it may have caused!

In the sixteenth century, the French army surgeon Ambroise Paré introduced the practice of lancing (cutting) the gum overlying the erupting tooth to "ease" its emergence [3]. This barbaric practice remained popular, albeit untested and unchallenged, throughout the next several centuries. Marshall Hall, a nineteenth-century British physician, claimed he "would rather lance a child's gums 199 times unnecessarily than omit it once if necessary" [3], although I doubt the baby would have the same preference. Vigorous objection to lancing gradually emerged later in the century, but the practice persisted at least until 1919 [4].

What Do Parents and Health Providers Believe About Teething?

Parents

I was able to locate only a single, recent systematic review and meta-analysis of published surveys of parental beliefs and practices about infant teething and the signs and symptoms it causes. Pereira and colleagues' 2023 systematic review included 29 studies involving over 10,000 parents from 16 different countries, including Africa, the Middle East, North and South America, Europe, and Australia [5]. The most commonly reported beliefs about signs and symptoms were excessive biting (median frequency reported, 78%), fever (76%), redness of gums (61%), general irritability (61%), excess salivation (60%), finger sucking (56%), and diarrhea (54%). The most common practices reported for treating those signs and symptoms were providing extra fluids (64%), taking the child to the doctor (55%), acetaminophen (51%), teething syrups or gels (44%), and teething rings or other hard objects (37%). Of note, the country in which the study was carried out was not significantly associated with the prevalence of these beliefs and practices.

Health Care Professionals

I was unable to find any systematic reviews of health care providers' teething beliefs and practices. I did, however, locate four individual studies among physicians and other health care professionals. In a survey from Florida, Correil and colleagues mailed a questionnaire to all 575 physicians who were members of the Florida Pediatric Society to assess their beliefs about "teething diarrhea" [6]. The use of that term, of course, strongly suggests teething as a *cause* of the diarrhea. Of the 575 mailed questionnaire, the authors received 215 (37%) usable responses; of those 215, 75 (35%) of the pediatricians responded positively to the existence of the teething-diarrhea association. Surprisingly to me, pediatricians who had completed their residency training more recently were slightly *more* likely to endorse the existence of teething diarrhea than those with more years in practice.

Barlow and coworkers surveyed parents' beliefs but also distributed their survey questionnaire to 100 randomly selected pediatricians and all 33 pediatric dentists practicing in the state of Iowa, of whom 45 and 25, respectively, responded [7]. Interestingly, the pediatric dentists' responses were similar to those of the parents, with over 80% agreeing that red, swollen gums and irritability, drooling, and sleep disturbance were caused by teething and around half agreeing that fever, decreased appetite, and diarrhea were also consequences of teething. Although the pediatricians agreed with the parents and dentists about the oral signs and symptoms, irritability, and reduced appetite, only 9% agreed that diarrhea was attributable to teething and only half agreed with fever as a consequence.

Wake and Hesketh compared beliefs about teething signs and symptoms among five groups of randomly selected health professionals in Victoria, Australia: 100 general practitioners, 100 maternal and child health nurses, 100 pharmacists, 100 dentists, and 100 pediatricians [8]. Questionnaires including a list of possible signs and symptoms of teething were mailed to those selected, with a very good (85%) overall response rate. The five groups of health professionals differed widely in the frequency with which they believed that all or most teething children demonstrated at least some signs and symptoms: 75% of the nurses, 60% of pharmacists, nearly half of general practitioners, but only about 25% of the dentists and pediatricians.

A more recent survey from New Zealand used a similar design and the same questionnaire as the Australian study but included two groups of nurses (regular practice nurses and maternal and child health nurses), as well as dental therapists [9]. The sample of practitioners was chosen primarily from the area where the authors were located (rather than a random sample), and the overall response rate (41%) was much lower than that of the Australian study. More than half of the dentists, practice nurses, and pharmacists believed that all or most children experience teething signs and symptoms; just under half of the maternal and child health nurses shared that belief, but only about a quarter of the general practitioners and *none* of the pediatricians adhered to the same belief.

In summary, as for parents, health care providers ascribe a number of signs and symptoms to teething. Unsurprisingly, they almost always attribute obvious local (oral) signs and symptoms like red and swollen gums and drooling to teething, but many also believe that more general, systemic problems like irritability, sleep disturbance, decreased appetite, fever, and diarrhea are caused by teething. The attribution of systemic problems varies among types of health care providers: more common among dentists, pharmacists, and nurses and less common among general practitioners and especially among pediatricians.

Key Evidence Points
- The pain and discomfort of teething in infants have been recognized for 5000 years.
- Primary ("baby") teeth eruption begins around 6 months and extends to 24–30 months, an age when infections and other causes of distress are very common.
- Sore gums, drooling, and biting behavior are well-established local (oral) signs and symptoms of teething.
- Many parents, and even health care providers, also believe that systemic symptoms like fever and diarrhea are caused by teething.
- It is extremely difficult to study whether systemic signs and symptoms are *caused* by teething, because tooth eruption cannot be randomly allocated.
- The best-designed observational studies have involved longitudinal follow-up of infants with frequent, intensive measurement of new tooth eruption and of potential signs and symptoms, but blinding of observers is difficult.
- The most rigorous of these observational studies show increased irritability and disturbed sleep associated with teething, but not diarrhea or true fever, although some have shown higher average temperatures within the normal range.

Systemic Consequences of Teething: Detailed Review of the Evidence[1]

Why have the health consequences of teething remained so controversial for so long? One of the main reasons is that during the first year or two of life, signs and symptoms like diarrhea, fever, sleep disturbance, and poor appetite occur quite commonly. They are often caused by viral infections like colds and gastroenteritis, which are extremely frequent among infants and toddlers—especially those who attend daycare and are therefore in close contact with other infected babies. Since teething is universal among babies between the ages of 6 and 24 months, the co-occurrence of teething and viral infection is very common.

In previous centuries, in fact, teething was often listed as the cause of *death* in infants, because many were teething at the time they died. Infant mortality rates were so high that half of all infant deaths in France between the sixteenth and nineteenth centuries were attributed to teething [10]. In 1839, teething was the recorded cause of death for over 5000 childhood deaths in England, constituting 12% of all deaths under the age of 4 years [10]. The Leeds (England) General Cemetery burial register contains over 450 child deaths for which teething is the listed cause of death [11].

So how can we distinguish cause from coincidence when systemic signs and symptoms co-occur with teething? For readers of this book who have not read Chap. 1, or read it long ago, I suggest reviewing it now. Randomized controlled trials (RCTs) won't work here, because we can't randomly assign babies to teethe or not teethe. But at the very least, observational studies must compare signs and symptoms among teething babies and non-teething babies of the same age—in other words, a control group. Those studies should also measure and control for potentially confounding factors like daycare attendance, the presence of young siblings at home, exposure to smokers at home, etc. An even stronger design would be to follow and assess the same babies prospectively over several months' time, using parent diaries and/or frequent examinations by health care providers to assess both emerging new teeth and the presence or absence of systemic signs and symptoms.

I was able to find three systematic reviews of observational studies. One of these was a narrative review (that is, without quantitative meta-analysis) reporting on multiple signs and symptoms [12], while the other two [13, 14] did include a meta-analysis, one of which was limited to studies of fever [14]. Unfortunately, none of the three systematic reviews restricted their analysis to studies that meet the methodologic criteria discussed in the previous paragraph and, in particular, the necessity of a non-teething control group to ensure that the presence of signs and symptoms with teething was not merely coincidental. Moreover, it is difficult to understand why the three systematic reviews included vastly different numbers of studies: 5 for Tighe and Roe [12], 16 for Massignan and colleagues [13], and 6 for Nemezio and coworkers [14]. The latter review's restriction to studies of fever

---

[1] Readers who prefer to skip the Detailed Review should proceed to the Summary at the end of the chapter.

cannot explain this discrepancy, since most studies of multiple systemic signs and symptoms have also included temperature and/or fever. This disparity is a poignant reminder that systematic reviewing is *not* an exact science!

I have therefore been forced to review, one by one, published studies that followed the observational design I discussed two paragraphs above, all of which involved the same group of infants and toddlers assessed over time (often daily!) before, during, and after teeth eruption. These studies were carried out in Tel Aviv, Israel; Cleveland, USA; Melbourne, Australia; and Diamantina, Brazil. I will summarize their methods and results in chronological order of publication. (I have omitted an older Israeli study from Jerusalem [15], because I am unable to interpret the data presented by the authors.) Unfortunately, all of the studies are prone to bias due to non-blinding, since parents or others who recorded the signs and symptoms also knew whether a new tooth had erupted.

Jaber and colleagues enrolled mothers of 46 young healthy infants who attended a single well-baby clinic in Tel Aviv and who had not yet experienced a tooth eruption [16]. The mothers agreed to record, on a *daily* basis (yes, every day!), their babies' rectal temperature and examined the baby's gums for evidence of tooth eruption and whether they were experiencing any diarrhea, convulsions, cough, or other systemic symptoms. The mothers were instructed to bring their baby to the clinic when they suspected a tooth eruption. The average temperature did not change during the period from 19 days to 4 days before the tooth eruption, remaining between 36.9 and 37.1 °C (98.4–98.8 °F), but rose gradually beginning 3 days before eruption to reach 37.6 °C (99.7°) on the day of tooth eruption. Fifteen babies had a temperature of 38 °C or higher (the usual threshold for defining "fever") on the day of eruption, versus five or fewer babies on the 19th to 4th days prior to eruption. No analysis was reported for the days following tooth eruption.

A study using a similar design enrolled parents of 125 healthy 4-month-old infants who were recruited during a routine check-up visit at a group practice in Cleveland, USA [17]. The infants were followed until the age of 12 months; the parents were asked to complete a daily log of 18 signs and symptoms, to record the baby's ear temperature twice per day, and to feel the baby's gums to determine if a new tooth had broken through that day and, if so, to record its location. Parents of 111 of the 125 infants complied with this intensive schedule of data collection. Of the systemic signs and symptoms studied, the following were statistically significantly associated with tooth eruption between 4 days before, the day of, or within 3 days after: irritability, reduced appetite (for solid foods), sleep disturbance, ear rubbing, facial rash, and high temperature (defined as at least one standard deviation above the average for that baby). Of the 2067 days on which the temperature was above 100 °F (37.8 °C), however, only 64 (3%) of those days also had a new tooth eruption.

The Australian study [18] was carried out among 21 babies between 6 and 24 months attending one of the three daycare centers in suburban Melbourne on weekdays during a 7-month period. It was published in the same year as the American study summarized in the previous paragraph but improved on the latter's design by having two independent assessors (parents and daycare staff) rate the babies' signs and symptoms. Moreover, a dental therapist who was unaware of the parents' and staff's symptom ratings took the child's ear temperature and assessed new tooth eruption. Signs, symptoms, and temperature were compared between the period of 5 days leading up to and including the day of tooth eruption and the periods more than 28 days before or after the eruption. The average temperatures were virtually identical (36.2 °C) in teething and non-teething periods. No significant differences were observed in systemic signs or symptoms between teething and non-teething periods, but the very small sample size (21 babies) was unable to exclude fairly large differences (a doubling or even tripling for bad mood, disturbed sleep, and diarrhea) with statistical confidence.

The Brazilian study [19] included 47 infants between 6 and 15 months of age who were assessed daily in their own homes. It incorporated one important design improvement over the above-mentioned studies: the examination of newly erupted teeth and measurement of both ear and armpit temperatures were carried out by specially trained dentists. Unfortunately, however, the dentists also interviewed the mothers about signs and symptoms, and no apparent attempt was made to blind the mothers to the dental examination. Temperatures, signs, and symptoms were compared on non-teething days to the day of, the day before, and the day after tooth eruption. Slightly but statistically significantly lower average ear temperatures (36.5 vs. 36.6 °C) were observed on non-teething days, as well as lower average frequencies of reduced appetite, sleep disturbance, runny nose, and rash.

Summary

The eruption of primary teeth ("baby teeth") has been recognized for thousands of years as a cause of pain and discomfort in infants and toddlers. It seems reasonable to infer that local signs and symptoms such as red, swollen gums around an erupting tooth, as well as drooling and increased biting behavior, are consequences of teething. The best studies also suggest that the systemic signs and symptoms of irritability and sleep disturbance are more common when a baby is teething, probably reflecting the pain and discomfort caused by the emerging tooth. The evidence is less convincing for fever and diarrhea, although a slight rise in temperature within the normal range has been observed in several of the better studies. Despite the intensive, daily follow-up of the high-quality studies, however, none of them is immune to bias due to non-blinding of teething status among the parents or professional staff who reported the signs and symptoms.

References

1. Radbill SX. Teething as a medical problem: changing viewpoints through the centuries. Clin Pediatr. 1965;4:556–9.
2. Day N. Morphine? Wolf's teeth? Hare brain? The endless quest to solve teething. Slate. 17 Apr 2013.
3. Ashley MP. It's only teething…a report of the myths and modern approaches to teething. Br Dent J. 2001;191(1):4–8.
4. McIntyre GT, McIntyre GM. Teething troubles? Br Dent J. 2002;192(5):251–5.

5. Pereira TS, da Silva CA, Quirino ECS, Xavier Junior GF, Takeshita EM, Oliveira LB, De Luca CG, Massignan C. Parental beliefs in and attitudes toward teething signs and symptoms: a systematic review. Int J Paediatr Dent. 2023;33(6):577–584.
6. Coreil J, Price L, Barkey N. Recognition and management of teething diarrhea among Florida pediatricians. Clin Pediatr. 1995;34(11):591–8.
7. Barlow BS, Kanellis MJ, Slayton RL. Tooth eruption symptoms: a survey of parents and health professionals. ASDC J Dent Child. 2002;69(2):148–50.
8. Wake M, Hesketh K. Teething symptoms: cross sectional survey of five groups of child health professionals. BMJ. 2002;325(7368):814.
9. Ispas RS, Mahoney EK, Whyman RA. Teething signs and symptoms: persisting misconceptions among health professionals in New Zealand. N Z Dent J. 2013;109(1):2–5.
10. Markham L. Teething: facts and fiction. Pediatr Rev. 2009;30(8):e59–64.
11. Gerard I, Root K. Teething. Leeds: University of Leeds General Cemetery Collection; 2017.
12. Tighe M, Roe MF. Does a teething child need serious illness excluding? Arch Dis Child. 2007;92(3):266–8.
13. Massignan C, Cardoso M, Porporatti AL, Aydinoz S, Canto Gde L, Mezzomo LA, Bolan M. Signs and symptoms of primary tooth eruption: a meta-analysis. Pediatrics. 2016;137(3):e20153501.
14. Nemezio MA, De Oliveira KM, Romualdo PC, Queiroz AM, Paula-E-Silva FW, Silva RA, Küchler EC. Association between fever and primary tooth eruption: a systematic review and meta-analysis. Int J Clin Pediatr Dent. 2017;10(3):293–8.
15. Galili G, Rosenzweig KA, Klein H. Eruption of primary teeth and general pathologic conditions. ASDC J Dent Child. 1969;36(1):51–4.
16. Jaber L, Cohen IJ, Mor A. Fever associated with teething. Arch Dis Child. 1992;67(2):233–4.
17. Macknin ML, Piedmonte M, Jacobs J, Skibinski C. Symptoms associated with infant teething: a prospective study. Pediatrics. 2000;105(4 Pt 1):747–52.
18. Wake M, Hesketh K, Lucas J. Teething and tooth eruption in infants: a cohort study. Pediatrics. 2000;106(6):1374–9.
19. Ramos-Jorge J, Pordeus IA, Ramos-Jorge ML, Paiva SM. Prospective longitudinal study of signs and symptoms associated with primary tooth eruption. Pediatrics. 2011;128(3):471–6.

No Tylenol? No Problem! Beliefs About Fever and Its Treatment in Children

23

Introduction

The 2022–2023 fall and winter season in the Northern Hemisphere was characterized by a very high incidence of viral respiratory infections, especially those caused by influenza, respiratory syncytial virus (RSV), and COVID-19. The high incidence was probably caused by the ending of the social distancing and wearing of masks previously mandated by public health authorities during the COVID-19 pandemic. The low incidence of influenza and RSV infection while those mandates were in effect almost certainly reduced the natural immunity that would have developed with normal levels of interpersonal contact prior to the pandemic.

In Canada, the most important consequence of the explosion of respiratory virus infections was an unprecedented number of babies and young children crowding hospital emergency departments and walk-in clinics. The result was a huge spike in hospital admissions for bronchiolitis (inflammation of the small airways of the lung) and pneumonia. But another consequence also received a great deal of publicity: Canada, the USA, and Europe experienced a severe shortage of medications used to treat pain and fever, especially the liquid formulations for babies and children. The most commonly used of these medications are acetaminophen (Tylenol, Panadol) and ibuprofen (Advil, Motrin). Pharmacies were shown on the evening news with bare shelves usually packed with these products, and pharmacists complained about back orders and delays. Journalists who interviewed parents, physicians, nurses, and pharmacists all expressed concern about the shortages and the potential grave consequences for children's health, and even for their survival!

I too was concerned about the severity of the respiratory virus epidemic. The Montreal Children's Hospital, where I worked in the Emergency Department for 25 years, even issued a call for retired pediatricians to come back temporarily to help manage the load. I considered offering to help out but then realized that by the time I retooled and received a temporary medical license, the epidemic would have subsided (which it did). My main reaction to the news coverage about the empty pharmacy shelves, however, was dismay that fever "phobia," which had been well

Fig. 23.1 A febrile infant
and her worried mother

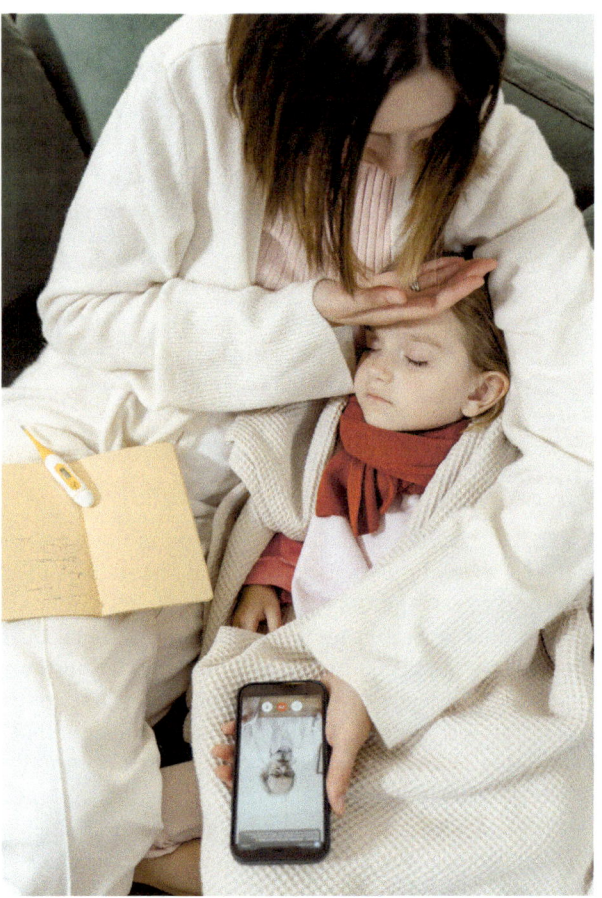

documented by me and other researchers since the 1980s, seemed to be as prevalent today as it was 40 years ago. In other words: *plus ça change, plus c'est la même chose* (the more things change, the more they stay the same). A sober reflection on how little impact research has on health beliefs and practices (Fig. 23.1)!

You might well ask why this Don Quixote would continue to stalk the windmills of erroneous beliefs and practices. I have no illusions that this chapter will eliminate misinformation or radically change how parents and health professionals react to and treat fever in children. But I also believe that if you have made it this far in the book, your mind is open to change if presented with convincing scientific evidence. If so, read on.

Historical Perspective

You may be surprised to learn that arguments about the dangers versus the benefits of fever have existed for thousands of years. Hippocrates and other ancients believed the humoral theory of disease, which postulated four bodily humors: blood, phlegm, yellow bile, and black bile. Balance among the four humors was believed to be essential for health, and fever was considered as a *favorable* sign that ill patients were "cooking" off an excess of phlegm or another of the humors—an indication that the body was combatting an infection or other illness [1, 2]. Conversely, fever was one of God's punishments for sins in the Old Testament (Leviticus 26:16 and Deuteronomy 28:22), and the Romans' goddess Febris was believed to either impose a fever or relieve it [1]. During the Middle Ages, fever was considered divine punishment among Christian believers, a curse by evil spirits among the less devout, and it was a frequent occurrence in victims of the bubonic plague and other severe infections [1, 3].

With the Enlightenment, medical practitioners again began to view fever as a favorable sign. Thomas Sydenham, the noted seventeenth-century English physician, wrote that fever is "nature's engine which she brings into the field to remove her enemy" [4]. Malaria-induced fever was used to treat gonorrhea and syphilis in the eighteenth and nineteenth centuries [1], although I am aware of no randomized trials that demonstrated its effectiveness. Experimental studies have shown increased mortality in animals prevented from developing fevers [5, 6], and laboratory studies in human blood samples have demonstrated improved immune function at febrile temperatures [1].

The renowned nineteenth-century French physiologist Claude Bernard observed that healthy animals died quickly when their body temperature was artificially raised by 5–6 °C (9–11 °F) [7]. That finding, however, relates to hyperthermia, that is, temperature *above* the set-point regulated by the hypothalamus (in the brain). Hyperthermia can lead to heat stroke in humans and is caused by physical activity in hot, humid conditions, or an inability to sweat. Fever, however, is a high temperature caused by an upward shift in the hypothalamic set-point and is caused by hormones released by the immune system. The important distinction between hyperthermia and fever was not recognized until well into the twentieth century, however, and remains poorly understood by the general public and even many health care professionals. Dangerous infections can cause *both* fever *and* brain damage or death. Fever and adverse health outcomes are consequences of infection; fever does not cause the adverse outcome.

Beliefs About Fever and Its Treatment in Children

Parents

In 1980, Schmitt coined the term "fever phobia" after documenting parents' unrealistic fears and over-treatment of fever in their children, based on a survey of 81 parents attending a university-based walk-in clinic in Denver, Colorado [2]. Most of Schmitt's study participants were of lower socioeconomic status, but my colleagues and I confirmed many of the same findings 5 years later in 202 parents of febrile children 6 months to 6 years of age attending a pediatric group practice in Montreal,

Canada [8]. Half of these parents considered temperatures below 38 °C (100.4 °F) to be a fever, over half reported that they would wake their child to treat a fever, and over 85% believed that a high fever that was left untreated could cause a seizure, loss of consciousness, stroke, other brain damage, or death.

In the 40 years that have passed, I would have hoped that fever phobia had diminished, that parents would have learned (or been taught by health care providers) to be less fearful of fever in their children and to be less aggressive in its treatment. Alas, the evidence suggests otherwise. Purssell and Collin's 2016 systematic review included 40 studies with a worldwide geographic distribution and a 35-year time span [9]. Fears of death, convulsions, coma, brain damage, and dehydration caused by fever were prominent, although highly variable across the included studies, and no significant trend toward reduced fear was observed over time for any of these adverse outcomes. The more recent systematic review by Clericetti and coworkers included 65 studies of fever phobia among over 26,000 child caregivers [10]. The authors found a statistically significantly greater degree of fever phobia among parents of low socioeconomic status; Latin American, Turkish, or Bedouin immigrants; parents of children with a previous history of febrile seizures (convulsions with fever); and younger mothers, but the authors did not analyze changes over time.

Health Care Professionals

Although fear of fever and its potential adverse consequences has been primarily studied among parents, several investigators have instead focused on health care professionals. After all, where does parental fever phobia come from? Do physicians, nurses, and pharmacists share the same fears as parents, or do they attempt to allay parental fear?

The above-cited systematic review by Clericetti and colleagues also included 15 studies in 4566 healthcare providers [10]. Although detailed data are not provided, fever phobia was common among all types of healthcare providers, with many of the same fears of adverse health outcomes and aggressive treatment practices as parents, especially among nurses. In one study from Lisbon, Portugal, nurses and general practitioners were more "phobic" about childhood fever than pediatricians [11]. Pediatricians were more likely to prescribe antipyretics to treat discomfort or irritability than to prevent seizures or other adverse consequences. A recent Australian study not included in the Clericetti review used Facebook to recruit 839 health professionals across the country, including nurses, general practitioners, pediatricians, and pharmacists [12]. Fear of death, seizures, and brain damage was highest among pharmacists, next-highest among nurses, and lowest among pediatricians.

Finally, Milani and coworkers recently used an online questionnaire to survey 121 final-year nursing students from five Italian university hospitals: 50% of those invited to participate [13]. More than 80% of them said they would use physical methods to reduce a child's fever. Respondents who felt knowledgeable about fever management were only one-third as likely to believe that high fever could cause brain damage as those who did not feel knowledgeable.

Do Educational Interventions Reduce Fever Phobia?

The stubborn persistence of parental fever phobia documented over the last 40 years suggests that educational interventions have not been effective. Perhaps they have not even been attempted, given that healthcare professionals seem to fear fever in children as much as parents! In this section, I will briefly review the scientific evidence bearing on the success of such interventions by health care providers, pharmacists, or public health authorities.

Before that review, I first wish to emphasize two points. First, as with any study of interventions, randomized trials, preferably with a placebo control intervention, are necessary to avoid confounding by factors that influence parents' receptiveness to the intervention, prior knowledge or fear of fever, health care-seeking behavior, and management of their children's fever. Randomization also facilitates blinding of the parents and observers to the assigned intervention. The second point relates to the study outcomes. Showing that an educational intervention increases parents' knowledge about fever is not very useful unless the intervention also influences how they treat the fever and their use of health care services. Do the parents awaken their febrile child to give acetaminophen or ibuprofen? Do they sponge their child in an attempt to bring down the fever? Do they take their child to an emergency department?

Young and colleagues published a narrative systematic review (without meta-analysis) that included ten studies of educational interventions in 1977 parents [14]. Only five of the ten included studies were randomized trials. A more recent narrative review by Peetoom and coworkers was restricted to eight randomized trials in well-child clinic settings and focused on changing parental behavior with subsequent episodes of fever, including visits to physicians or emergency departments, telephone consultations, home visits, and medication management [15]. Follow-up periods ranged from only 1 to 12 months. Variations in types and definitions of outcomes across trials prevented the authors from meta-analyzing the reported results. A reduction in the frequency of physician consultations was seen in six of the seven trials reporting that outcome; two of three trials observed a significant reduction in home visits. Only those trials with multi-component interventions (involving reinforcement of a single intervention or more than one type of intervention) achieved a reduction in telephone consultations and improved medication management.

The evidence I have just reviewed suggests that educational interventions to reduce fever phobia *can be effective*, if they use multiple types of intervention (such as information leaflets, one-on-one sessions with parents, videos or other communication aids) and multiple occasions to reinforce the message. Given the costs and logistical challenges of such interventions, however, it is not surprising that no overall impact on the parent population has been detectable [9]. That is especially true in light of the fever phobia documented among pharmacists, nurses, and some physicians—the very health care professionals to whom parents are likely to turn for advice. In the case of pharmacists, selling antipyretic medications like acetaminophen and ibuprofen while advising customer parents about what to do for fever in their children creates an obvious conflict of interest!

Key Evidence Points
- Fever has been recognized as a cardinal sign of infection for thousands of years, but opinions have varied widely as to whether children are better off with or without it.
- "Fever phobia," that is, unjustified fear of high fever and its potential consequences, has been repeatedly documented over the past four decades—not just among parents, but also among health care professionals.
- Much of the unjustified fear of fever in children is due to a failure to understand the difference between fever (an upward shift in the body's temperature set-point to a safe level) and hyperthermia (a dangerous rise in temperature above the set-point).
- Despite effective educational interventions, fever phobia has not improved over time.
- Antipyretics like acetaminophen (Tylenol) and ibuprofen (Advil) are not effective in preventing febrile convulsions but do make children more comfortable, whereas physical methods such as sponging and bathing often lead to shivering (discomfort).
- Despite studies demonstrating that antipyretics can increase mortality in animals artificially infected with serious bacterial infections, no adverse effects on duration or severity of viral infections have been found in randomized trials in children.

Detailed Review of Evidence on Treating Fever in Children[1]

The Biology of Fever

Earlier in this chapter, I reviewed the history of beliefs about whether fever is harmful or helpful. Fever is almost always a consequence of infections, most of which are caused by viruses, of short duration (a few days), and not dangerous. Nor is the fever itself dangerous. Much of parents' fear of fever stems from their confusion (unfortunately shared by many health care personnel) of fever with hyperthermia. As I discussed earlier, a fever is an upward regulation of the body's temperature set-point. The set-point is adjusted by a region of the brain called the hypothalamus in

---

[1] Readers who prefer to skip the Detailed Review should proceed to the Summary at the end of the chapter.

response to hormones released by cells of the body's immune system when confronted with a bacterial, viral, fungal, or parasitic "invader." Temperature up-regulation may well be beneficial in helping the immune system fight off the infecting microbe [1].

Moreover, temperatures during fever have a ceiling. Fever-induced temperature elevations rarely exceed 40 or 41 °C (104–106 °F) and almost never exceed 42 °C (107.6 °F). As rare and as scary as those temperatures are, they do not cause death or brain damage. During hyperthermia caused by heavy exercise in hot, humid conditions or when the body's ability to sweat is impaired (as in the elderly), temperatures can rise above that scary level, and heat stroke (brain damage due to overheating) can indeed occur. In contrast, the immune system has evolved over tens of millions of years to ensure that febrile temperatures do *not* rise that high.

Seizures (convulsions) can indeed be a consequence of fever in children, especially babies and toddlers between 6 months and 2 years of age. Febrile seizures are scary for parents, even though they almost never last longer than several seconds or minutes and do not cause brain damage. It may surprise you to learn that scary febrile seizures do not require scary temperatures. Febrile seizures can occur even at 38.5 or 39 °C (101–102 °F) and often arise during the development of the fever—before the parents are even aware that the child is ill! It may also surprise you to learn that antipyretics have *not* been shown to prevent febrile seizures. The same is true for sponging and bathing, which can also make the child shiver from cold if the body temperature is reduced below the elevated set-point. Shivering is one of the body's mechanisms to raise its core temperature. If the child hasn't convulsed by the time the parents take her temperature, she is very unlikely to have a convulsion afterward. As documented in Offringa and colleagues' 2021 Cochrane review, the only treatment that has been convincingly shown to reduce the risk of a febrile seizure is anticonvulsant medication [16]. This medication can be used to prevent a recurrent seizure in a child with a past seizure history but leads to adverse behavioral side effects that outweigh any benefit of preventing another febrile seizure. Antipyretics (acetaminophen or ibuprofen) are ineffective in preventing recurrence of febrile seizures [16].

In summary, fevers in children are limited in how high the temperature can rise and are not dangerous for the child's brain, nor do they threaten the child's life. Obviously, febrile seizures are scary for parents, and it would be great if we could prevent them with safe and effective measures. But the measures that are safe and effective for lowering the child's temperature do not prevent febrile seizures, nor do they speed recovery from the underlying infection that causes the fever. The anticonvulsant medications that are effective in preventing recurrence of febrile seizures should not be used in an attempt to prevent a first febrile seizure, because the seizure is likely to occur before the medication is administered.

In other words, we need to refocus the *goal* of treating a child with fever. If fever is a natural manifestation of the immune system's attempt to fight an infection, then lowering the child's temperature could theoretically do more harm than good by increasing the severity or duration of the illness. Children with infection and fever are often uncomfortable and cranky; some do not sleep well. It is important to avoid the trap of blaming those symptoms on the fever. Adults and older children with infections and fever often experience headache, sore throat, sore muscles, general malaise, fatigue, and reduced appetite. It is reasonable to assume that the same is true for babies and toddlers who are too young to verbalize their complaints or to understand why they have them.

It is therefore reasonable to target the young child's comfort and mood when prescribing antipyretic (fever) medications. Both acetaminophen and ibuprofen have dual effects: they are both pain relievers and antipyretics. Parents tend to blame the child's discomfort and crankiness on the fever and to credit the resulting lower temperature after administering Tylenol or Advil with the improved comfort and mood. But parents tend to treat the thermometer instead of the child and often seem relieved by a falling temperature even if the other symptoms continue unabated!

Review of Published Evidence

With these introductory remarks in mind, I can now proceed with reviewing the published scientific evidence bearing on achievable benefits (improved comfort and behavior) and possible risks (increased severity or duration of illness) of treating fever in babies and young children. I will restrict my review to double-blind, placebo-controlled randomized trials, so as to avoid the obvious biases inherent in observational designs: confounding differences between children receiving active medication versus controls, especially differences in the severity of accompanying symptoms; non-blinding of the parents and care providers to the treatment received; and reverse causality (children given active medication at the peak of their fever or other symptoms are likely to improve sooner than those treated earlier in the course of their illness).

In 1991, my colleagues and I published a double-blind, placebo-controlled randomized trial of an antipyretic (Tylenol) in febrile children 6 months to 6 years of age [17]. The children presented to a group pediatric practice or a university-based emergency department with a fever of at least 38 °C (100.4 °F) lasting 4 days or less and had no evidence of a bacterial infection such as meningitis, pneumonia, ear infection, Strep throat, or urinary tract infection. I emphasize this trial not because I was the lead researcher, but to relate how difficult it was to recruit parents into a study in which they agreed to provide a syrup every 4 h while the fever persisted, a syrup that had only a 50% chance of being "real" Tylenol, rather than a placebo. Parents' reluctance to enroll their child in the study was so powerful that we ran out of funds to support the research assistants to recruit participants at the two study sites long before we reached our target sample size of 210 participants. Several years later we applied for, and received, additional grant support to complete the trial in 1990, 8 years after we had begun! In other words, I understood why it was so difficult to get parents to agree to such a trial and why even after 8 years, no other group of researchers had published a trial like ours!

Parents were asked to keep a diary of rectal temperature and other symptoms four times per day until the child had been fever-free for at least 24 h, as well as to record each administration of study medication. They were asked to rate the change in the child's behavior (separate questions on activity, alertness, mood, comfort, appetite, and fluid intake) 1–2 h after each dose of study medication, using a five-category scale ranging from much worse to much better. They received telephone support from the research assistant every 2–4 days and were asked to mail in their diaries to the trial investigators after the child had recovered. Our primary outcome was the duration of the underlying infection, measured as the time after randomization that the fever resolved and the time that symptoms other than fever had also resolved. The mean durations were virtually identical in the Tylenol and placebo groups. Changes in the child's behavior favored those receiving active Tylenol, with a significantly higher proportion rated as having at least a one-category average improvement in both activity and alertness, but no significant differences for mood, comfort, appetite, or fluid intake. The parents remained blinded to the treatment received (Tylenol vs. placebo), since only half in each treatment group correctly guessed the treatment at the final telephone interview. In summary, Tylenol did not prolong the duration of fever or other illness symptoms but did improve several aspects of the child's behavior. No febrile seizures occurred in either group.

A 2002 Cochrane review included 12 randomized trials, but only 7 of the 12 compared acetaminophen with placebo, and our above-mentioned trial was one of only two that compared duration of fever or other illness symptoms or behavioral signs and symptoms [18]. No significant differences were observed in time to healing of chickenpox rash in the other trial. Unsurprisingly, one trial of a single dose reported that children receiving acetaminophen had a much higher proportion without fever 2 h later than those receiving placebo. The same authors published a second review 1 year later in which they analyzed three randomized trials comparing acetaminophen alone versus acetaminophen plus tepid sponging [19]. Although a higher proportion of children in the combined treatment group had no fever 1 h after a single dose, children in the combined group were also five times as likely to experience shivering and goose bumps as those receiving acetaminophen alone.

Finally, Wong and colleagues' 2013 Cochrane review analyzed six trials that compared the use of a single antipyretic (acetaminophen or ibuprofen) to a combination of the two medications, either in alternating sequence or combined at each administration [20]. Unsurprisingly, combined treatment resulted in lower temperatures after 4 and 6 h of follow-up. One of the trials comparing alternating to single-agent antipyretics reported lower scores on a pain and discomfort scale on days 1, 2, and 3 of the trial, but no placebo was used, and thus the parents (who used the rating scale) were not blinded to which treatment was received.

Summary

In summary, fever has been recognized as a sign of illness (especially infectious illness) for millennia. Opinions have varied widely, however, as to whether infected patients are better off with or without it. The distinction between fever and hyperthermia, and in their risks, is poorly understood by the general public and by many health care providers. Fever phobia is highly prevalent in parents of young children and even among the professionals who provide care to such children and advice to their parents. Despite laboratory studies demonstrating improved immune function at febrile temperatures, human studies have not demonstrated any adverse effects of antipyretic medications on the duration or severity of the underlying infection. Babies and young children appear more alert, active, and comfortable after receiving antipyretic medications, although those benefits may well be effects of pain relief from the medications, rather than fever reduction. Unfortunately, most parents and many health care providers seem more focused on treating the thermometer than the child.

References

1. El-Radhi AS. The role of fever in the past and present. Med J Islam World Acad Sci. 2011;19(1):9–14.
2. Schmitt BD. Fever phobia: misconceptions of parents about fevers. Am J Dis Child. 1980;134(2):176–81.
3. LaFrance A. A cultural history of the fever. The Atlantic. 16 Sept 2015.
4. Payne JF. Thomas Sydenham. London: T Fisher Unwin; 1900.
5. Kluger MJ. Fever: its biology, evolution, and function. Princeton: Princeton University Press; 1979.
6. Kluger MJ, Ringler DH, Anver MR. Fever and survival. Science. 1975;188(4184):166–8.
7. Bernard C. Leçons sur la Chaleur Animale. Paris: Ballière; 1976.
8. Kramer MS, Naimark L, Leduc DG. Parental fever phobia and its correlates. Pediatrics. 1985;75(6):1110–3.
9. Purssell E, Collin J. Fever phobia: the impact of time and mortality—a systematic review and meta-analysis. Int J Nurs Stud. 2016;56:81–9.
10. Clericetti CM, Milani GP, Bianchetti MG, Simonetti GD, Fossali EF, Balestra AM, Bozzini MA, Agostoni C, Lava SAG. Systematic review finds that fever phobia is a worldwide issue among caregivers and healthcare providers. Acta Paediatr. 2019;108(8):1393–7.
11. Martins M, Abecasis F. Healthcare professionals approach paediatric fever in significantly different ways and fever phobia is not just limited to parents. Acta Paediatr. 2016;105(7):829–33.
12. Gaffney GR, Bereznicki LR, Bereznicki BJ. Knowledge, beliefs and management of childhood fever among nurses and other health professionals: a cross-sectional survey. Nurse Educ Today. 2021;97:104731.
13. Milani GP, Corsello A, Fadda M, Falvo I, Bianchetti MG, Peroni D, Chiappini E, Cantoni B, Sannino P, Destrebecq A, Marchisio P. Approach to fever in children among final-year nursing students: a multicenter survey. BMC Nurs. 2023;22(1):119.
14. Young M, Watts R, Wilson S. The effectiveness of educational strategies in improving parental/caregiver management of fever in their child: a systematic review. JBI Libr Syst Rev. 2010;8(21):826–68.
15. Peetoom KK, Smits JJ, Ploum LJ, Verbakel JY, Dinant GJ, Cals JW. Does well-child care education improve consultations and medication management for childhood fever and common infections? A systematic review. Arch Dis Child. 2017;102(3):261–7.
16. Offringa M, Newton R, Nevitt SJ, Vraka K. Prophylactic drug management for febrile seizures in children. Cochrane Database Syst Rev. 2021;6:CD003031.
17. Kramer MS, Naimark LE, Roberts-Bräuer R, McDougall A, Leduc DG. Risks and benefits of paracetamol antipyresis in young children with fever of presumed viral origin. Lancet. 1991;337(8741):591–4.

18. Meremikwu M, Oyo-Ita A. Paracetamol for treating fever in children. Cochrane Database Syst Rev. 2002;2:CD003676.
19. Meremikwu M, Oyo-Ita A. Physical methods for treating fever in children. Cochrane Database Syst Rev. 2003;2:CD004264.
20. Wong T, Stang AS, Ganshorn H, Hartling L, Maconochie IK, Thomsen AM, Johnson DW. Combined and alternating paracetamol and ibuprofen therapy for febrile children. Cochrane Database Syst Rev. 2013;10:CD009572.

Index

A

Acceptable daily intake (ADI), 133
Acesulfame potassium (Ace-K), 132, 135
Acetaminophen, 221, 225, 226, 228, 229
Acne
    chocolate, 70
    closed comedones, 67
    dietary supplements, 68
    fatty or oily foods, 75
    glycemic index carbohydrates, 70
    identical *vs.* non-identical twins, 68
    omega-3 LCPUFAs, 72
    open comedones, 67
    overview, 67
    prevalence of, 69
    vitamin D, 72
    vitamin E, 74
    zinc, 74
Advil, 228
Aloe vera plant, 61
    burn treatment, 62
    history of, 61
    randomized controlled trials (RCTs), 63
    topical antibiotics, 63
Antibiotic resistance, 152
Antihistamines, 119
Antioxidant nutrients, 160
Antipyretics, 224, 226–229
Aroma therapy, 126, 127
Artificial sweeteners
    Ace-K, sucralose, and aspartame, 135
    ADI, 133
    body weight, fat, cardio-metabolic risk
        factors, 137–138
    cancer, 139
    consumption, 134, 135
    dental health, 138
    during pregnancy, 140

glucose and fructose, 131
    history, 131–133
    principles, 136, 137
    sucrose, 131
Ashwagandha root, 123, 124
Aspartame, 132, 135
Astigmatism, 90
Attention deficit hyperactivity disorder
    (ADHD), 144, 145
Autism, 205–207
Autoimmune diseases, 208
Ayurveda alternative medicine
    system, 115, 123

B

Bacillus Calmette-Guérin (BCG), 207
Beneficial chance occurrence, 4
Biting behavior, 215
Body weight, 137, 138
Brain damage, 223–225, 227

C

Caloric restriction, 105
Campylobacter, 158
Chamomile, 122, 123
Child behavior
    confounding and reverse causality,
        146, 147
    food additive, 143
    hyper behavior, 144, 145
    sleep and diet, 147
    sugar intake, 145, 146
Childhood vaccines
    autism, 205–207
    history, 199, 200
    immune system, 207, 208
    qualitative studies, 201, 202
    quantitative studies, 202–205

Common cold
  adenoviruses, 19
  antiviral medications, 19
  chill theory, 24
  coronaviruses, 19
  definition, 19
  historical origins, 20
  home-based remedies, 48
  immune response, 25
  indoor crowding and ventilation, 26
  outdoor temperatures, 25
  seasonality, 23
  symptoms, 19
  viral replication, 25
Treatment of common cold, 45
  bedrest and exercise, 49
  historical origins, 46
  humidifiers and vaporizers, 47, 51
  nasal irrigation, 47, 51
  placebo effect, 49
  supplemental fluids, 50
Confirmation bias, 4, 23
Confounding, 146
Convulsions, 224, 227
COVID-19 pandemic, 199, 202, 204, 207,
    208, 221
Crocetin, 125
Crohn's disease, 208
Cyclamate, 132, 134, 135

D
DDT, 152
Dental caries, 138
Dental health, 138
Diabetes mellitus (DM), 136, 137, 139
  glucose, 183
  history, 184
  sugar consumption, 185–188
  sugar-sweetened beverages (SSBs), 185
  type 1 diabetes, 183
  type 2 diabetes, 184
Dietary supplementation, 126
  Canadian Community Health
      Survey, 34
  Consumer marketing survey data, 33
  EPIC, 34
  micronutrient supplement, 35
  NHANES surveys, 33
  nutritional supplements, 33
  nutrition and infection, 30–32
      LCPUFAs, 32

  stomach flu, 31
  probiotic supplementation, 40
  scientific evidence, 35
      flavonoids, 38
      gastrointestinal infection, 39, 40
      omega-3 fatty acids, 38
      probiotics, 39
      vitamin A, 36
      vitamin C, 37
      vitamin D, 36
      vitamin E, 38
      zinc, 38
Digital eye strain (DES), 91, 93
Duct tape, 55

E
E coli contamination, 158
Essential oils, 126, 127
European Prospective Investigation into
    Cancer and Nutrition (EPIC), 34
Exchangeability, 6
Eye strain
  asthenopia, 90
  astigmatism, 90, 94, 95
  lazy diagnosis, 89
  optical defect, 90
  optical stressors, 94

F
Feingold diet, 143
Fermented milk, 125
Fever
  biology, 226, 227
  child's comfort and mood, 228
  educational interventions, 225, 226
  health care professionals, 224, 225
  historical perspective, 222, 223
  parents, 223, 224
  respiratory virus infections, 221
  seizures, 227
  temperature, 227
Food additive, 143, 148

G
Generally regarded as safe (GRAS), 127
Genetically modified organisms (GMOs),
    152, 153
Gestational age, 195–197
Gestational duration, 195
Guillain-Barré syndrome, 208

H

Hangover
  adverse economic impact, 112
  alcohol-induced dehydration, 109
  beliefs and practices, 111
  biological mechanisms, 110
  cognitive function, 110
  dose of alcohol, 113
  historical and cultural overview, 110–111
  placebo-controlled crossover trials, 111
  preventive and therapeutic interventions, 114
Headache
  ciliary muscle, 91
  DES symptoms, 96
  monofocal lenses, 96
  presbyopia, 96
  refractive errors, 91, 95
Heat stroke, 222
Human papilloma virus (HPV), 204
Hyperthermia, 222

I

Ibuprofen, 225, 226, 228
Immune system, 207, 208
Influenza, 204
Inhaled oils, 127
Insomnia
  aroma therapy, 126, 127
  definition, 119
  dietary supplements, 126
  herbal teas and extracts
    Ashwagandha root, 123, 124
    black and green tea leaves, 124
    chamomile, 122, 123
    crocetin, 125
    East Asian multi-herb tea, 124
    Guizhi gancao longgu muli, 123
    montmorency tart cherries, 125
    passionflower, 124
    rosemary, 124
    saffron, 124, 125
    shumian capsule, 123
    valerian, 122, 123
    wuling capsule, 123
  milk, 125
  prevalence, 120
  Z-drugs, 119
Intermittent fasting
  beliefs and practices, 103
  during pregnancy, 106
  medical benefits, 102
  online cross-sectional survey, 104

J

Jet lag
  biological clock, 176
  history, 175
  pre-flight measures, 177
  prevention, 178–180
  symptoms, 175

L

Listeria, 158
Liver cancer risk, 139
Long-chain polyunsaturated fatty acids
    (LCPUFAs), 32, 70, 72–73
L-theanine, 124

M

Magnesium, 126
Malaria-induced fever, 222
Measles-mumps-rubella (MMR),
    203, 206
Melatonin, 119, 177, 179, 180
Milk, 125
Multisystem inflammatory syndrome in
    children (MIS-C), 208
Muscle mass and strength, 165
Myocarditis, 208

N

National Health and Nutrition
    Examination Survey
    (NHANES), 33, 81
Natural remedies, 3
Nearsightedness (myopia), 94
  contact lenses, 85
  degree of, 79
  elongation, 84
  environmental factors, 80
  ethnicity, 81
  focus groups, 82
  overview, 79
  prevalence of, 80
  temporal trends, 80
  treatment, 85
  wearing glasses, 82
Neonatal deaths, 195, 196
Neuromyths, 145
Non-steroidal anti-inflammatory drugs
    (NSAIDs), 110
Nutrition, health, or risk reduction
    (NHR), 153

O

Omega-3 long-chain polyunsaturated fatty acids (LC-PUFAs), 38, 160
Organic foods
  bacterial contamination, 158
  taste, 156, 157
  chemical contamination, 157
  definition, 151
  health improvement, 159, 160
  NHR, 153
  non-consumers, occasional consumers, and regular consumers, 154
  nutrient content, 158, 159
  organic farming, 152, 153
Organicopónicos, 153

P

Passionflower, 124
Penicillium, 4
Pertussis, 200
Pesticides, 152, 157, 159, 160
Physical performance, 170, 171
Polio vaccines, 200, 207
Pregnancy, 193–195
Prematurity, 195
Preterm birth, 195, 197
Propionibacterium acnes, 67
Protein supplementation
  confounding factors, 168
  definition, 163
  in elderly, 170–172
  in healthy adults, 168–170
  history, 165
  muscle mass, 163
  prevalence, 165, 166
  protein shake, 166

R

Repeated low-level red light (RLRL), 85
Resistance training, 168–172
Respiratory virus, 221
Reverse causality, 147
Rheumatoid arthritis, 208
RotaShield, 200
Rotavirus, 200

S

Saccharine, 131, 132, 135
Saffron, 124, 125
Salmonella, 158

Scientific evidence, 11
  benefits and risks, 15
  cherry picking, 12
  conventional reviews, 11
  expert judgment, 12
  health belief and practice, 14
  journals and publications, 11
  randomized controlled trial (RCT), 12
  systematic review, 12, 14
Scientific inference, 4
  bias and precision, 7
  causal inference, 5
  confounding, 8
  controlled experiment, 6
  ethical difference, 6
  exchangeability, 6
  health beliefs, 5, 9–10
  observational studies, 7
  precision, 9
  randomization, 6
  reverse causality bias, 8
Self-fulfilling prophecy, 197
Shumian capsule, 123
Sleep time, 126
Smallpox, 207
Sorbitol, 138
Sucralose, 132
Sucrose, 131
Sugar-sweetened beverages (SSBs), 187, 188
Systematic vs conventional review, 13

T

Teething
  definition, 213
  hard rubber/plastic, 213
  health care professionals, 215, 216
  historical perspective, 213, 214
  parents, 215
  signs and symptoms, 217–219
Tylenol, 228, 229
Type 1 diabetes, 183, 184, 186, 208
Type 2 diabetes, 183, 184, 186–188

U

Ulcerative colitis, 208

V

Valerian, 123
Vitamin D supplementation, 126

W
Warts
   cryotherapy, 57
   duct tape, 55, 56
   medical treatments, 58
   overview, 55
   topical treatments, 57
Wuling capsule, 123

X
Xylitol, 133, 138

Z
Z-drugs, 179